SAVING THE HEART

SAVING THE HEART

The Battle to Conquer Coronary Disease

Stephen Klaidman

OXFORD
UNIVERSITY PRESS

2000

OXFORD
UNIVERSITY PRESS

Oxford   New York
Athens   Auckland   Bangkok   Bogotá   Buenos Aires   Calcutta
Cape Town   Chennai   Dar es Salaam   Delhi   Florence   Hong Kong   Istanbul
Karachi   Kuala Lumpur   Madrid   Melbourne   Mexico City   Mumbai
Nairobi   Paris   São Paulo   Singapore   Taipei   Tokyo   Toronto   Warsaw

and associated companies in
Berlin   Ibadan

Copyright © 2000 by Stephen Klaidman

Published by Oxford University Press, Inc.,
198 Madison Avenue, New York, New York, 10016
http://www.oup-usa.org

Oxford is a registered trademark of Oxford University Press

Library of Congress Cataloging-in-Publication Data
Klaidman, Stephen
Saving the Heart : the battle to
conquer coronary disease /
Stephen Klaidman.
p. cm.   Includes bibliographical references and index.
ISBN 0–19–511279–2
1. Coronary heart disease—Treatment—History.
2. Coronary heart disease—Surgery—History. I. Title.
[DNLM: 1. Thoracic Surgery Biography.
2. Coronary Disease—history.
3. Coronary Disease—surgery.
4. Thoracic Surgery—history.
WZ 112.5.S8 K63h 2000]
RC685.C6K53   2000   617.4'12059—DC21
DNLM/DLC   for Library of Congress   99–28930

9 8 7 6 5 4 3 2 1
Printed in the United States of America
on acid-free paper

*This book is dedicated
to the memory of Yakov Eren,
Kitty's brother,
who became the brother I never had.*

One prescription cannot suit all. The concern of medicine
should be, while not losing sight of general principles, to
fit the treatment to the patient.

Let those humble themselves too who live by their pre-
scribings, and cease from attributing to the groping, vanity
and tricks of their calling results solely to be laid . . . at the
door of God, of nature in her wisdom and of moderation
and temperate living.

These are the words of Don Diego de Torres Villarroel (1693–1770),
mathematician, priest, soldier, prognosticator, and picaró, who taught himself to be a physician in thirty days and in these excerpts displays learning
greater than most of his contemporaries and some of ours. Both quotations
are from *The Remarkable Life of Don Diego: Being the Autobiography of
Diego de Torres Villarroel* (London: Folio Society, 1958), pp. 168–69 and
173, respectively.

Contents

Acknowledgments

I could not have written this book without the help of a great many people who were kind enough to share their time and resources with me. I cannot thank them all individually because they were too numerous. They, of course, know who they are, and I thank them collectively here. A smaller group of people contributed knowledge, judgment, and wisdom that substantially affected the book's content. Foremost among these were John Kirklin, Spencer B. King III, Richard Myler, and Valentin Fuster. I would also like to give special thanks to the surgeons who allowed me to come into their operating rooms and watch them work.

These were Paul Taylor, Paul Corso, Greg Ribakove, and Valavanur Subramanian; and to the patients who shared their stories with me: David Allison, Stan Hinden, and the pseudonymous Lewis Hollander.

A number of other cardiologists, surgeons, and entrepreneurs were especially generous with their time. These include John Simpson, Paul Yock, Edwin Alderman, Wes Sterman, J. Willis Hurst, Tom Fogarty, Wil Sampson and Michael Mack. Special thanks are also due to the librarians at the American College of Cardiology, especially Gwen Pigman. Much of my research was done at "Heart House," and life would have been much more difficult without their support. My thanks also to LeRoy Walters and the Kennedy Institute of Ethics at Georgetown University for intellectual and logistical support, and to Doris Goldstein, Martina Darragh, and the other librarians at the institute who helped me find crucial material. I am also indebted to Daniel Ein, a wise physician and dear friend, who read part of the manuscript and gave me good advice and much support. This book, like my previous two, owes a great deal to Jeffrey House, my editor at Oxford, who knows how to save me from myself. And as always, I thank my wife, Kitty, and my children, Daniel and Elyse, for their ideas and support.

Finally, I want to give very special thanks to two cardiologists who made themselves, their insights, their deep knowledge, and their good judgment available to me almost on demand. Stuart Seides spent many hours answering my questions, many of which, at least early in the project, must have seemed naive and tedious. At no time, however, did he show impatience, and I learned something every time I called him or went to see him. And Mitchel Sklar educated me to the point where I was not embarrassed to begin requesting interviews with busy practitioners and researchers who had no reason to be patient with me. Mitch, a longtime friend who was enthusiastic about the project from the start, was an inspired teacher, a critical reader of the manuscript, and a constant resource.

By way of postscript, I owe the book's title to the fertile mind of Edward Luttwak.

Foreword

Medicine comes under more scrutiny from outsiders than most professions. Like lawyers, engineers and teachers, we tend to agree that outsiders, lacking our years of specialized training and experience, are incapable of judging our actions. However, because in medicine human life is at stake, it would be inappropriate as well as imperious for physicians and surgeons to resist the scrutiny of others. Medicine has to accept and even welcome external scrutiny across the spectrum from managed care to journalists.

Stephen Klaidman is a senior research fellow at the Kennedy Institute of Ethics at Georgetown University who spent 23 years as a journalist with The New York Times, The Washington Post and the International Herald Tribune. He has applied his reporting and analytical skills to examining cardiology as representative of how technology has changed the practice of medicine. While not a physician, Klaidman has educated himself about cardiology remarkably well. Many if not all of the cardiologists who were interviewed by him will likely applaud the author's knowledge about heart disease.

It is appropriate for him to focus on cardiology not only because it exemplifies more than any other specialty the points that he wishes to make about medicine, but also because it treats the nation's number one killer, coronary heart disease. Despite the advances discussed in this book, heart disease's number-one ranking is likely to persist for many decades. Although heart disease is not solely a disease of the elderly, an individual's risk for suffering a heart attack increases with age. And with an aging population, both heart disease and its sibling disease, stroke, will increase dramatically in the United States and in many countries of the world.

Klaidman's book primarily focuses on the technological—the origins and current uses of angioplasty and bypass surgery as well as potential imaging methods for diagnosing subclinical atherosclerosis and vulnerable plaques. After reading—or hearing about—the book, many of my cardiology colleagues may wish that the author had focused on oncology, neurology, or any specialty other than our own because the book brings into the open troubling observations, complaints and concerns that many of us have voiced to each other. It is unsettling to read his conclusions about self-interest, conflict of interest and ego of physicians. It is embarrassing to be reminded how medicine's inherent conservatism has resulted in excessive delays in the acceptance of new findings that eventually changed the cardiology landscape and saved patients' lives. It is easy to forget sometimes that we are human beings as well as doctors.

This is a book that offers valuable lessons for members of the specialty—clinical cardiologists, interventional cardiologists and cardiac surgeons—other physicians, and, perhaps most importantly, patients. It is nuanced in its awareness of the difficulty of clinical decision-making in an era in which both technology and understanding of the underlying causes of coronary artery disease are advancing rapidly. For practitioners it should serve as a reminder to approach new technologies and new theories about the etiology of the disease with a carefully balanced blend of skepticism and open-mindedness.

Klaidman is also sensitive to the pressures under which physicians must operate in an age of managed care. But he is properly critical of those who overuse high-tech procedures because they are lucrative and insurers will pay for them. He makes clear as well that some of the newer, minimally invasive and beating-heart procedures are not appropriate for everyone and should not be done except in the best hospitals, by the most skilled surgeons, with state-of-the-art equipment and experienced, highly trained surgical teams.

While not under-rating the importance of objective evidence in medical decision-making, he points out that clinical trials to test devices and surgical procedures may cost tens of millions of dollars and yield findings that are of little or no use in helping patients select a form of treatment. Klaidman also notes that treatment choices are often not obvious, that each patient is an individual, not a statistic, and that practitioners frequently differ in what they think is appropriate treatment for a particular patient. Indeed, depending on the cardiologist, the same patient might be seen as a candidate for surgery, angioplasty, angioplasty with a stent, or drug therapy.

Coronary patients, or anyone who may in the future be a coronary patient, will be far better prepared to participate with their physicians in the stressful decisions that must be made—where to get a second opinion, selecting a form of treatment, choosing a surgeon—if they have read this book.

As for those of us in cardiac medicine in particular, and medicine generally, I hope that Klaidman's book will help us overcome self-interest, conflict of interest and ego and be more open to new findings and ideas. Not only will we benefit, but more importantly, so will our patients.

Valentin Fuster, M.D., Ph.D.
Past President, American Heart Association,
Director, Zena and Michael A. Wiener
Cardiovascular Institute, and Dean for
Academic Affairs, Mount Sinai Medical Center

Preface

If there is a twentieth-century plague, it is coronary artery disease. Even though the death rate for this illness has declined by more than 50 percent since 1963,[1] coronary artery disease still kills more people in the United States and in the Western world than any other single illness, and it is the number one consumer of health-care dollars in the United States, at more than $90 billion a year.[2]

At the end of the final decade of the twentieth century, 14 million Americans are suffering from coronary artery disease. It causes 1 of every 4.7 deaths in the United States. Someone has a heart attack every twenty seconds in this country. An American dies of a heart attack every minute. About 500,000 die from this disease annually. By comparison, in 1994 AIDS caused 42,000 deaths, breast cancer caused 44,000, and lung cancer caused 58,000.[3]

Until thirty years ago all doctors could do to treat coronary artery disease was precribe drugs to relieve the pain of angina, but in the past three decades a variety of treatments have been developed. The story of these discoveries and the names of their ambitious, farsighted, and often larger-than-life discoverers are unknown outside of medicine. To take just two examples:

Mason Sones, the visionary inventor of coronary angiography. Sones was driven beyond the point of obsession. He sacrificed his family to his work and experimented on patients without asking their permission. But his contribution made bypass surgery and angioplasty possible.

Andreas Gruentzig's appetite for life—women, flying, car racing, mountains of sausage, and rivers of wine—and his talent for promoting a radical new treatment—blowing up balloons in arteries—were as big as his gift for science. Today the procedure he invented and its progeny are used more often than bypass surgery.

The stories of these men's lives embody more than just the excitement of medical discovery and the intellect, energy, and courage of the discoverers. In their complexity, they also shed light on conflicts of interest that sometimes produce risks for research subjects and patients. Because cardiology and cardiac research are particularly lucrative fields, and because they are so technology driven, conflicts of interest are more tempting than in many other areas of medicine and more prevalent.

This book is about these men and their legacy. It is about what happens at the intersection of medical practice, clinical science, technology, and entrepreneurship. And it is about the benefits and pitfalls of entrepreneurial, technologically driven medicine.

Stephen Klaidman
Berkeley, California
January 1999

SAVING THE HEART

1

A Heart Attack

His arteries silted up like an old river.[1]

Early in 1984, David Allison, a 41-year-old political consultant in Juneau, Alaska, went to the hospital with pain in his chest. He saw the only cardiologist in town, who did an electrocardiogram and concluded that the probable cause of his pain was stress, not coronary disease, and that he was not at risk for a heart attack.

Allison's primary-care physician, a stereotypically thorough and authoritarian German woman, thought the diagnosis was reasonable. But she had taken a medical history during which she discovered that Allison's father, mother, and older brother had all had heart attacks. As a precautionary measure, she ordered him to reduce his consumption of salt and fats and to monitor his cholesterol.

Despite his family history, Allison, like many Americans at the time, was only vaguely aware of cholesterol's potentially destructive effects. And he didn't make the connection between smoking and heart disease. When he asked her if he could step outside her office for a smoke, she lectured him severely: "You vill not smoke in zis hospital and you vill stop smoking," which he did, although it took him two years.[2] Until that day Allison had never focused on the fact that by virtue of genetic predisposition he might be at greater risk than most people for a heart attack.

Heart attacks occur when a blood clot, a bit of fatty plaque, or more likely both block blood flow through one or more of the three main coronary arteries and their branches. These tiny vessels wind sinuously around the heart's surface, sometimes burrowing into the muscle, which they supply with blood. A blockage in a coronary artery can deprive part of the heart muscle of oxygen and nutrients, causing tissue to die. Dead tissue cannot contract and therefore the heart's pumping capacity is compromised. This is the event physicians call a myocardial infarction and the rest of us know as a heart attack.

But Allison was a marathon runner. He was convinced that his heart was

3

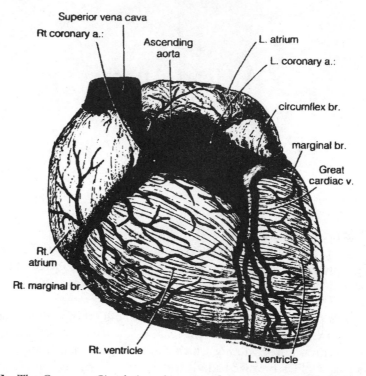

Superior vena cava

Rt coronary a.:

Ascending
aorta

L. atrium

L. coronary a.:

circumflex br.

marginal br.

Great
cardiac v.

Rt.
atrium

Rt. marginal br.

Rt. ventricle

L. ventricle

1.1. The Coronary Circulation: A crown of arteries encircles the heart to supply its muscular walls with oxygen and nutrients (fats and carbohydrates). Two main trunks spring from the aorta, the great vessel arising out of the left ventricle through which blood that has been cleansed and oxygenated in the lungs is pumped to all of the body's cells. The left coronary artery divides into two branches, the left anterior descending (LAD) and the circumflex, almost as soon as it emerges from the aorta. The LAD runs down the front of the heart, branches out and feeds the right and left ventricles. The circumflex artery winds around to the back of the heart and feeds the left ventricle and the left atrium. The right coronary artery supplies blood to the walls of the right atrium and ventricle through its marginal branch on the front surface of the heart, and to both ventricles through its posterior branch. The main arteries spread like trees with their smallest branches plunging into the muscle where they subdivide still further, first into tiny arterioles, and then into capillaries that are no more than two ten/ thousandths of an inch in diameter. Each capillary nourishes one of the roughly three billion heart cells. Cardiac veins, following roughly the same path as the arteries, carry deoxygenated, waste-hauling blood back to the coronary sinus from where it enters the right atrium and then the right ventricle, which pumps it back into the lungs to be oxygenated and cleansed again. It takes about 5 percent of the body's blood to nourish the heart. Only the brain requires more.

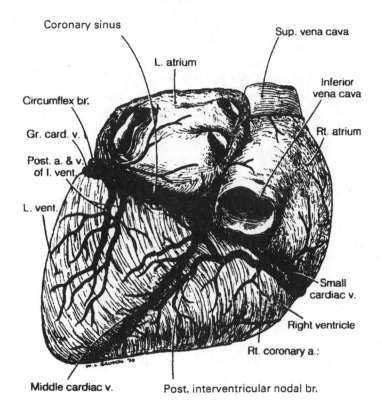

a strong, healthy pump. And so it seemed to be for the next twelve years, during which time he remained symptom-free.

In 1996, Allison was working as an environmental lobbyist in Washington, D.C. Over several weeks he noticed that during physical activity he would get a kind of sludgy feeling in his upper chest; his lungs didn't seem to fill with as much air as they always had; it was harder to breathe. The air seemed thicker, somehow. These physical changes worried him, but he didn't do anything about it. "I didn't have insurance," he said. "I waited too long. I think I was in denial."[3]

At Christmastime Allison drove from Washington to Miami, where he took a boat to the Bahamas to go scuba diving. It was a bad trip from beginning to end. He got seriously seasick during the rough sailboat crossing to the islands. And he had a couple of panic attacks while diving, after which he quit. On the rainy, fogbound drive back to Washington he slept only a few hours in the car, overdosed on steaks, eggs, bacon, sausage, and alcohol, and arrived in Washington exhausted. But he was happy to be home in time to spend a quiet New Year's Eve with his girlfriend Cindy.

The next night, after making love, he got up in the early morning hours to put on a pot of coffee for her. He got a few steps from the bed and suddenly felt a tightness in his chest and then pain in his stomach. He went to the bathroom and took an antacid. He also felt the familiar heaviness, the thickness in his breathing. Not knowing what else to do, he took a couple of aspirin. He was afraid that it might be his heart.

Then he broke into a cold sweat. Within seconds his entire body was drenched. "My chest felt like it was collapsing in on me," he said. "I took a deep breath and lay down. I took another deep breath and it hit me again. I had a pain like somebody had attached a 220 electric line to my chest. I curled up on the bed. I had pulled a blanket up over me because I was chilling. I looked at a clock and it was 6:20 A.M. I'm lying there looking at the digital numbers and I thought: 'Well, this is really interesting; it's 6:20 A.M. and I'm having a heart attack.' "[4]

He called out for Cindy, who saw his obvious distress. She asked if he needed to go to the hospital. He hesitated for a moment, but it quickly dawned on him that if he didn't get to a hospital fast he might die, right there on the floor of his house. He had taken a bus a few days before that went by the nearest hospital, D.C. General, so he knew where it was, only seven blocks away. He gave directions to Cindy, who drove him to the emergency room.

"I walked in," Allison said, "and there was a woman sitting at the desk. I ran over and said, 'Help me, help me, help me, I think I'm having a heart attack, help me please,' and fell on the desk. I described pain in my jaw, my neck, my back, my arm was completely numb, clavicle was on fire. I didn't know at the time these were classic symptoms. I was crying. She asked me if I had insurance, I said, 'No, I don't have insurance.' She never stopped. She was asking me questions and moving me to the emergency room. I was on the table and had a team on me I think within two minutes of coming through the door.

"A resident or a doctor said, 'Tell me what your pain is, had I had a heart attack before, what's your level of pain from one to ten?' 'It's horrible, one to ten, man, it's like a twelve or fourteen.' They were injecting me with something, asked me if there was anything I was allergic to. 'We're gonna get rid of your pain, we're gonna give you morphine'; asked me if I'd taken any drugs. Kept asking me, 'What's your level of pain?' They injected me with twelve units of morphine. I know that at five minutes of seven I was lying there and at ten after seven they were asking me for permission to use drugs that might be able to clear the blocked artery. 'Where do I sign? Yes, do whatever to make this stop.' They asked me if they could do a cardiac catheterization. I said whatever you need to do. Pain is still a ten and coming in waves. I'm twisting around on the table. A doctor said, 'Now this is what we call the twister response to MI [myocardial infarction].' Everybody laughed."

Allison's pain finally began to subside; he felt he was able to breathe normally, "shallow and relaxed." Because of his twisting, the medical team couldn't do emergency angioplasty, the cutting-edge procedure they thought would be best, which involves inserting a catheter and blowing up a balloon inside the artery to unblock it. They gave him a clot-busting drug intravenously instead. This is slightly more dangerous because it is more likely to loosen bits of arterial plaque, which can migrate to the brain and cause a stroke.

The next thing Allison remembers is being in an operating room under a bright surgical light. Someone was shouting, " 'Get the [defibrillator] paddles, I think we're losing him.' I'm clear as a bell. My mind's working fine. Now, this is silly. They're not losing me. I've just got to tell them I'm okay. I'm using every bit of energy I've got. I'm trying to peel my eyes open. And they open. And there's this guy standing there in all kinds of blue. And I feel like I'm in a TV show or something, all these people standing around looking at me and someone says, 'It's coming back up,' and there's this guy standing there with these freaking paddles.

"No, this is not something that's happening, and I moved my head and I looked up and I wasn't in an operating room. I was still sitting in the emergency room. There was no operating room light there." The defibrillator was real, though. Allison's blood pressure and heart rate had dropped precipitously, bringing him close to death.

The D.C. General staff had not called Matthew Parker, Allison's personal physician. "When I called him and told him" what had happened, Allison said later, "he was livid. He told me to get out of D.C. General as quickly as I could." Parker wanted Allison transferred to the Washington Hospital Center, which has a world-class cardiology and cardiac surgery program. "I said I didn't have any insurance. He said, 'Get out. We'll make arrangements. The important thing is for you to be alive.' But I was really scared of leaving the doctors who had been taking care of me. I had all these students and this intern. I was afraid to leave and go to someplace new. I wanted to stay for the [angiogram] they wanted to do. I felt very comfortable. I felt a great deal of confidence. They seemed confident."

A couple of days later, a cardiologist at D.C. General performed the angiogram. In this procedure, radio-opaque dye is squirted into the arteries, making blockages visible when X-ray pictures are taken. The cardiologist told Allison that he had had a total blockage of the left anterior descending coronary artery, which courses down the front of the heart and supplies blood to the left ventricle, the heart's main pumping chamber. Even after injection of the clot-busting drug tissue plasminogen activator (tPA), this artery still was about 80 percent blocked.

Allison was also told that there were 40 percent and 25 percent blockages in two other arteries and that an area of his heart muscle had died. Since the part of the muscle supplied by the major blocked artery had died, they said, they had no plans to do angioplasty or bypass surgery.

Two days later, Allison was sent home. He went to see Parker, who sent him to Cardiology Associates, a large group that practices out of the Washington Hospital Center. They did an electrocardiogram and scheduled him for a thallium stress test, a procedure that measures blood flow through the coronary arteries and heart. Meanwhile, Parker told him he'd had a major loss of heart function resulting from his heart attack and asked him to call his office before nine each morning to report on how he felt. "I was scared again after that discussion," Allison said. "I was told that I'd lost the functioning of about a third of my heart after the stress test. I didn't want to believe that this was a permanent condition.

"They told me that the lost function meant blood was pooling and therefore there was a potential for clotting and that I would have to take Coumadin [a blood thinner] for the rest of my life." This meant that Allison, an outdoorsman and fitness enthusiast, would have to avoid risky physical activities because an injury could result in uncontainable bleeding. Allison was also told by a physician at Cardiology Associates that there was to be no interventional procedure—not surgery and not angioplasty—because the area of heart muscle normally supplied by the still badly blocked artery was dead; it no longer could contract and pump, therefore there was no use supplying it with blood.

Allison, glad to be alive, took the Coumadin and other medications and was fine for several months, but then symptoms began to recur. The doctors at Cardiology Associates were concerned and ordered him back into the hospital. Surprisingly, an angiogram showed that there were pockets of viable heart muscle in the area supplied by the clogged left anterior descending artery, which was why he was having symptoms. Because this vessel was still supplying blood to some living tissue, they did an angioplasty to open it to 50 percent or more and increase the supply.

The procedure was successful. Allison was taken off Coumadin and told he could exert himself in any way he wanted, even train to be a triathlete. But it was important for him to remember that he had suffered a heart attack, as had both of his parents and his brother. He still had a high-risk profile. Moreover, there is no cure for coronary artery disease. There is only palliation. He would have to watch himself for the rest of his life.

David Allison's experience is instructive because he was a possible candidate for each of the three groups of treatments available for coronary artery disease at the end of the twentieth century—bypass surgery, interventions such as angioplasty and stenting, and drug therapy.

The pertinence of Allison's case becomes obvious when viewed against a decade-by-decade timeline. Had he had his heart attack in 1976, he probably would have had open-chest bypass surgery through a foot-long incision. Had it occurred in 1986, he would have had open-chest bypass surgery or angioplasty. In 1996, as we know, he was given clot-busting drugs and later angioplasty. But if he had been taken directly to the Washington Hospital Center instead of D.C. General Hospital he might just as easily have had bypass surgery done through a three-inch incision without the use of a heart-lung machine while his heart continued to beat, or perhaps angioplasty combined with the insertion of a tiny metal scaffold called a stent to keep his artery from shutting down.

But if David Allison had had his heart attack in 1966 or earlier, he would have been put to bed and given frequent doses of nitroglycerine to relieve his pain. At that time, by way of treatment, that's essentially all there was.

What follows is the story of how clinical scientists, biomedical engineers, and entrepreneurs working together developed today's generally effective treatments—not cures, but life-enhancing and sometimes life-extending treatments—for this devastating condition. It begins with a brief historical sketch of medicine's quest to understand and respond to coronary artery disease, from Galen, a great second-century Greek physician, to John Gibbon, the patrician Pennsylvanian who invented the heart-lung machine.

2

The Revolution of 1912

What a mystery the heart is. The mind is simple by
comparison.

Mary Gordon[1]

Throughout literature, the heart turns up in a thousand guises. In Yeats's
"The Lake Isle of Innisfree," for example, it is portrayed as the place where
subtle tones of feeling, unregistered by the intellect, resonate:

> I hear lake water lapping with low sounds by the shore;
> While I stand on the roadway, or on the pavements gray,
> I hear it in the deep heart's core.[2]

In Edgar Allan Poe's classic horror story "The Telltale Heart," a "low,
dull, quick sound" throbs insistently in a murderer's mind, driving him
mad.[3] Is the pulse he hears entirely psychological, or is it the physiological
reality of a heart beating after all other signs of life have ceased? In either
case, the heart is the instrument of his torment.

In the Egyptian Book of the Dead the sign of Truth was placed in one
pan of a balance, a human heart in the other.[4] Aristotle believed the heart
was the seat of pain, pleasure, and all sensation.[5] Richard I, the great
knight-errant of the Third Crusade, was dubbed lion-hearted to symbolize
his courage and strength. And Pascal, who lived two thousand years after
Aristotle, attributed a quality of mind to the heart that he intimated the
brain lacked when he wrote, "The heart has its reasons, which reason does
not know."[6]

The heart has been cast not only as the source of virtues such as truth,
intelligence, valor, and love, but also of evil and vice. Here, for example,
is Jeremiah (17:9): "The heart is deceitful above all things, and desperately
wicked." In *Richard III* (act 1, scene 2, line 15), Anne, daughter of Henry
VI, "Cursed the heart that had the heart" to murder her father. That
duplicitous heart, of course, belonged to Shakespeare's darkest villain, the
duke of Gloucester, soon to be Richard III.

10

An evil person is called black-hearted, someone who lacks compassion is labeled heartless, a moral person is portrayed as pure of heart, and the hearts of lovers are said to become one. To what other organ, or organism, or object or idea, has humankind attributed such diverse and vital content, such varied and consequential capacities, such magical and magisterial qualities?

But for the cardiologist, the cardiac surgeon, the clinical researcher, when working as designed, the heart is a marvelously efficient three-quarter-pound pump. Each day its muscle, pulsing to a steady, neurologically induced electromechanical beat, propels more than seven thousand quarts of blood through a complex network of hundreds of major arteries and veins, thousands of lesser ones, tens of thousands of arterioles, and billions of capillaries. It drives carbon dioxide-laden venous blood into the lungs, where there is a minute-long gas exchange across a membrane of three hundred million air sacs. During this exchange, waste is expelled and the blood absorbs oxygen, turning from blue to crimson as a result. Then it is routed into the heart's left ventricle, which pumps it through the arterial side of the circulatory system to all of the body's cells. On this journey it continuously deposits life-sustaining oxygen and collects noxious carbon dioxide and other waste. Blue once again, the blood is returned through the veins to the heart, which pumps it back into the lungs, where once more waste is expelled, oxygen is absorbed, and so on for a lifetime.

Despite—or more likely because of—all we have invested in it emotionally, the animating secret of this fist-sized, four-chambered, involuntary muscle, suspended deep inside the chest in a balloonlike sac, went undisclosed until early in the twentieth century. It was only then that the neurological genesis of the heartbeat, the source of so much of the organ's mystery, was properly understood by medical science.[7]

The heart has been studied for millennia. A three-thousand-year-old Olmec figurine depicts a heart with several anatomically correct features.[8] Its muscle has been well characterized in medical literature since perhaps the fourth century B.C. And by the mid-sixteenth century, the tiny coronary arteries, wound like wires around the heart, had been accurately depicted—although their function was not understood—by skilled anatomists such as Andreas Vesalius, who among other things proved Galen wrong about bone and muscle structure by doing what the great second-century Greek physician apparently had never done—probing inside a human body. Vesalius's anatomical masterpiece *De humani corporis fabrica* (On the Fabric of the Human Body) (1543), with fine drawings by Jan Stephan van Calcar, is arguably the most important single work on medicine of the Renaissance. The coronaries had also been drawn by another sixteenth-century anatomist of note—Leonardo da Vinci.

Also in the mid-sixteenth century, as an aside in a theological tract taking issue with the doctrine of the Holy Trinity,[9] the Spaniard Michael Serve-tus—trained as a physician but a theologian by avocation—described how blood flows from the right side of the heart through the lungs to the left side of the heart. His essentially correct view of the pulmonary circulation contradicted Galen, who believed that blood crossed from one side of the heart to the other through invisible pores in the septum (wall) dividing the two sides. Unfortunately for Servetus, his work was deemed heretical— for its religious rather than for its physiological speculations—and he was burned at the stake at Champel outside of Geneva on October 27, 1553, after having been betrayed by an acquaintance who saw him attending church in Geneva.[10]

Early in the seventeenth century, William Harvey made one of the greatest discoveries in the history of medicine when he demonstrated ir-refutably, using quantitative methods, that blood circulated continuously through the body. Harvey also showed that the coronary arteries carried blood to the heart to nourish it with oxygen.[11] Moreover, he recognized a link between the pulse and a patient's symptoms as early as 1628. But he wrote nonetheless that ". . . I almost believed . . . that the motion of the heart was to be understood by God alone."[12]

Later in the seventeenth century, in a leap of the imagination foreshad-owing the invention of the stethoscope, which made it possible for phy-sicians to hear the heart's rhythm,[13] Robert Hooke wrote poetically, "who knows but that as in a Watch we may hear the beating of the Balance and the running of the Wheels, and the striking of the Hammers and the grat-ing of the Teeth. . . ."[14]

In 1761, Giovanni Battista Morgagni described hardening of the coronary arteries.[15] And in 1768, William Heberden, who later attended Samuel John-son at his death, defined in evocative detail the recurring chest pain and re-lated symptoms caused by this so-called hardening. He named the condition angina pectoris.[16] But unlike his British contemporaries Edward Jenner and Caleb Parry, both of whom speculated that angina might result from disease of the coronary arteries, Heberden had no idea what caused it.

Until the late nineteenth century, no one made an unequivocal connec-tion between Morgagni's observation of clogged arteries and Heberden's description of angina pectoris, the constricting chest pain that is the classic symptom of coronary heart disease and a frequent precursor of heart at-tacks. And heart attacks themselves were not described with enough detail and precision to make the medical profession recognize them as an acute indication of a treatable disease until just before World War I.

The cardiologist-historian W. Bruce Fye believes that one reason almost 140 years separated the first published descriptions of angina pectoris and

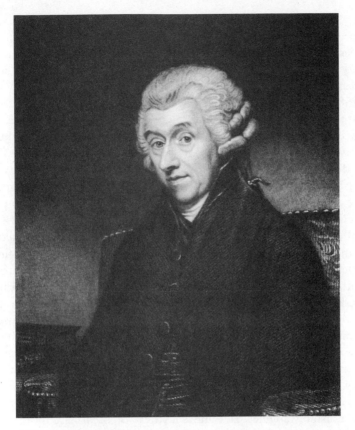

2.1. William Heberden described angina pectoris.

those of heart attacks might have been a "failure to examine the coronary arteries and myocardium [heart muscle] routinely at autopsy."[17] Fye is unsure why these arteries were rarely if ever examined in cadavers, but he said that despite Harvey's identification of the function of the coronary circulation, little if any research was done on them.[18]

Although it was first thoroughly described some 230 years ago, the twentieth-century American cardiologist Paul Dudley White wrote that angina pectoris probably first afflicted a "prosperous cave man who very likely dropped dead . . . after gorging himself with a roast of venison and on his way to a date with one of his harem." While he thought that coronary artery disease began in prehistory, White also concluded that blockages of the coronary arteries, and heart attacks, were probably rare until "the automobile came in in the 1920s and the population at large became more prosperous and overnourished. . . ."[19]

But White's view was not universally held. Another well-known cardiologist, H. B. Sprague, wrote that coronary artery disease is probably no more prevalent today in the industrialized West than it was in the same countries several hundred years ago.[20] Nobody knows for sure whether coronary disease has become more prevalent in the twentieth century, but fatty plaque has been found in the arteries of an Egyptian mummy dating from 1580 B.C.[21]

What is clear is that there is still no cure for coronary artery disease and that effective palliative treatments began to be developed only in the mid- to late twentieth century. This is so even though much had been discovered and published a century or more earlier about the mechanisms of the disease. Between 1840 and 1890 numerous articles appeared on the devastating effects of blocked coronary arteries. By 1881 the German pathologist Julius Cohnheim had speculated correctly, despite the lack of pathological evidence, that many heart conditions were due to obstruction of the coronary arteries. Moreover, recognizing the link between the findings of Harvey and Morgagni, Cohnheim, correctly albeit obliquely, attributed the death of muscle tissue that causes heart attacks to oxygen deprivation.[22]

Nevertheless, despite these physiological insights, at the turn of the twentieth century the means available to treat coronary heart disease consisted entirely of bedrest and three basic types of drugs—the digitalis variety, which increase the pumping force of the heart; nitrates such as nitroglycerin, which expand the arteries and veins, thereby reducing the heart's work; and opiates such as morphine, which improve blood flow and relieve pain. None could offer more than temporary relief from symptoms such as crushing anginal pain and shortness of breath. A more effective form of treatment was needed, but at the time virtually no one believed it could be found.

Of course, workable treatments were eventually devised. And from the perspective of the late twentieth century it is easy to see that Wilhelm Roentgen's discovery of X rays in 1895 was the first in a series of discoveries leading to bypass surgery and angioplasty. These treatments made long-term relief and in some cases longer life possible. But these developments were far from obvious at the time.

In 1895, the heart was still inviolate. It could be studied at autopsy and *in vivo,* but neither cut nor sutured. For more than two thousand years, Aristotle's maxim that the heart "is the only one of the viscera" that cannot withstand injury[23] was taken as gospel. Theodor Billroth, Europe's leading surgeon in the early 1880s, said at a meeting of the Vienna Medical Society that "Any surgeon who wishes to preserve the respect of his colleagues, would never attempt to suture the heart."[24]

As late as 1896, fear of touching the pulsing organ surgically was so pervasive that Sir Stephen Paget, author of one of the most respected thoracic surgery textbooks of the time, still reflected the conventional view when he wrote: "Heart surgery has probably reached the limits set by nature." To his knowledge, Paget noted, no one had ever successfully sutured a human heart.[25] Later in his text Paget added, however, that the Norwegian surgeon Ansel Cappelen had tried but that his patient had died. Technically, Paget wrote, suturing of the heart is "at least not impossible."[26]

Paget was dead wrong when he said heart surgery had reached its limit. He was right when he said no one had ever successfully sutured the heart—although several had tried—but had he said it a few months later, he would have been wrong about that, too. On September 9, 1896, in Frankfurt, Germany, Ludwig Rehn, using three silk sutures, became the first surgeon to successfully close a wound in the heart. His twenty-two-year-old patient, who had been discharged from the army with "advanced heart disease," had been stabbed in the heart during a brawl.[27]

In 1902, Luther L. Hill, whose son, U.S. Senator Lister Hill of Alabama, was instrumental in founding the National Heart Institute, became the first American to successfully suture a wound in the heart. The beneficiary was a thirteen-year-old boy who had been stabbed five times. The operation was done by the light of kerosene lamps on a kitchen table.[28]

Rehn's courageous—and successful—operation did not, however, quickly lead to other kinds of heart surgery, for many reasons. Among other things, there was as yet no way to keep the heart alive for more than a few minutes, anesthesia techniques were inadequate, there were problems involving blood banking and blood typing, the right diagnostic equipment had not yet been developed, and there was no way to reverse the often fatal electrical disturbance of the heart called ventricular fibrillation, which could be accidentally induced by manipulating the organ during surgery.

In the 1950s surgeons found ways to do quick repairs of congenital heart defects and faulty valves, and then the heart-lung machine was invented, which made longer operations possible. But the first, sustained surgical assault on coronary artery disease began a full seventy-one years after Rehn's operation. To operate on the beating heart's tiny arteries, which can be as small as two millimeters in diameter, presented what seemed like an insurmountable technical challenge, as did identification of the blockages.

But the technical obstacles were not the whole story. There was an equally daunting conceptual barrier. The conventional wisdom of a powerful medical establishment was that heart attacks were undiagnosable, fatal events identifiable only on autopsy. Therefore, only a small number of physicians paid attention to the provocative evidence that some heart attacks were survivable and could be diagnosed in living patients. As the philosopher-historian Thomas S. Kuhn and others have observed, in science as in other areas of life, it takes more than facts to topple conventional wisdom.

Kuhn theorized that fundamental change occurs in science only when a radically new way of thinking about old problems emerges that throws into question all relevant propositions. He called this a paradigm shift, from which flows a scientific revolution based on the new paradigm.[29] Kuhn's theory has been challenged in recent years,[30] but it does seem that in this case, as a result of an entrenched but mistaken view, progress in treating coronary artery disease was substantially slowed.

At the same time, however, the tools that would eventually make treatment of coronary artery disease possible were beginning to be developed. Francis H. Williams, America's first radiologist, had used X rays to diagnose an enlarged heart less than a year after their discovery.[31] "It is interesting to note," Williams observed, "that the heart could be made out through the man's waistcoat and two shirts."[32] And at the turn of the twentieth century the Dutch physician Willem Einthoven, using a quartz "string" one ten-thousandth of a millimeter in diameter, invented a machine that even by today's standards made superb electrocardiographic tracings.[33] Einthoven received the Nobel Prize in 1924. But a revolution in thinking about the role of blocked coronary arteries in causing heart attacks was needed before real progress could be made. And even then, for this conceptual revolution to yield better treatment, it would have to be followed by dramatic technological advances.

During the first decade of the new century there were substantial advances made by an unusually inventive experimental surgeon, but no change in the conventional wisdom regarding surgical approaches to the human heart. Early in the second decade, however, a research-oriented cardiologist challenged the establishment's myopic view. This challenge led to the emergence of modern clinical cardiology, and, drawing on the work of the experimental surgeon, invasive cardiology and cardiac surgery. Here's how it happened.

In 1912, the experimental surgeon, thirty-nine-year-old Alexis Carrel, who left France after having been told he would never get a job there, became the youngest person ever to win the Nobel Prize for Physiology or Medicine.[34] The operations on animals for which he won the prize included grafting veins onto dogs' arteries, and bypassing a coronary artery in a dog using a section of carotid artery to connect the aorta to the left coronary artery. These operations laid the groundwork for coronary bypass surgery in humans. The year he won the Nobel Prize, Carrel also made the first known attempt at stenting—keeping a blood vessel from closing by inserting a rigid tube into it.[35] Moreover, he identified tissue rejection in organ transplantation.[36]

Two events early in Carrel's life probably set him on course for a career in experimental surgery. During his medical training in Lyon, the president of the French Republic, Sadi Carnot, was stabbed in the stomach by an anarchist. An important vein was severed, which surgeons at the time had no way of repairing. As a result, Carnot died, providing the initial thrust for Carrel's interest in experimental vascular surgery, which led to his devising an ingenious way to suture together the ends of severed blood vessels. Carrel's interest could easily have brought a Nobel Prize to France rather than to the United States, had he not, out of curiosity, gone to Lourdes with a group of pilgrims.

Like almost everyone else at the time, Carrel had twice failed the examination to qualify for a surgical faculty position. While waiting to take

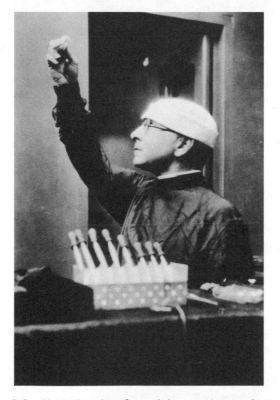

2.2. Alexis Carrel performed the experiments that paved the way for surgical treatment of coronary artery disease.

the exam a third time, he traveled to Lourdes, the world-famous Roman Catholic shrine in southwestern France, where, according to believers, miraculous cures have occurred. At Lourdes he witnessed the recovery of a young girl said to have been dying of tubercular peritonitis, an inflammatory disease of the walls of the lining of the abdomen and pelvis.[37] Back in Lyon he reported what he saw and speculated that the cure might have resulted from a placebo effect. He was immediately skewered simultaneously by the Catholic Church for his skepticism about miracles, and by the medical establishment for his gullibility.

Shortly thereafter he was told that whatever chance he once had of getting a faculty post in France was now gone. So he made his way to Chicago by way of Montréal and began an extraordinarily productive career as an experimental surgeon in the United States, first at the University of Chicago and then at Rockefeller University in New York.

While carrying out his dog experiments using vein segments to reroute blood around arterial blockages, Carrel and the aviator Charles Lindbergh, with whom he shared fascist political leanings and racist views, joined forces to develop a pump that was a forerunner of the heart-lung machine. Moreover, Carrel did the world's first recorded heart transplant—also in a dog—in 1905. But animals are not people, and as impressive as Carrel's work was, no one was ready to transfer it from the dog lab to the operating room.

Only once in all of his years in the United States did Carrel leave the dog lab to operate on a human being. He saved a five-day-old girl dying of a disease that causes hemorrhaging by stitching an artery in her father's wrist to a vein in her leg, thereby giving her a transfusion. The operation, like Luther Hill's, was done on a kitchen table.[38]

Carrel was a renegade of sorts, already working outside the boundaries of what Kuhn called normal science, or a mature paradigm, in which, according to Kuhn, science consists mainly of forcing "nature into the preformed and relatively inflexible box that the paradigm supplies."[39] But in Carrel's pre-Nobel years, no new paradigm had begun to take shape yet. It is not always possible to pinpoint precisely what sets the change in motion, but the revolution in understanding coronary artery disease began with an identifiable event in 1912, the year Carrel won the Nobel Prize.

In that year, on the seventh of December, an article appeared in the *Journal of the American Medical Association (JAMA)* titled, in the bland style typical of such publications, "Clinical Features of Sudden Obstruction of the Coronary Arteries."[40] The five-and-a-half-page text was modest in tone, cautious in its approach, and advertised no strikingly new discoveries. At the same time, it drew conclusions, based on ample evidence, that were breathtakingly at odds with the existing paradigm. James Herrick, by careful comparison of the symptoms of living patients to those who died and were shown to have blocked arteries, demonstrated that coronary artery disease was recognizable in living patients. He also offered compelling although not conclusive evidence that a totally blocked major coronary artery need not cause death, or even a heart attack; that heart attacks were very likely caused by blood clots in the coronary arteries; and that some heart attacks were survivable.

Herrick understood the implications of what he had done: He had identified as diagnosable and potentially treatable, a disease proclaimed by the medical establishment to be undiagnosable and, in its acute form, inevitably fatal.[41] Unsurprisingly, no one believed him. The old paradigm was not ready to topple. Herrick said that when he delivered the paper, "It fell like a dud."[42]

In 1918, however, he delivered a paper subsequently published in *JAMA* that provided additional evidence, including comparative animal and human electrocardiographic tracings that helped identify the existence of blocked coronary arteries[43] and "offered hope that it might reveal the location of the resulting . . . damage" to the heart muscle.[44] He also added to the evidence presented in the 1912 article that blood clots were the major cause of heart attacks. The livelier minds in the medical profession finally began to take notice.

It was not until 1980, however, that an American physician named Marcus DeWood, using a diagnostic technique unavailable to Herrick called selective coronary angiography, showed that blood clots in the coronary arteries, as opposed to the slow accretion of atherosclerotic plaque, caused most heart attacks. This proved Herrick's theory, which had stood as the conventional wisdom from about 1920 until 1960, when for lack of proof it began to be questioned. DeWood's contribution restored it to favor.[45]

Carrel and Herrick had created templates for what could and would be done in cardiology and cardiac surgery. From before Aristotle until the end of the nineteenth century, the maxim that one must not suture the heart went virtually unchallenged. But in the second half of the twentieth century, in the wake of these seminal figures, surgeons not only sutured it but also stuck tubes into it, pumped dye into it, abraded it with talc and asbestos, tunneled arteries deep into it, replaced bits of it with plastic and metal, attached it to internal and external pumps and pacemakers, stopped it from beating by dumping ice all over it or injecting it with drugs, shocked it electrically to start it up again, drilled holes in it with lasers to get blood to flow from the inside out, grafted veins and arteries from elsewhere in the body to its native arteries, threaded radionuclides through its vessels, and replaced it with human hearts from the recently dead, with baboon hearts, and even with machines. The revolution was in full swing.

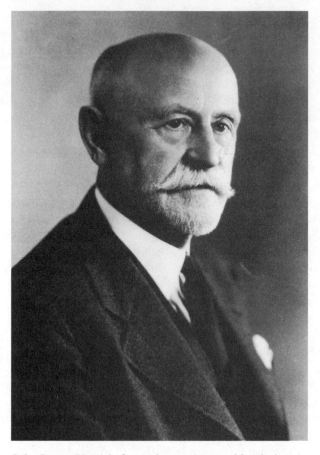

2.3. James Herrick focused attention on blood clots in the coronary arteries as the cause of heart attacks.

To make treatment practical, scientists, clinicians, and engineers had to work together to overcome all kinds of formidable obstacles, such as how to stop the heart from beating without killing the patient—and then start it again—and how to find life-threatening blockages without fumbling blindly inside the patient's chest.

Over a half century, a series of pharmacological and technological discoveries were made, each of which removed an obstacle to surgical treatment of coronary artery disease. And a few years after the last obstacle was removed, coronary bypass surgery became a reality. None of the discoverers, however, started out with bypass surgery in mind. Indeed, some had nothing in mind, but rather were the lucky beneficiaries of accidents. Of course, chance, as Pasteur has said, favors only the prepared mind.[46] Had the favored researchers not understood the significance of these accidents, cardiac surgery would have been set back years.

Physicians and historians of medicine may differ on the relative importance of these discoveries, of which there were a great many, but few would disagree that the three recounted in the next chapter belong on any short list. They are the stories of Werner Forssmann, an intern in a German provincial hospital who disregarded his chief's orders and snaked a ureteral catheter into his heart to find a safer way to get drugs to it and to learn about its physiology; Jay McLean, a onetime mucker in a California gold mine who isolated a chemical that prevents heart attacks and strokes during surgery; and John Gibbon, a poet manqué who spent a quarter century developing a machine to substitute for the heart and lungs so that surgeons could work delicately, for long periods, in a still, bloodless environment.

3

Creating the Platform

Jay McLean was born into a medical family in the shadow of gold mines and oil derricks. He was the son and nephew of Old West physicians who were trained at the frontier University of California in the second half of the nineteenth century. He also had a physician cousin in the East, then on the staff of the Johns Hopkins University Medical School and destined to become one of the world's leading endocrinologists.[1] Young McLean wanted to be an academic surgeon, and his cousin convinced him that rather than study surgery at Berkeley, he should come to Baltimore. There were just two problems: money and getting accepted.

Money was a problem because the 1906 San Francisco earthquake had destroyed his family's home and his stepfather's workplace. But McLean was strong-willed and hardworking. Hopkins required a third year of premedical education, which he couldn't afford, so he dropped out of college and worked for a year and a quarter at everything from mucker to millhand in a gold mine. This got him through the premed third year, but he was broke again, so he worked fifteen months drilling oil wells. He then applied to Hopkins while attending the University of California as a first-year medical student. But when the letter from Hopkins came, it was a rejection.

McLean, however, was not easily deterred. In 1915 he bought a railroad ticket to Baltimore, crossed the country, introduced himself to the dean of the medical school, and by virtue of an unexpected opening, was accepted the next day. But he was admitted for the following year, which meant he had a year to kill. He applied to William H. Howell, a Hopkins physiologist, for what, in effect, was a one-year research assistantship, and got it. Howell assigned McLean to follow up on a study he had first reported in 1912 on what caused blood to clot. Howell thought one clotting agent might be a brain extract called cephalin, and he instructed McLean to try to purify it and determine whether it had clotting properties, and if it did, to measure them. Remembering some German medical literature he had read, McLean suggested to Howell that he also test extracts from other organs. One of these was heparphosphatide, from the liver.

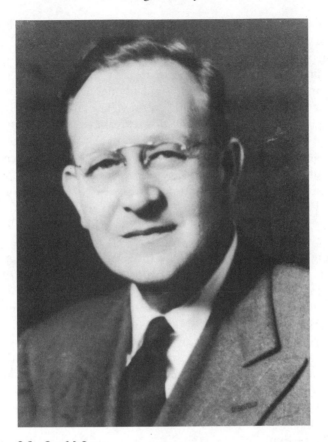

3.1. Jay McLean.

In testing the various extracts, McLean noticed that two substances appeared to slightly retard rather than promote coagulation. This was an entirely unexpected result, but confronted with the experimental evidence, McLean retested the substances several times, eventually demonstrating that the liver extract was a powerful anticoagulant.

McLean went to Howell's office and announced that he had "discovered antithrombin."

Howell smiled and asked: "Are you sure that salt is not contaminating your substance?"

McLean was not sure, so he took cat blood, put it in a beaker, and added a batch of pure heparphosphatides. He set the beaker on Howell's desk and asked him to keep an eye on it to see when it clotted. It didn't. Inexplicably, McLean's 1916 publication on his experiment mentions only that the other extract, cuorin (from an ox heart), "possesses an anticoagulating power."[2] After publishing his paper, McLean finished his medical education and moved on to other areas. Howell named McLean's liver extract heparin and continued work on its purification. Clinical-grade heparin was first produced in Toronto in 1937.[3]

Without heparin, or other anticoagulants developed at about the same time[4] or later, vascular surgery was too risky. The chance of a clot forming and clogging an artery, or moving downstream to cause a blockage elsewhere and possibly a stroke, was simply too great to take. Moreover, the heart-lung machine, which would come along decades later and make heart surgery substantially easier to do, could not function without heparin or something like it to prevent clotting in the plastic tubing through which the blood flowed. Even now, as the twentieth century comes to an end, heparin is still used to prevent clotting when blood passes through the machine's tubing.

Clotting was the big problem—life-threatening and unpredictable—but it was not the only obstacle on the road to a treatment for coronary heart disease. If they were going to treat clogged coronary arteries, surgeons had to know exactly where the blockages were. This meant injecting dye into the arteries so that they would show up on X rays. The trouble was, at the time everyone thought that if you injected enough dye to make the artery visible, it would cut the oxygen supply to the heart and kill the patient. Decades later this belief would be proved false, leading directly to the final discovery that made bypass surgery and angioplasty viable forms of treatment. But before this could happen, there had to be a crucial intermediary step.

Catheters—thin, flexible, atraumatic tubes of the kind that would be needed to inject dye into coronary arteries—had been threaded into the hearts of living animals but not into the hearts of living humans. Unless the coronary arteries could be safely catheterized and radio-opaque dye safely injected, blockages could not be seen and therefore could not be removed. And this could not be done without a blood thinner such as heparin to prevent clots induced by the presence of the catheter in the artery.

Jay McLean had no inkling of open-heart surgery or angioplasty when he discovered "antithrombin." Neither did Werner Forssmann when he became the first medical researcher to document catheterization, not of the coronary arteries, but of the right side of a human heart—his own. Forssmann was looking for safe and better ways to inject medicine into the heart, to study its physiology, and to diagnose heart disease. Like McLean, he was a very young man when he made his contribution. But unlike the Californian, who talked his way into one of America's elite medical schools,

Forssmann was trapped in a highly authoritarian, hierarchical system in Germany.

In 1929 Forssmann, then twenty-four years old, got a job as an intern at a regional Red Cross headquarters in Eberswalde, a small town northeast of Berlin noted today mainly for racist attacks on immigrants. He reported to Dr. Richard Schneider, a surgeon, and the public health officer in Eberswalde.[5] Unlike the typical martinet *Herr Professor* surgeon of the time, Schneider was avuncular, and under his guidance Forssmann was soon performing simple operations on his own. Perhaps because his chief was so encouraging, at age twenty-five Forssmann took an astonishing initiative—he ignored a direct order and changed the course of cardiology. However, because of the conjunction of various circumstances, including German medical politics, the outbreak of World War II, a sojourn of convenience as a member of the Nazi Party, and his subsequent consignment to provincial backwaters, it would take him twenty-seven years to win international recognition for his experiments on himself.

Forssmann and his young colleague Peter Romeis were insulated in the sleepy Prussian town of Eberswalde from much of the Nazi-inspired po-

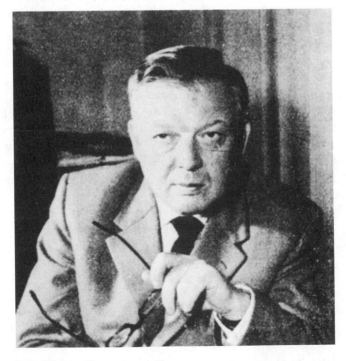

3.2. Werner Forssmann.

litical turmoil then sweeping Germany. Like most interns, they worked hard—sometimes twenty-four hours without a break—but they had few distractions and enough energy for late-night medical debates. A recurring theme of these nocturnal discussions was dissatisfaction with the means available for diagnosing heart disease. At the time these consisted of tapping the chest while listening for telltale sounds, listening with a stethoscope, trying to interpret blurry X-ray images without the benefit of radio-opaque dyes to sharpen contrast, and relatively primitive electrocardiograms.

Time and again autopsies had shown these techniques to be limited or unreliable in diagnosing coronary artery disease. Forssmann had also noticed that in cases of cardiac arrest, injections of resuscitating drugs directly into the heart were avoided until the last minute for fear of lacerating an artery; collapsing a lung; or causing blood to seep into the pericardium, the sac of thin tissue that contains the heart.

In explaining much later his intense interest in probing the heart, Forssmann described an image that he said haunted him day and night. The illustration that made such a profound impression appeared in a nineteenth-century French physiology book. It was a reproduction of an engraving showing Stephen Hales, a British clergyman with a bent for physiology, observing his assistant holding a long glass tube about as thick as a finger that had been inserted through the jugular vein into a supine horse's heart. It is not visible in the engraving, Forssmann said, but "the tube ends in a small inflated rubber balloon inside the ventricle which registered the changes in [blood] pressure," which were then transcribed onto a graph.[6]

This engraving captured a signal example in a long tradition of animal experiments in which tubes were inserted directly into chambers of the heart to study the cardiovascular system.[7] In 1929, however, there was no history of this procedure ever having been done in a human being. Forssmann believed that the ability to thread a tube into a human heart would eventually improve the quality of diagnosis and in an operating room emergency allow drugs to be channeled directly into the heart, avoiding potentially dangerous blind injections through the chest wall. Initially, however, it would contribute to the understanding of how the cardiovascular system works.

Forssmann was convinced not only that it could be done, but that it could be done safely and therefore, he reasoned, ethically. This belief, however, was to be challenged at the highest levels of German medicine, especially since the subject of his experiment could not benefit from the research. Although it seems surprising today, at that time, almost two decades before the brutal experiments conducted by Nazi doctors on concentration camp inmates, the German medical profession had established standards of medical ethics that were equal or superior to any in the world.[8]

Forssmann did not believe that the horse experiment was a good model for human experimentation because it would leave a visible scar on the neck where the tube was inserted, and there was a risk of an air bubble forming and blocking the flow of blood. The chances of the latter happening were far less than he thought, but his judgment was prudent based on what was known at the time. By the summer of 1929 he had decided that the way to do it was through a vein in the elbow.

Forssmann, even at twenty-five, was not entirely naive about the conservatism of German medicine, nor about how politically risky it was to carry out an experiment as innovative as the one he was proposing on a human subject. Therefore he was not surprised when Schneider rejected his request. In the tradition of great medical researchers, he offered to do the experiment on himself, but Schneider vetoed this proposal, too, telling Forssmann, "Imagine how it would be if I had to inform [your mother], who's already lost her husband in the war, that her only son had died in my hospital as a result of an experiment which I had approved."[9]

But Forssmann went ahead anyway. The first things he needed to carry out the experiment were sterile instruments, so he recruited a nurse who had access to them. "I let a few days go by," he wrote in his autobiography, "and then started to prowl around Nurse Gerda Ditzen like a sweet-toothed cat around the cream jug. . . . Gradually, carefully, I steered the conversation round to my hobbyhorse, and found she was interested. She was an attentive listener and wanted to know every detail—not only how the experiment was to be carried out but also what its ultimate purpose was. . . . When, about a fortnight after my conversation with Schneider, she said with a sigh, 'What a pity we can't do the experiment together,' I decided the time had come."[10]

The next day Ditzen volunteered to be his subject. "You'll be the first person in history to undergo such an experiment," Forssmann told her, but it was a lie. He never had any intention of inserting the catheter into Ditzen. Rather, he realized that it was an opportunity to get the instruments with a minimum of fuss so that he could do it on himself. Ditzen prepared the operating room. Then she sat down and held out her left arm. Forssmann told her to lie down on the operating table for the anesthetic. He strapped her legs and hands down tightly so she could not see what he was doing, anesthetized his own left elbow, then went back and began to disinfect hers. He put a sterile cloth over it and killed time while waiting for his anesthetic to take effect. Once it did, he made an incision in the crease of his elbow, inserted a large-caliber needle into the vein, and then pushed the catheter through the needle about a foot into his vein. He then packed the incision with gauze and laid a sterile splint over it, released Ditzen's right hand, and loosened the straps around her knees.[11]

Ditzen accepted the deception with the minimum amount of outrage dignity would permit; then she and Forssmann headed for the X-ray room. With a technician's help, she positioned Forssmann behind a fluoroscope screen. Forsmann's friend Romeis then burst in, said, "what the hell are you doing?" and tried to pull the catheter out of Forssmann's arm.[12] "I had to give him a few kicks on the shin to calm him down," Forssmann wrote.

"I had a mirror placed so that by looking over the top of the screen I could see in it my thorax and upper arm," Forssmann continued. "As I'd expected the catheter had reached the head of the humerus [the long bone of the upper arm]. Romeis wanted me to stop at this point and remove it. But I wouldn't hear of it. I pushed the catheter in further, almost to the two-foot mark. Now the mirror showed the catheter inside the heart."[13]

The technician took some X-ray pictures to record the event and Forssmann withdrew the catheter, unaware that what he had done could easily have caused his heart to fibrillate and kill him. Almost before the catheter was out, he was summoned by Schneider, his chief, who gave him a perfunctory dressing down for disobedience, then shook his hand and told him three things: that he had made a great discovery; that he no longer belonged in the provinces; and that he had damn well better publish fast. He also gave him permission to insert a catheter into the heart of a patient who was dying of a septic abortion. Forssmann's account of this procedure, which, like the one he performed on himself, had no potential for therapeutic benefit, makes no mention of obtaining permission of any kind from the patient. He catheterized his own heart nine times, but this dying woman appears to have been the only other living person into whose heart he inserted a catheter.

It took Forssmann only about two weeks to prepare his paper.[14] Although he considered the potential for treatment the least important outcome of his experiment, he emphasized therapy in his journal article because Schneider warned him that if he didn't, the conservative medical establishment would crucify him on ethical grounds.[15] In 1980 James V. Warren wrote in the *American Journal of Medicine* that "Had [Forssmann's experiment] not occurred until today rather than fifty years ago, modern constraints on investigation of the human subject might have blocked medicine's ability to capitalize on this technique."[16] Warren seems to have had in mind the same thing Schneider did fifty-one years earlier—the ethics of the trade-off between the benefits such experiments may provide for society and the rights of the experimental subject, for whom they provide no benefits.

Forssmann's contribution is the foundation on which modern invasive cardiology is built. It made possible innovations that provide a much more detailed understanding of the heart and the central circulatory system based on observable data. When Forssmann did his experiment, knowledge of how the beating heart functioned was much less precise than it is now. His work opened the way to measurements of pressure in the heart's chambers and the major blood vessels using a special catheter that makes possible diagnosis (and ultimately repair or replacement) of damaged valves, blockages in the aorta, and congential conditions such as holes in the wall separating the two sides of the heart.

It also made possible angiography—mapping of the arteries on movie film—and thereby the pinpointing of blocked vessels; the assessment of the functioning of the left ventricle, the heart's main pumping chamber; a more thorough understanding of the circulation of blood through the lungs; and a means of determining the cause of life-threatening fluid overload in the lungs. And without the quasi-surgical techniques based on Forssmann's 1929 experiment, bypass surgery, the gold standard for treating complex coronary artery disease, would be virtually impossible because finding the blockage that needs to be bypassed would be guesswork.

Forssmann sent his article with accompanying X-ray photographs to the *Klinische Wochenschrift*, which published it on November 5, 1929, and, with an assist from Schneider, moved on to the pinnacle of German surgery, the Charite hospital in Berlin. All the conditions seemed right for the launching of a brilliant career in medical research, but ironically this prized appointment turned out to be the beginning of a protracted decline: a series of professional struggles and setbacks; a pragmatic accommodation to Nazism, including party membership from 1932 on; endurance of harsh conditions in the Wehrmacht; a period during which he was forbidden to practice because of his Nazi past;[17] and finally, a small-time career in urology.

But before fading from sight altogether, Forssmann carried out one more series of experiments that was to have a major impact on cardiology, and radiology as well. After a brief and disappointing interlude at the Charite, where the publication of his article in the *Klinische Wochenschrift* was treated scornfully and challenged as unoriginal, although no one else could document having done what he did, he returned to Eberswalde. Schneider was supportive as always and this time was eager to help his young protégé pursue his research agenda.

Forssmann was impressed by the way in which introduction of a radio-

opaque dye made it possible to produce relatively high-quality X-ray images of the stomach at work. He concluded that the same should be possible with the heart, which, like the stomach, is a hollow organ. The
hospital in Eberswalde had no facilities for animal experiments and an inadequate X-ray lab. But through a contact made at the Charite, Forssmann
was able to get access to an up-to-date radiology department.

He did the experiments on dogs, which his mother kept in her apartment. In effect, he rented the dogs, which were returned to the breeder
after their wounds healed. The fact that the dogs did not die and were
returnable meant he paid 15 marks instead of 20 per dog, which, given
his straitened circumstances, was not an inconsequential difference.

Forssmann gave each dog a shot of morphine at his mother's house, put
it in a potato sack, and took it to the hospital in a taxi. Once at the hospital,
he dosed the animal with ether, shaved the operating area, and inserted a
catheter into the jugular vein. He then injected dye into the heart through
the catheter and took X-ray pictures. Once done, he put the dog back into
the sack, returned to his mother's apartment, and put it in the bathtub.
The animal was alert again within half an hour. His mother changed dress-
ings, removed stitches, and otherwise cared for the animal over the next
ten days.[18] Then Forssmann repeated the process, this time making the
incision on the other side of the neck, after which he took the dog back
to the kennel and brought another one home. Forssmann did these experiments on half a dozen dogs, determining that highly concentrated contrast medium could be introduced into the central circulatory system without harming the dog and that clear pictures could be taken.

The next step was obvious to Forssmann: He would have to experiment
on himself again. He mixed a contrast medium, which he tested for toxicity
by holding the mouth of a test tube filled with the dye against the mucous
membrane inside his cheek for several hours. When the contrast medium
did no harm, he subjected it to several additional tests and concluded it
was safe enough to inject into his heart. After injecting the dye he felt a
slight haziness and his vision blurred momentarily, which he attributed to
the concentrated fluid flowing through his brain. The results, however,
were disappointing because the X-ray machine at Eberswalde was not powerful enough to produce sharp images. Nevertheless, he had proved that
the human heart could tolerate a substantial dose of contrast medium. He
published his results in the *Münchner Medizinische Wochenschrift.*[19]

After the contrast medium experiments, Forssmann dropped into obscurity, although he conducted one last—and highly risky—experiment on
himself while serving in the urology department of the Rudolf Virchow
Hospital in Berlin. More precisely, Forssmann and his chief, Karl Heusch,
agreed to conduct this experiment on one another. They were interested

in contrast radiography of the aorta, the main trunk from which the arterial system branches to the entire body.

"Heusch injected me between the shoulder blade and the spine," Forssmann wrote. "When the tip of the needle reached the wall of the aorta, which he could feel throbbing, an excruciating pain shot through me like an electric shock, probably because the nerve plexus which lines the vessel had been touched. It was the kind of stabbing pain that I imagine comes with tabes, a kind of tertiary syphilis that can be extremely painful. After three unsuccessful attempts, we abandoned the session and I had to go to bed, exhausted. Half an hour later I started to get violent headaches and stiffness in my neck which continued for three days. Elsbet [Forssmann's wife] and Heusch were both very anxious. Her expression was a mixture of worry and anger. When I muttered 'I wonder if it was a vegetative reflex!' she exploded, 'There'll be no more of your crazy experiments.' "[20]

And there were no more. Shortly thereafter, Forssmann began eight weeks of military training at Fort Hahneberg in the Spandau military district. After completing the course, he served as a civilian at hospitals in Mainz and Dresden, then as an army surgeon, and after the war as a urologist in private practice in Bad Kreuznach in the Black Forest, his name if not his accomplishments forgotten by all but a few. Even today, there remains some controversy over whether he was the first person to catheterize a human heart. What is uncontroversial is that he alone has the documentary evidence in the form of X-ray photographs, and, thanks to Schneider, the first publication—in one of Germany's premier medical journals. He also has the Nobel Prize in Medicine or Physiology.

In the years between the late twenties and midfifties, others, such as André Cournand and Dickinson W. Richards, who shared the 1956 Nobel Prize with Forssmann, were rapidly transforming the fields for which Forssmann had laid the groundwork and that would come to be known as cardiac surgery and interventional cardiology. Cournand and Richards had used cardiac catheterization to significantly advance knowledge of cardiovascular functioning. Using blood samples taken directly from the heart and complicated mathematical formulas, they were able to calculate the amount of blood pumped. This made possible sophisticated diagnostic judgments. The Cournand and Richards formulas are still used today.

The advances made by Cournand and Richards were so substantial and complex that Forssmann no longer had the will, or perhaps the strength, to catch up and contribute again. But Forssmann lived until 1979, long enough to witness, or at least read about, some of the dramatic developments for which he laid the foundation: bypass surgery, coronary angioplasty, stenting, and the use of clot-busting drugs, which proved that catheterization had a direct role to play in therapy, not just in diagnosis and research. One of the most critical advances foreshadowed by Forssmann's experiments made it possible to locate blockages in coronary arteries and thus do bypass surgery. But before this could happen, two other problems had to be solved.

First, it was difficult to perform delicate surgery on the coronary arteries while the heart was filled with blood and pumping; this was because of the movement and because bronchial and coronary blood flow obscured the surgeon's vision. A way was needed to empty its chambers, stop it from beating, keep its muscle alive while it was being deprived of oxygen, and start it up again when the operation was over. And second, a mechanical means had to be found to keep the brain and other organs supplied with oxygenated blood during the operation.

Stopping the heart (and starting it up again) was first reported in Britain in July 1955 by Denis Melrose, but in dogs.[21] Melrose injected a metabolic poison, potassium citrate, into the ascending aorta, causing cardiac arrest, which stopped the heart's motion, thereby reducing its need for oxygen and allowing it to be emptied of blood and manipulated. He was able to restart the heart simply by releasing the clamp he had placed on the aorta to keep the chambers empty. The resumed blood flow washed out the potassium citrate and allowed the coronary arteries to resume perfusing the muscle. A couple of months later he succeeded in stopping and restarting a human heart with potassium citrate.[22]

A team at the Cleveland Clinic led by Donald Effler and Willem Kolff began testing Melrose's method almost immediately. And in February and March 1956 they used the technique on three humans, publishing their results in April 1956.[23] Like Melrose, they stopped the heart by injecting potassium citrate in a blood solution into the ascending aorta and restarted it by releasing the aortic clamp.

There was, however, a learning curve for putting the Melrose method into practice. It involved, first, figuring out how much potassium to use— Melrose had used too much—and second, how much to cool the solution to further reduce the heart's need for oxygen. During this time, powerhouses of medicine such as Denton Cooley, Michael DeBakey, and C. Walton Lillehei raised all sorts of legitimate objections to cardioplegia, as this chemical means of cardiac arrest was called. The most serious of these was that on occasion it was impossible to restart the heart.

Melrose's technique was shelved for a number of years while several others were tried, including replacing potassium with the neurotransmitter acetylcholine, or dumping icy saline slush directly onto the heart. But by the mid-1970s the Melrose method made a strong comeback. At the end of the twentieth century a combination method using general lowering of body temperature and injection of a cold blood solution of potassium was one state-of-the-art means of achieving cardiac arrest. The principal alternative method used a crystalloid solution of potassium. In both cases the solution is oxygenated, an addition that increases the heart's ability to resume normal contractions.

There were other important developments in the 1950s, such as the introduction of cardiac intensive-care units and learning how to use banked rather than freshly drawn blood for surgical purposes. But of all the obstacles confronting the handful of early-twentieth-century physicians who were dreaming of an invasive solution for coronary artery disease, or at least relief of its symptoms, the biggest was this: If the heart stopped pumping oxygenated blood to important organs—first and foremost the brain—people died within minutes. Since most surgeons believed you couldn't safely perform complicated coronary surgery without stopping the heart from pumping, a mechanical substitute had to be found for both the pump (heart) and the oxygenator (lungs), a technological feat that most doctors thought was impossible.

It was well into the 1930s before anyone began to attack this problem systematically, although an early attempt was made in 1929, when the aviator Charles Lindbergh's sister-in-law was diagnosed with rheumatic heart disease. An operation was not feasible because "The heart could not be stopped long enough for surgeons to work on it." Why, Lindbergh wondered, was it not possible to build a pump that could substitute for the heart during surgery?[24]

Lindbergh was introduced to Alexis Carrel, who was then at Rockefeller University working on a perfusion pump to preserve organs outside the body. Carrel told Lindbergh that what he wanted done was harder than he thought; that more than a pump was needed to keep patients alive. The machine would have to add oxygen and remove carbon dioxide from blood without significantly damaging its cells, tasks the lungs normally handle with highly sophisticated natural equipment, namely six hundred million capillaries and three hundred million air sacs. Lindbergh quickly saw the difficulties involved, but his interest was sufficiently engaged for him to work with Carrel on his perfusion project. In 1935 the experimental surgeon and record-breaking flier produced a Pyrex pump that oxygenated perfusion fluid and kept a cat thyroid gland alive for eighteen days. Preservation of other organs followed. On June 13, 1938, Lindbergh, Carrel, and their glass device, an important forerunner of the heart-lung machine, made the cover of *Time* magazine.[25]

When Carrel and Lindbergh were beginning to work on their pump, John H. Gibbon, Jr., was a twenty-seven-year-old research fellow at Massachusetts General Hospital. He was speculative, precise, and intellectually curious, qualities that were already evident by the time he was five and asked his mother, "If God is everywhere, but we can't hear Him or see Him, why can't we feel Him?"[26] Later, like his mother, he was fond of reading philosophy, especially William James.

On October 3, 1930, he was one of several members of a team keeping a nervous watch at the bedside of a woman who had suffered a massive pulmonary embolism, a blood clot with the potential for shutting down her blood supply. His assignment was to check her blood pressure and pulse rate every fifteen minutes to determine whether the clot had totally blocked her pulmonary artery, in which case his mentor, Edward D. Churchill, would immediately attempt to remove the clot. For seventeen hours nothing much happened. Then "the patient became unconscious, had no palpable pulse, and stopped breathing." It took Churchill just six minutes and thirty seconds to remove the clot and close the artery. It was fast and elegant surgery, but not fast enough. The woman died.[27]

Churchill had tried pulmonary embolectomy, a last-ditch procedure. It had been invented in Germany by Friedrich Trendelenburg but had been done successfully only 9 times out of 140 attempts,[28] and never in the United States. Like almost everyone who had attempted this operation, he was too slow. When deprived of blood, the brain dies in about six minutes and sustains irreparable damage even sooner. Gibbon, like Carrel when he heard about President Carnot's death, was deeply disturbed by the experience, by medicine's impotence. He kept thinking, while in his own words "helplessly watching the patient struggle for life as her blood became darker and her veins more distended," that lives such as this one could be saved by a machine that would do "part of the work of the patient's heart and lungs outside the body."[29]

Had he followed his own lights, Gibbon, whose father was a professor of surgery and the second American to try to suture a wound in the heart,[30] and whose grandfather, great-grandfather, and great-great-grandfather were also physicians, would not have been at that bedside thinking those frustrating thoughts. And the heart-lung machine undoubtedly would have been longer in coming.

While an undergraduate at Princeton, where he developed a lifelong fondness for hard liquor and cigarettes, Gibbon declared openly that he wanted to break with the family tradition: to be a poet, or perhaps a painter. But his father gently disabused him of these notions in the age-old tradition of fathers, by assuring him that poetry and painting were fine careers as long as one didn't mind cold and hunger. The argument apparently impressed young Gibbon, who had been reared in privilege—a French governess, private schools, country properties, trips to Europe—so he enrolled in medical school.

However, he was quickly bored by the rote learning typical of the first two years, and told his father he wanted to quit. This time his father told him that if you don't practice medicine, that's your business, but once you start something, you should finish it. Again he took his father's advice, and graduated from Jefferson Medical College, where the elder Gibbon taught.[31] He accepted a two-year internship at Pennsylvania Hospital, during which he assisted a physician carrying out a hypertension study. The exposure to research captured his imagination, led to his fellowship under Churchill, and evolved into a lifelong passion.

After completing his fellowship in Boston, Gibbon returned to Philadelphia with a new wife and collaborator, Mary (Maly) Hopkinson, and a nagging, unarticulated desire to invent a machine that would oxygenate and circulate blood. For the next three and a half years at the University of Pennsylvania, he operated in the morning and did research in the afternoon—and at home, on weekends and in evenings. Years later he described some of this after-hours research:

> My wife and I carried out . . . slightly bizarre experiments on ourselves and our friends. . . . We were particularly anxious to learn how slight a shift in body temperature would cause vasoconstriction [tightening of vessels in the circulatory system] or vasodilation [relaxing of circulatory vessels] of the extremities. We got a very sensitive mercury thermometer about three feet long, which would measure temperatures to a hundredth of a degree Centigrade. The bulb of this thermometer would be stuck into my rectum or that of a friend, and the subject would then swallow a stomach tube, down which we poured as much ice cold water as could be tolerated, measuring the effect on skin temperature of the fingers. I also once got my wife to give me an ice-cold intravenous solution for the same purpose.[32]

But no matter how interesting he found his research, he still had the same deep sense of frustration. Nothing he was working on would prevent patients like the woman with the pulmonary embolism from dying. Therefore, in 1934 Gibbon returned to Boston with a second research fellowship under Churchill, who was unenthusiastic about the heart-lung machine but nevertheless willing to give his young protégé a chance to work on it. A more skeptical colleague at Massachussetts General Hospital warned Gibbon that the machine probably wouldn't work and that he would have nothing to show for his time and trouble. But Gibbon was unwavering, and thirty-three years later his invention became the platform from which coronary artery bypass surgery was launched.

Gibbon assembled his prototype heart-lung machine in the lab from bought components and parts, including a secondhand air pump that cost just a few dollars. When he couldn't find what he needed, he made it. Among other things, he produced one-way valves for the original pump using a razor blade, rubber stoppers, and glass tubes. First, he cut little flaps on the sides of a stopper. He then inserted a glass tube through its center and fitted the stopper into a slightly larger tube, creating what he called "a very adequate valve."

But the pump was the easy part. Gibbon knew that the biggest challenge was figuring out how to build an artifical lung that could remove carbon dioxide and add oxygen without seriously damaging human blood cells. Attempts had been made before, but they were uniformly traumatic to the blood. Gibbon reviewed the literature and also consulted a professor of steam engineering at Harvard, who suggested "a slightly cone-shaped vertical revolving cylinder on which the blood would film and then emerge from the top of the cylinder, like a cream separator."[33] It was necessary to make the blood into a thin film so that the oxygen could penetrate in an osmosislike process to the hemoglobin, the oxygen-carrying element of the red blood cells. Two Germans, Max von Frey and Max Gruber, had figured this out in 1885 and built a rather sophisticated device similar to the one Gibbon finally came up with. They used it for the same purpose that Carrel and Lindbergh used their Pyrex pump, to perfuse isolated organs.[34]

Gibbon modified the engineer's design, coming up with a vertical revolving cylinder inside a stationary cup. The blood was filmed on the inside of the cylinder, where it absorbed oxygen before being collected in the cup for return to the body. The thin bottom edge of the cylinder and the cup were placed in a relationship designed to minimize damage to fragile blood cells, which is caused by abrupt changes in the rate or direction of blood flow. He also was careful to use materials and design features that would minimize damage to blood cells and would not promote clotting.

Gibbon chose cats for his experiments, in part because they were cheaper than dogs. Indeed, sometimes they were free because he and his wife would often catch strays at night. He also used cats because they were smaller and therefore less blood was needed to prime the pump.[35] To test the machine, he compressed the animals' pulmonary arteries, thereby simulating massive emboli and cutting off their circulation. He then put them on artificial circulation and respiration.

In his first operation, Gibbon removed a piece of a cat's breastbone, exposed the pulmonary artery, and clamped it. Then, by means of thin-walled metal tubes inserted into the jugular vein in the neck and the femoral artery in the groin, he hooked up the cat to the jerry-rigged heart-lung machine. A crude piston-type pump drove the cat's dark, venous, oxygen-depleted blood into the artificial lung, which removed carbon dioxide and restored oxygen. Then the blood, now bright red, was pumped back through the animal's arterial system, with heparin added to prevent clotting.

Gibbon worried that as a result of using the newly available anticoagulant,[36] fatal hemorrhaging might result, but this turned out to be a negligible concern. The experiment succeeded, and within months he was able to keep a cat alive on the machine for more than three and a half hours. But a cat wasn't a human. Moreover, the machine needed to keep a cat alive was the size of a concert grand piano, it required "buckets of blood" to prime it, and it often leaked blood all over the floor during use.[37]

In 1935 Gibbon returned to the University of Pennsylvania and continued his experiments on cats. He soon recognized that success could mean tremendous advances in cardiac surgery, including the possibility of repairing damaged heart valves. At that time, no one had yet conceived of the possibility of doing coronary artery bypass surgery on humans. Over the next several years Gibbon worked on improving the machine. His ultimate goal was to build one that was roughly twenty times bigger than his concert grand and that would work on humans.

But this critical phase of his life's project would have to wait. Within weeks of the Japanese attack on Pearl Harbor on December 7, 1941, Gibbon began four years of service in the Army Medical Corps, more than half of which was spent at a hospital in New Caledonia, in the Coral Sea between Australia and the Solomon Islands. He was so impressed by the army's system of medical care that when he returned after the war he wrote an article for *Harper's* magazine in which he advocated that civilian medicine adopt important features of the military system, such as careful monitoring of physician performance. He also recommended a program of universal health care and insurance that at the time was widely and pejoratively labeled "socialized medicine."[38]

Once out of the army, Gibbon was determined to redouble his efforts to invent a heart-lung machine. These efforts kept him away from home and appear to have reinforced his children's feeling, formed during the war, of being functionally fatherless.[39] Early in 1946 he took a job at Jefferson Medical College that would allow him to work long hours in the lab. Over the next couple of years two things happened that, while not guaranteeing him success, improved his chances substantially. He got the first of a series of grants from the new National Heart Institute that would support his work from 1949 until 1962. But even before that, in 1946, a freshman medical student at Jefferson was able to arrange a meeting for him with Thomas J. Watson, Sr., chairman of International Business Machines.

The two men got together, Gibbon explained that he needed the engineering know-how to build a machine that could oxygenate blood without damaging blood cells and that would not be the size of a ballroom, and Watson immediately agreed to supply it, providing an early example of productive cooperation between a medical researcher and a high-tech industrial corporation. IBM donated the engineering help and materials Gibbon needed to develop a heart-lung machine of manageable size that would work on humans and forswore all future profits.[40] Such collaborations between physicians and industry were common by the 1980s, but by then nobody was forswearing profits, not the companies and not the medical researchers.

The original heart-lung machine, delivered to Gibbon by IBM in 1949, was by today's standards a huge apparatus with its own air-conditioning system and a panel of highly complicated controls. The valveless pump, of a type first introduced in 1927 and modified by Michael DeBakey in 1934, used rollers to compress the flexible tubes through which the blood passed. To avoid damaging blood cells the rollers did not completely compress the tubing. The artificial lung, although larger than the original, was the

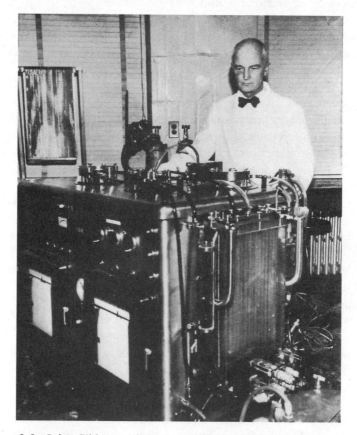

3.3. John Gibbon with his heart-lung machine built with the help of IBM engineers.

same revolving-cylinder type that Gibbon had invented for his first cat experiments.[41]

While testing the new machine to work out bugs such as the introduction into the circulation of tiny but potentially fatal emboli from donor blood, two workers in Gibbon's lab made an important discovery: Turbulence significantly increased the amount of oxygen the blood absorbed. As a result, Gibbon and his coworkers tested different kinds and different configurations of mesh screens to create just the right amount of turbulence inside the cylinder. Eventually IBM built an updated machine with a series of stainless steel mesh screens inside a clear plastic chamber as the oxygenator. This apparatus kept a twenty-pound dog alive for an hour and thirty six minutes in April 1951.

For the next year or so Gibbon used this machine to keep dogs alive while he operated on congenital defects of the type commonly known as holes in the heart. Then, one day in the spring of 1952, he quietly made the momentous decision to hook up the machine to an eleven-pound, fifteen-month-old baby girl suffering from severe congestive heart failure. Other doctors who had studied the case attributed the disease to an "interatrial septal defect," a hole in the wall that separates the two upper chambers of the heart. But the diagnosis was wrong and, as a result, the incision was made in the wrong place. The baby died shortly after the operation through no fault of the heart-lung machine.

At about the same time as Gibbon's first attempt to operate on a human patient using the heart-lung machine, two surgeons at the University of Minnesota, John Lewis and Mansur Taufic, were experimenting with a different method of making the heart operable. They wrapped a five-year-old girl named Jackie Weeks in a cooling blanket, bringing her temperature down to eighty-one degrees Fahrenheit, and successfully closed a hole in her heart. Lewis and Taufic put into practice what a Canadian surgeon named Wilfred Bigelow had reported in 1950 based on studies of hibernating animals: Cooling reduces the body's need for oxygen, which gives the surgeon a few added minutes to finish suturing while clamps isolate the heart. But cooling does not add enough time to do lengthy procedures such as valve and bypass surgery.

Just over a year later, Gibbon was ready to try again. The patient was eighteen-year-old Cecilia Bavolek, who was suffering from heart failure, and this time the cause really was a septal defect, although it was not clear whether the hole was between the atria or the ventricles. Bavolek was an ideal candidate for surgery using the heart-lung machine. Gibbon told the young woman and her mother that the "only previous time the [heart-lung machine] had been used in a human patient, the apparatus had performed satisfactorily but the child had died because of an unrecognized cardiac lesion which was not corrected."[42] Bavolek and her family agreed to the surgery, and on May 6, 1953, Gibbon operated on her to close a hole the size of a silver dollar while her blood was oxygenated and circulated by his machine. Here's his matter-of-fact description of the first successful operation ever on a human with mechanical cardiopulmonary bypass:

> The patient was connected with the apparatus for forty-five minutes and for twenty-six minutes all cardio-respiratory functions were maintained by the apparatus. She had a large interatrial septal defect which was quite easily closed with a continuous silk suture. The patient's postoperative convalescence was uneventful. She was readmitted to the hospital in July 1953. At that time, cardiac catheterization showed that the septal defect was completely closed. . . . The cardiac murmur had completely disappeared and she was in good health.[43]

Gibbon was so enervated after the surgery that for the only time in his career he did not write the postoperative note describing the operation himself. He was also deeply relieved. That evening he telephoned two great surgeons to tell them what he had done: Alfred Blalock at Johns Hopkins and Clarence Crafoord in Stockholm. But Gibbon's next two patients died, and he never did open-chest heart surgery again.[44] John Kirklin, a renowned heart surgeon who later improved on Gibbon's design with a team at the Mayo Clinic, speculated that these deaths occurred because Gibbon failed to appreciate "some of the technical aspects of cardiac surgery."[45] Although the machine was not at fault, Gibbon was dejected and decided to spend the following year trying to correct defects involving clotting, to increase pumping capacity, and to provide a more uniform flow of blood.

Despite Bavolek's complete recovery, and improvements on the heart-lung machine made by Kirklin's team, for several years there were as many failures as successes using pump-oxygenators. This included machines such as Gibbon's, one developed by Denis Melrose in England that used rotating disks to create a thin film of blood that could easily absorb oxygen, and others that bubbled oxygen through the blood. Moreover, experiments using animal lungs as oxygenators continued around the country. Gibbon wrote in 1970 that for some time after the heart-lung machine was in general use he disliked reading about open-heart operations in surgical journals for fear that he "had opened some kind of Pandora's Box."[46]

C. Walton Lillehei, who had been working on heart-lung bypass at the University of Minnesota, was also concerned about the machine's safety. He decided less than a year after Gibbon's operation on Cecilia Bavolek that it would be safer to hook up a patient to another human being and "cross-circulate" their blood. His colleagues Morley and Joan Cohen, and a resident named Herbert Warden, had been experimenting with cross-circulation, or pumping blood directly from the circulation of a donor through the patient's circulation. The technique was not new. Apart from Carrel's kitchen-table case, it had been used in physiological experiments, in open-heart experiments on animals, and in treating end-stage uremia in a human patient.[47] But Lillehei and his associate Richard Varco were the first to use it on human open-heart patients.

Between 1954 and 1955 Lillehei and colleagues used this procedure forty-five times at the University of Minnesota, with severely ill infants or children as the patients and with parents generally as the donors. Although the surgeon George J. Haupt said this was the only known operation with a potential 200 percent mortality,[48] two-thirds of the patients survived the surgery, and there was only one donor complication and no donor fatalities, which seems remarkable considering the immunological problems that might have resulted.[49]

In perhaps the most publicized of these procedures, a child named Michael Shaw was referred to Lillehei to correct a complicated congenital defect. In the absence of an acceptable parental donor, an altruistic local gravedigger named Howard Holtz volunteered to serve as the living heart-lung machine. The operation was successful, and Shaw went on to live a full life.[50] Nonetheless, the risk of killing a donor seemed too high, and concern over possible malpractice suits, although there had been only one in the series of forty-five cases, compounded the concern.[51] The heart-lung machine, while not risk-free, looked like a better bet.

In 1963 Cecilia Bavolek's picture was taken with Vice President Lyndon Johnson as the American Heart Association's Heart Queen. By then newer machines were getting better results than Gibbon's early models. In Texas, Denton Cooley built a workable machine mostly out of parts from local hardware stores and a restaurant supplier that came to be known as Cooley's Coffee Pot.[52]

The heart-lung machine vastly improved the ability of surgeons to do long, complicated operations, but it did not solve all the problems. It did not, for example, produce a perfectly blood-free operating field, which surgeons need to see what they are doing.[53] And it didn't stop the heart from beating, which makes precise suturing difficult. Over the next decade, however, modern heart surgery became possible because Gibbon's machine and its improved successors were used in combination with cooling of the body, chemical cardiac arrest, or both. These additional techniques reduced the heart muscle's need for oxygen, thereby giving heart surgeons the time they need to do their delicate work.

4

Groping in the Dark

The heart is the last great northwest of surgery.

Harvey Cushing

Claude Beck was a bright young man from the anthracite belt of eastern Pennsylvania. As a youth he was handsome, with a sensitive mouth and caring eyes. In later life he grew to resemble W. C. Fields. During a long, distinguished career he made important contributions to cardiac surgery and cardiac care generally. His experimental operations were among the first attempts to surgically restore restricted blood flow to the heart muscle, the same goal as bypass surgery. His work also exemplifies a number of ethical issues in surgery, some of which remain controversial today.

In 1923–24 Beck was the Arthur Tracy Cabot Fellow in Surgical Research at Harvard Medical School. While at Harvard he worked on finding a way to reopen blocked mitral valves, a condition that can cause heart failure and death. The mitral valve, so named because it resembles a bishop's miter, is one of four one-way gates that keep blood flowing through the heart in the right direction. It regulates blood flowing from the left atrium into the left ventricle. A valve known as the tricuspid, for its three toothlike projections, controls the flow from the right atrium into the right ventricle. The other two valves, the aortic and pulmonary, direct flow respectively from the left ventricle into the aorta, from which it circulates throughout the body, and from the right ventricle into the pulmonary artery, from which it enters the lungs to be purified and oxygenated.

Blood freshly oxygenated by the lungs passes through the mitral valve into the left ventricle before being driven through the circulatory system by the contraction of the ventricle. Beck devised an instrument to open this valve by removing a piece of it, but the operation was a dismal failure. Years later, Samuel Levine, who had worked on an earlier unsuccessful attempt to open blocked mitral valves, said cryptically of the ill-fated series: "The patients were admitted through the front door of the hospital. They were discharged through the back door [as cadavers]."[1] All seven died.

Elliott Cutler, the senior surgeon who actually performed all of these mitral valve operations, acknowledged failure in his final report but concluded that "[T]he mortality figures alone should not deter further investigation, both clinical and experimental, since they are to be expected in the opening up of any new field of surgical endeavor."[2] Beck, who was the second author of the final report, agreed fully.[3]

Cutler and Beck's attitude is still common among surgeons who do clinical research. In 1996 Paul Corso, a Washington, D.C., surgeon, asked rhetorically: "Is there any way to prove whether a particular technique is going to be successful without doing a bunch of patients? Nope," he answered, "there isn't."[4]

In an article published in 1989 on his early efforts to operate on the heart using the newly invented heart-lung machine, the distinguished heart surgeon John Kirklin wrote: "We had decided to do all eight patients, determined to do the eighth patient even if the first seven died. All of this was planned with the knowledge and approval of the governance of the Mayo Clinic."[5] And in 1996 Cleveland Clinic heart surgeon Paul Taylor said: "Surgeons try things out, sometimes on animals, sometimes on clinical patients. And if they like what they see, even if the early mortality rates are very high, they continue with the new procedure."[6]

Is Corso right that there is no better way to advance surgery, no more humane way, no way to benefit future generations of patients while still treating the subject of the experimental operation ethically? Tom Fogarty, a Stanford surgeon turned inventor, says he is. According to Fogarty:

> Once you've got [surgical] technology you . . . have to use it in a whole bunch of different clinical situations before you know what it's most appropriate for. And that is a process you can't avoid. Now after you document what's appropriate it's very easy to look back and say, "That was inappropriate." The fact is that it made sense to test the limits of what you were doing relative to the outcome.[7]

About a decade after the mitral-valve operations, Beck provided another example of this surgical ethos. He operated on a fifteen-year-old boy to remove a compression scar from his heart. When Beck pinched the scar between his left thumb and index finger so he could excise the scar with the scalpel in his other hand, he curtailed blood flow to the heart. This caused left ventricular fibrillation, a disruption in the heart's electrical circuitry marked by a rapid, chaotic rhythm that devastates the organ's ability to pump and makes the ventricle feel, in a well-known analogy, like a bag of wriggling worms. The boy died.

"I accepted responsibility for his death," Beck said, "but he did not die in vain. He is one of the unsung heroes of medicine."[8] Beck's point, like Cutler's, was that the boy's death contributed to knowledge, in this case about the nature of ventricular fibrillation, and that as a result other lives would be saved. Beck knew that the death of the fifteen-year-old had implications for understanding fibrillation, and he went on to invent the first life-saving defibrillation technique using a strong electrical shock to restore the normal rhythm of a fibrillating heart.

More than sixty years later, about one-third of those who suffer heart attacks die from left ventricular fibrillation. As many as 175,000 deaths a year could be prevented by placing defibrillators, which are relatively inexpensive and easy to use, in public places and training people to operate them.[9] In the late 1990s three U.S. airlines—American, Delta, and Alaska—followed the lead of Qantas, the Australian national carrier, and began putting the $3,000 machines on their planes.[10] In November, 1998, Michael Tighe, who was flying from Boston to Los Angeles on American, became the first person to have his life saved in flight by one of the booksize devices.[11]

Cutler and Beck were grappling with a conflict that still bedevils surgeons. The scholar Jay Katz characterized it as balancing society's interests in a way that "will protect the individual's well-being and right to self-determination and encourage the acquisition of knowledge through scientific investigation."[12] The two surgeons took an academic, population-centered view, which is typical of many clinical researchers: While not indifferent to the fates of their patients, they were primarily dedicated to answering research questions.

Most bioethicists take a more clinical, patient-centered view: While not indifferent to solving research problems, they contend that the surgeon's primary commitment should always be to his patients. Cutler was right to conclude that mortality figures alone should not be allowed to retard surgical progress. And in a sense Beck was also right that his young patient did not die in vain. But even two or three deaths should be seen as evidence of a need to stop and reconsider. And the social utility attributed to the boy's death probably did little to console his parents. Both men's comments, though typical for the time, and understandable even today given the imperatives of research and the nature of surgery, show a lack of respect for the rights of individual patients that is incompatible with personal dignity and human rights.

Quite apart from moral considerations, Beck's experience with the fifteen-year-old had consequences for cardiac surgery. Once he realized that uneven blood flow had caused his teenage patient to fibrillate, Beck began to look for the responsible mechanism. Using electrocardiography, he discovered that where heart muscle that was well supplied with arterial blood touched muscle that was poorly supplied, there was electrical instability. The effect of this instability was the same as shocking the heart with a live wire. It caused fibrillation.

In the course of his work Beck noticed that the oxygen-deprived muscle was bluish in color and the fully oxygenated muscle was pink. A heart that was all one color, he determined, was more stable electrically than a two-color heart. But if it happened to be all blue rather than all pink, it would soon die from lack of nourishment. One job, then, was to figure out how to convert a two-color heart to an all-pink heart. The way to do it, Beck concluded, was by "the surgical production of collaterals—connections between one coronary artery and another—so that [an oxygen-carrying] red blood cell could go where it was needed most."[13] The idea was promising. But how could it be done?

As he continued his research on dogs, Beck noticed that when he severed a natural adhesion between the heart and the pericardium, the sac that contains it, both ends bled profusely.[14] This suggested to him the possibility of bringing blood to the heart muscle by purposely adhering its surface to tissue outside of it, such as the fatty surface of the pericardium. With this in mind, he consulted with Alan Moritz, a pathologist at Western Reserve who was studying blood vessels that developed naturally within such adhesions. Eventually Beck settled on two fairly primitive ways of attempting to coerce the heart into forming collaterals, or perhaps opening preexisting but previously unopened collaterals.

First he roughened with a burr the surface of the heart and the lining of the pericardium in the belief that inflammation would stimulate collaterals. Then he chemically irritated the heart by coating its surface with finely ground animal bone. Beck believed that this, too, would stimulate collateral development through inflammation. Later he switched to powdered asbestos.

He also concluded that he could stimulate collateral formation from outside the heart and pericardium by adhering a pectoral muscle to the heart. And finally, in a second part to the procedure, he narrowed the coronary sinus (the terminus of the coronary vein) to slow the flow of venous blood through the heart, on the theory that this would increase oxygen absorption by the heart muscle.[15] His main goal, however, was not to provide additional blood to the heart muscle, but to reroute oxygenated blood to areas that were not getting enough, which Beck believed would relieve anginal pain and protect against death from future heart attacks.

After an additional series of dog experiments by his colleague David Leighninger, Beck, a slow, meticulous surgeon, performed his operation for the first time on a human. The patient was a Cleveland man named Joseph Kritchmar, who was incapacitated by chest pain. The operation was done on February 13, 1935, at Lakeside Hospital. Beck used bone dust as the irritant, and he grafted pectoral muscle to the heart to see if collateral vessels would grow across the muscle from arteries on the interior of the chest wall. It is not clear whether they did or didn't, but Kritchmar recovered and lived for about fifteen years. He worked as a gardener after the surgery.[16]

Beck performed his operation, which became widely known as Beck I, 37 times between 1935 and 1942, the year he entered the army. Toward the end of the series he dropped the pectoral graft. After the war he developed another operation, known as Beck II, which was designed to force arterial blood through the veins and also to stimulate the development of collaterals between coronary arteries. He did 124 of these technically demanding operations between 1948 and 1954 before returning to Beck I, a simpler procedure. In the late 1950s about 50 surgeons were doing Beck I operations in the United States, and some were predicting that they would become as common as appendectomies.[17] They did not. Between 1954 and 1968 Beck performed about 1,000 Beck I operations using the burr, asbestos, and sinus-narrowing techniques.[18] The hospital mortality rate was 5.7 percent.[19] Today the best hospitals that accept all comers for bypass surgery have mortality rates half of Beck's.

Although studies in the 1960s suggested that patients had benefited from the operation, the consensus now is that this was never proved and that any benefit very likely resulted from a placebo effect. One Cleveland Clinic surgeon, moreover, contends that "about half of Beck's patients had no coronary disease. If you had a pain in the chest," he said, "for Beck you were probably a candidate" for surgery.[20]

Meanwhile, as late as the 1950s, other respected thoracic surgeons were seeking different solutions to the problem of supplying the heart muscle with enough oxygen. These included tieing off patients' internal mammary arteries in the belief that this would force more blood into the coronaries, thereby relieving angina. Some reported success.[21] But most physicians were skeptical. The skeptics were sure that in this operation, too, the relief was due to a placebo effect. So a physician named Leonard Cobb and some of his colleagues from the University of Washington set up a small trial in which they compared the attempt to reroute blood to a sham operation.[22]

Cobb's study was double-blind, which meant that neither patients nor physicians who handled postoperative follow-up knew which patients received the treatment and which just a skin incision to make it look like they had had their internal mammary arteries tied. Indeed, the patients were only told they were participating in an evaluation of the treatment, not that they might or might not get it. Although they were told the effectiveness of the procedure had not been proved, many of them had read or heard of a *Reader's Digest* article that had reported enthusiastically on it.[23] The physicians maintained what the study referred to as "a reasonably optimistic attitude."

Seventeen patients, all of whom had seriously limited lifestyles as a result of angina, agreed to participate. Eight were randomly selected to have their arteries tied and nine to have the sham operation. Two patients died during follow-up, one from each group. A patient whose arteries were tied died of a heart attack two months later. A patient whose arteries were not tied died eight months later, probably of a heart attack. The follow-up period ranged from three to fifteen months. Here is what the authors concluded:

> During the first six months, five out of eight of the ligated patients [those whose arteries were tied off] and five out of nine of the nonligated [those whose arteries were not tied] reported "significant" subjective improvements. Striking improvement in exercise tolerance occurred in two patients whose internal mammary arteries were not ligated; one of these patients failed to demonstrate the abnormal electrocardiographic changes that occurred preoperatively with the same exercise test.
>
> Internal mammary artery ligation probably has no effect on the pathophysiology of coronary artery disease.[24]

Two things stand out about the Cobb study. One, of course, is the primitiveness of knowledge, as late as 1959, about treating coronary artery disease. Most of the population at risk for this disease at the millennium were already working adults in 1959. Today there is an armamentarium of invasive and noninvasive treatments available to them that in some cases can give them twenty years of angina-free normal living. In 1959 there was little more than nitroglycerin tablets, sometimes swallowed at the rate of more than forty a day, and prolonged bed rest. Care for coronary artery disease is still mainly palliative, but medicine has come a long way.

The other noteworthy feature of this study, at least from an end-of-century perspective, is that patients were unwittingly subjected to a sham operation. They were cut, under local anesthetic, perhaps permanently scarred, and led to believe that they were receiving a treatment that had at least some potential to do them lasting good. Under current ethical norms the Cobb study would be impermissible because there was no informed consent, the subjects were misled about the purpose of the study, and the researchers did not believe there was a potential for benefit. But sham operations, with informed consent, are being done again in 1999 and a new debate is brewing over the ethics of asking even willing patients to submit to a surgical procedure that cannot do them any good.

The protection of the rights of research subjects remains problematical. How well do patients understand, for example, the purpose of clinical trials in which they enroll? Consider the case of a microbiologist well versed in the life sciences who, while in the hospital for bypass surgery, was enrolled in a study of which he said he had only a sketchy understanding. He agreed to participate even though the study required him to undergo an otherwise unindicated angiogram. One of his motives, he said, was altruistic, but on what basis did he conclude that the study was likely to benefit humanity? The other motive was that he believed, although no one told him so, that he would get better treatment from doctors and nurses as a study subject than he would otherwise receive. There is no evidence that he did.[25]

And how well do clinical researchers balance the conflict of interest inherent in caring for patients while pursuing research goals? Recruitment for trials, including pressure to enroll patients quickly, is always a problem, which makes credible this allegation made by Leonard Golding of Cleveland Clinic: He said he knew—although he would not name—a head of cardiology at an academic hospital who instructed his staff that no patient was to pass through the cardiology service without becoming a subject in a clinical trial.[26] Surely some among these patients, if fully informed, would have elected not to participate. Another cardiologist, who did not want to be identified, said that based on his personal experience, Golding's assertion was "not surprising."

While clinical trials for drugs and new medical devices began about fifty years ago, this has not been the case with surgery. And it certainly was not the case more than fifty years ago when Beck and Arthur Vineberg, a Canadian working at McGill University in Montréal, were independently attacking the problem of the ischemic myocardium—the oxygen-starved heart muscle—in an attempt to relieve angina and possibly extend life. While there is virtually unanimous agreement among today's surgeons that Beck's operations were failures, Vineberg's case is more complicated. There is no doubt that sometimes his operation did supply new blood to the heart muscle, relieving the angina and probably extending the lives of some patients.

Beck had tried Vineberg's procedure on dogs, but did not pursue it in humans because he believed it was an uncertain source of blood and unacceptably risky because it involved too much manipulation of the heart.[27] The strategy was implantation of an internal mammary artery into a tunnel gouged into the heart muscle. The internal mammaries, which feed blood to the chest wall and several organs situated between the pleural sacs, are now the conduits of choice in bypass surgery. Not only are they a good size matchup for the heart's main vessels—the left anterior descending, circumflex and right coronary arteries—but also, after surgery, they remain open for fifteen years or more about 95 percent of the time. Saphenous vein grafts taken from the leg match up less well and clog sooner.

But in 1945, the year Vineberg began animal experiments using the internal mammary arteries to bring oxygenated blood to the heart muscle, bypass surgery had only been done on dogs, and there is nothing in the literature to suggest that anyone was considering trying it on a human being. Indeed, it was generally believed at the time that when coronary artery disease became symptomatic, the heart muscle was already so scarred that it would be useless to try to increase its blood supply.

Once more, however, as was the case with Herrick's 1912 article on heart attacks, the conventional wisdom was undercut by a careful reading of the literature. Vineberg came across an obscure article published in 1941 showing that even when blockages exist in coronary arteries, the network of tiny vessels within the heart muscle are usually disease-free. The article also pointed out that each of the three coronary artery systems—left, right, and circumflex—supplies a specific zone of the heart muscle, and that in 9 percent of normal hearts, and in almost all diseased hearts, collateral channels connect these zones.[28]

This information led Vineberg to conclude that you could route blood around a blocked coronary artery by plugging a big, high-pressure, high-flow artery directly into the muscle of the heart's main pumping chamber, the left ventricle. The idea was to get the artery of choice, the nearby internal mammary artery, to grow tiny branches, or force open existing but closed branches, that would connect with the equally tiny arterioles inside the muscle. These branches would then provide oxygenated blood to the muscle through the arterioles.[29]

Vineberg's crude-sounding idea was to dig a small tunnel in the muscle of the left ventricle, bury the internal mammary artery inside it with its end tied shut, and hope it would sprout collaterals. Although Vineberg's operation was different from what we now know as bypass surgery, the principle was the same: Get blood beyond the blockage, to where it was needed. The latest spin on the Vineberg approach involves injecting a growth factor into a blocked coronary artery, which coaxes the vessel into growing collaterals to bypass the blockage.

In 1945 Vineberg began experimenting on dogs. The first two years were discouraging. Of 104 dogs operated on, only 49 survived, and of those 49, in 41 the implanted internal mammary arteries shut down and failed to develop these collateral connections. Vineberg was ready to give up. But before abandoning revascularization surgery altogether, he took a last look at the protocols of the eight animals in which the internal mammary arteries remained open and developed connections. He discovered that these dogs were all small, as were their arteries. More relevantly, he noted that because the arteries were small, he had not bothered to tie off their even-smaller side branches, so they bled directly into the muscle. With this lesson absorbed, he tried again, this time implanting all of the internal mammary arteries, irrespective of size, with their side branches bleeding. The results were gratifying. Connections formed, and hematomas, or blood clots, didn't.

Further improvements were introduced, and by April 1950 Vineberg was ready to answer the big question: What would happen when a bleeding artery was implanted in a diseased area of human heart muscle? The answer came quickly. The operation, performed at Royal Victoria Hospital in Montréal, was a success, but the patient died. The implanted internal mammary artery was wide open, but sixty-two hours after surgery a blood clot closed off the patient's circumflex artery, which feeds a different part of the heart muscle, causing a fatal heart attack.

Over the next four years Vineberg performed his operation on thirty-one patients. The operative mortality rate was a grim 25 percent. But with an attitude similar to that of Cutler and Beck, he persisted, and between 1954 and 1962 only two patients died out of sixty-three, a rate of 3.2 percent. During the same period two other surgeons did Vineberg operations, one reporting 2.2 percent operative mortality with forty-five patients, and the other eleven cases with no operative deaths.[30] Vineberg reported that of the last sixty-three patients in his series, 64 percent were improved and 75 percent returned to work.

But most of his colleagues, in the words of René Favaloro, the Argentine surgeon who made bypass surgery practical, remained "totally skeptical."[31] One major objection was that it usually took about three months for collateral vessels to develop after the operation, during which time the patients were at risk of having a heart attack and dying. Although there was no tradition of clinical trials in surgery, they wanted to see some objective proof, not just Vineberg's clinical observations. This was because Beck and others had made claims that had not panned out about renewing blood supply to the heart and relieving angina.

By 1962 there was a way of getting such proof.[32] Mason Sones, a pint-sized, irascible, angry, innovative iconoclast from the hinterlands, devised the method in 1958 but did not report it in the literature until four years later. His discovery, together with those of McLean, Forssmann, and Gibbon, made possible all of the invasive treatments for coronary artery disease—bypass surgery, angioplasty, and stenting.

Sones was by all accounts "a rough diamond." One surgeon who knew him said, "If he thought someone was an asshole, he'd tell 'em to their face, in the middle of a meeting if necessary."[33] He was the antithesis of the polished, privileged, Harvard-, Yale-, or Johns Hopkins-trained physicians who typically flourished in the medical establishment. He was graceless, sharp-tongued, and curmudgeonly; a graduate of a tiny college and an unheralded state medical school who, perhaps because he read little and wrote less in the prestigious medical journals of the day, was less influenced by the conventional wisdom than were his elite colleagues.

Despite his undeniable brilliance and self-confidence, Sones likely would have been beaten down by today's relentlessly bureaucratic system of medical science, and very likely even by his own institution, the Cleveland Clinic, which has ballooned into a glittering, world-class medical megacenter in the past forty years. In the judgment of Leonard A. R. Golding, the Australian-born surgeon who called him a rough diamond, "there's no way he'd survive today."[34] But in the 1950s, the place he worked was just a private clinic—albeit a good one—in a run-down neighborhood of a midsize city often parodied for its provincialism. And in that place, at that time, without benefit of either charm or diplomacy, it was still possible for a brilliant but unpolished clinician to reject an unexamined stereotype and, with a modicum of institutional support, make a radical leap.

In the United States today, for better or for worse, increased bureaucracy, risk aversion in public policy and greater attention to ethical concerns discourage radicalism in medicine. Many physicians, especially those engaged in research, argue that safety and ethics regulations are overly restrictive leading to an unfavorable balance between protections for patients and the rapid development of life-saving treatments. This is a difficult hypothesis to test, but what is undeniable is that many drugs and medical devices that previously would have been subjected to clinical trials in the United States now undergo trials in the less-restrictive environments of Europe, Asia and Latin America.

The story of Mason Sones is a classic example of a significant medical advance achieved by a researcher obsessed with the idea of personal integrity who used what are now considered ethically unacceptable methods, although they were common at the time, to accomplish his goals. Without his contribution there would be no coronary bypass surgery or angioplasty, treatments that have helped millions of disabled patients worldwide to resume productive lives and that probably have extended the lives of a million or more patients.

But to test his new diagnostic procedure, for almost four years he conducted experiments of uncertain risk on just over a thousand patients, many of whom had no idea they were being used as research subjects. Sones, meanwhile, knew that none of these patient-subjects would themselves benefit from the procedure. Three of them died. By contrast, in 1997 the National Aeronautics and Space Administration suspended participation in a research project because a rhesus monkey died of a heart attack.[35]

Mason Sones's family moved from Noxapater, Mississippi, to Baltimore when he was a young child. His father was a machinist at Continental Can Company, and his mother was a homemaker. Sones went to a small college called Western Maryland, where he was a drum major at football games, and then to medical school at the University of Maryland in Baltimore. He married Geraldine Newton in his third year.

To support himself and his new wife, Sones took a low-paying job available to medical school seniors that came with housing in a mental institution. To earn his keep he had to take night calls at the hospital. "It was touch and go at times," Geraldine Sones said. "I went to work on a bus. He went to school on a bus. And sometimes [we had] to see how many Pepsi bottles [there were for] the bus fare."[36]

Sones was already a three-pack-a-day smoker, but to save money, Geraldine carefully rolled his cigarettes from Bugler tobacco. She could make him a pack for a nickel. "I'd watch when he would offer them to people," she said. "I wouldn't want him to give them away because I would sit there and trim the ends and everything."[37]

After medical school Sones did a year-long internship at the University of Maryland and then went into the air force and served in the Pacific for eighteen months. When he returned he entered a cardiology residency at the Henry Ford Hospital in Detroit, where he learned to do cardiac catheterization, the technique Werner Forssmann pioneered and that requires threading a tube through a peripheral artery to the heart. At the time it was used mainly to measure blood flows and pressures, or to inject radio-opaque dye so that X-ray images of the heart's chambers could be made to diagnose valve disease or congenital heart defects. Few physicians were trained to do this invasive procedure. In 1950 Sones was hired as director of pediatric cardiology and of the cardiac laboratory at the Cleveland Clinic.

As a pediatric cardiologist he was especially interested in an operation developed a few years earlier by the surgeon Alfred Blalock and the cardiolgist Helen Taussig to correct the multiple heart anomalies that caused blue-baby syndrome, a hemoglobin disorder that inevitably led to death at an early age. Often after an operation Sones, out of concern for his patient, would spend the night in the infant's room.

He remained interested in heart catheterization, which provides much useful physiological information and which, he believed, might one day provide a road map to the coronary arteries. But there was no catheterization laboratory at the Cleveland Clinic, so Sones, a man of boundless energy and drive, created one in the bowels of the hospital. And to keep it on cardiology turf, he fought off the radiologists who may have sensed that it was on the verge of becoming an important and lucrative diagnostic tool.

Sones was universally regarded as fair, honest, dedicated to medicine, and, although he often kept them waiting for hours, to his patients, especially the children. His sensitivity with young patients was familiar to everyone who worked with him. Elaine Clayton, for many years Sones's secretary, described how gently he would "put his forehead against the forehead of a Down syndrome child and calm him down."[38]

But everyone who knew him also agreed that he was a tyrant: volatile, demanding, domineering, and insensitive to the needs of just about anyone who wasn't a patient, including his fellows and office staff. And he was equally difficult with his colleagues. For a year the cardiologist William Proudfit was assigned to conduct a weekly meeting with Sones, Donald Effler, the chief of thoracic surgery, and Willem Kolff, a leading cardiologist who had developed a heart-lung machine and a method of stopping the heart during surgery. The purpose of the meeting was to keep open lines of communication among Sones and his two colleagues, all of whose egos and tempers made this difficult.[39]

But the ones who suffered most from Sones's single-mindedness, ego, and temper were his wife and his own four children. His widow, Geraldine, whom he divorced to marry another woman, but who returned to nurse him through a final devastating bout with lung cancer, said that Sones usually left the house at seven-thirty in the morning, almost never came home for dinner, and sometimes didn't come home at all. Weekends were no different from weekdays. And when he was home, he spent his time dictating or catching up on written work. She said he knew he was depriving his family, but he always said "he had to do it because there were all these people who would not be alive, except for him."

Geraldine Sones used to tell him, "Yes, but there are these four people, with names, who are alive because of you, and need you." It didn't do any good, though, she said, because "it [always] got interpreted that I was fighting [against] medicine instead of fighting for the family. I heard him say in a psychologist's office where we were taking one of our children that he just figured I would pick up the slack. We used to jokingly say that to get attention from Dad you had to have your head hanging by a thread." When asked whether any of the Sones children had gone into medicine, Mrs. Sones said, "No, they knew how it hurt the family life, so no one even thought about it." Today one son lives in a tepee in the woods near Taos, New Mexico, and builds adobe houses; a daughter lives in Sedona, Arizona, and works in an inn; another son works in a garden and pet store, and the third son works in commercial real estate.[40]

Elaine Clayton, who was Sones's secretary for seventeen years, said, "Geraldine put up with an awful lot. There were lots of problems with the kids. It was his fault." Like many of those who worked with and for Sones,

Clayton felt intense admiration for him and frustration bordering on resentment for his inconsiderateness and insensitivities. Sones "was an unqualified genius," she said, "[who] communicated a sense of 'we have something to do and I need you to do it with me.'"

Clayton said Sones, who often worked in a T-shirt, was addicted to coffee and cigarettes and never stopped coughing. He used to keep his secretaries from going home, often sitting around doing nothing, just in case he might have work for them later. "He'd kick the bathroom door when he wanted to get a secretary out and back to work," she said. "At one point, I quit from overwork. I was putting in eighteen-hour days, twelve minimum. I was eating nonstop and losing weight. I erased part of a disk once. He didn't yell. When I asked, 'Why?' he said, 'You'll feel worse that way.'" Another secretary in the office, Jo Rolphe, once asked Clayton how come her mother had christened her "Goddamn Elaine."[41]

Professionally, Sones was unusual because of the seemingly equal intensity of his compassion for his patients and his passion for research. Since his patients were in a sense the raw materials for his biomedical investigations, there was an obvious conflict of interest: What comes first, an individual patient's rights and interests, or the pursuit of an answer to a research question? Sones might have argued that the two are not incompatible, but in practice he used his patients' bodies to test a procedure—the insertion of a catheter into their coronary arteries—that had no potential for benefiting those patients. Moreover, he did not tell them he was planning to do it.

For several years Sones's curiosity had been piqued by reports from Sweden of "incidental visualization of the coronary arteries" that occurred when small amounts of dye entered the coronaries during X-ray studies of the aorta.[42] For one thing, he paid attention to the fact that nothing happened to patients when these small amounts of dye entered their coronary arteries. They didn't die, or even get sick. So he tried various ways, short of injecting directly into the coronaries, to get consistently clear pictures, but was never satisfied with the results. He also had been working on improving ways to image the heart—including the hearts of infants—so as to be better able to diagnose congential heart conditions and defects in patients with rheumatic heart disease.

During this time a young Welshman named Royston Lewis, who had graduated with honors from St. Mary's Hospital Medical School in London, where Alexander Fleming discovered penicillin, showed up at the Cleveland Clinic to begin a fellowship in cardiology. He had seen the job advertised in the *Journal of the American Medical Association,* applied for it, and got it. On his first day, Lewis reported for an interview with Sones, who by then was an internationally known pediatric and invasive cardiologist.

Lewis remembers the stubby, chain-smoking Sones, eyes obscured by thick lenses, as physically unimpressive. But once he began talking, Lewis said, he was unmistakably charismatic. Lewis also remembers that Sones put him to work quickly, peremptorily.

"There's a baby over in the pediatric ward in heart failure," Sones said, his voice disarmingly tinged with southern softness but his words characteristically blunt. "Go over and digitalize the hell out of it."[43]

"My heart dropped," Lewis said, but "I found out what to do and went and did it."[44]

For the next eight months Lewis worked closely with Sones. During that time he became an ardent admirer, later calling Sones "one of the three men who had the most profound influence on me in my life." "Mason Sones had enormous foresight," Lewis continued, "and he was one of the fairest men I'd ever met. As long as you did two things with Mason, you were fine. You worked hard and you were always truthful. If you followed those two principles and your work was just average he would forgive that."[45]

By the time Lewis joined him as a fellow, the hard-drinking Sones and a sober, soft-spoken, gentlemanly colleague, Earl Shirey, had established themselves in the dingy basement of the clinic's main hospital building in an area known as B-10. Sones occupied a large room with a big horseshoe-shaped desk, Shirey a smaller office, and the secretaries sat in a corridorlike area lined with glass-doored cabinets. Clayton said that Sones and the bombastic surgeon Paul Taylor would sometimes have shouting matches about patients in their narrow work space that threatened to shatter the glass.

The lab was just down a hall lined with brown metal lockers like ones you might find in an inner-city high school. It was a drab, windowless room, about thirty feet by sixteen feet, with beige glazed tiles and plain brown wooden cabinets on the walls and hospital green linoleum on the floor. The centerpiece of the room was a radiolucent table with an X-ray tube suspended above it and an awkward-looking six-foot-long, six-hundred-pound image intensifier positioned in a pit below.

Sones had installed a smaller intensifier in 1956, but he decided it was inadequate for making the quality pictures he needed and therefore set off to Baltimore to consult with an expert at Johns Hopkins named Russell Morgan. Following Morgan's guidance, introducing a few ideas of his own, and with the help of engineers from the Dutch company Phillips and a few thousand dollars from a private benefactor, Sones devised and installed a larger amplifier.

This involved digging a four-foot-deep hole in the floor, which, as it happened, was directly over a creek. Every time the workmen swung a shovel or a pick, water spurted up into the lab. Eventually, though, they were able to dig the hole and line it with concrete, which kept the water out. Lewis estimated years later that the job should have cost a few hundred dollars but ended up costing $10,000.[46] As for the image intensifier, the resolution was so poor with the larger device that Sones soon went back to the smaller version.

The way Sones's system worked, someone had to get into the pit and look through a kind of periscope to see a mirror image of the heart. It had been used many times, mostly uneventfully. But October 30, 1958, was different. The large image intensifier was still in place. Sones was in the pit, and Lewis was with the patient, waiting for Sones's command to inject dye.

"The man we were catheterizing was Otis Dickey," Lewis said, "and he came from West By God, Virginia. He had rheumatic heart disease. He was about twenty-seven or twenty-eight."[47]

They had just shot some film of the patient's left ventricle, and Sones instructed Lewis to pull the catheter tip back from Dickey's main pumping chamber and leave it resting in his aorta, the large artery through which oxygenated blood is returned from the heart to the rest of the body.

Then Sones said, "Let's have a smoke." The two men lounged on the edge of the pit in their lead aprons and surgical gowns, as they often did in the middle of a procedure, and relaxed with a cigarette while waiting for the dye to clear. To smoke while working, Sones kept a special sterile forceps on his tray solely to pick up and put down cigarettes.[48]

After a while Sones said, "Let's get on in," and Lewis got up and loaded the mechanical injector with dye. They both thought the catheter was positioned in the patient's ascending aorta, through which the dye was supposed to go into the left ventricle for a standard catheterization of roughly the kind that Werner Forssmann had done on himself in 1929. Sones asked, "What kind of pressure pulse are you getting?" and Lewis said, "It looks very good."

Lewis fiddled around with the injector a bit and said, "I'm ready." Then Sones, relying on the pressure reading rather than actual visualization for assurance that the catheter was where it belonged, turned on the 35mm X-ray camera and said, "Okay, fire!" Lewis hit the button, and a high-pressure shot of dye flashed down Dickey's right coronary artery, lighting up the fluoroscopic screen. Sones realized instantly what had happened: The catheter had whipped out of the aorta and into the aortic sinus, sending dye into the coronary circulation instead of into the ventricle. He yelled, "PULL IT OUT!" which Lewis did in a couple of seconds.

Sones expected Dickey to go into ventricular fibrillation when the dye displaced blood in his coronary arteries, cutting off the heart muscle's oxygen supply. This chaotic heartbeat, which prevents the heart from pumping blood throughout the body, is fatal unless it is stopped within minutes. Sones scrambled out of the pit and raced around looking for a scalpel to cut open the patient's chest so he could apply the paddles of an AC defibrillator directly to his heart, shocking it back into a normal rhythm.[49]

Then something caught Sones's eye. It was an oscilloscope readout of Dickey's electrocardiogram. It was flat, which meant that he wasn't fibrillating but was in cardiac arrest. Knowing that an explosive cough could produce enough pressure in the aorta to drive the dye out of the coronary artery and into the systemic circulation, Sones frantically pounded on Dickey's chest and shouted, "COUGH! COUGH!" which Dickey, who was under local anesthetic, was able to do. Three or four strong coughs forced most of the approximately 30 cc of dye out and got Dickey's heart going, first too slowly, then, during fifteen or twenty seconds of acceleration, too rapidly, but eventually at a normal rate.

"We sewed up the [incision in his chest]," Lewis said years later, "and sent him back to his room, after which Sones said, 'You watch that sonofabitch through the day [because] if anything happens to him, it's back to Mississippi for me.' "[50]

It is not clear whether Dickey would have fibrillated and died without the cough, but even if he had, it is unlikely that Sones would have lost either his job or even much of his reputation. It is likely, however, that the discovery of coronary angiography would have been set back, perhaps for years. Dickey's death would have been seen as proof that enough dye in a coronary artery to produce a clear image is enough dye to kill the patient by disrupting the heart muscle's blood supply. At that time this view was gospel among cardiologists. The next day, however, Otis Dickey was fine, and an excited Mason Sones told a few colleagues that he thought it was possible to inject enough dye directly into the coronary arteries so they could be clearly and consistently imaged, which eventually would make it possible to identify blockages and treat them surgically.

Sones said to Shirey, "Look at what we did, Earl. And the patient survived. Why can't we inject just a small amount" of dye?[51] The answer, Sones went on to prove, was that they could, and that it would produce a clear picture. The accident in B-10, and Mason Sones's ability to grasp its significance, meant Scripture would have to be rewritten. Sones excitedly told Elaine Clayton that he and Lewis had revolutionized cardiology. Clayton said Sones used to always say that but this time it was true.[52]

Standard practice in those days, in a era when there were no hospital ethics committees looking out for patients' rights, would have been to quickly test the procedure on ten or twenty patients and, assuming favorable results, publish in a medical journal as soon as possible. Medical researchers are, of course, no different from anyone else in their desire to claim credit for their work. But this was not Mason Sones's style. He didn't want to be wrong. He worried that he didn't know enough about the coronary circulation. He also hated to write. But Sones resisted publishing mainly because he wanted to be absolutely certain that his new procedure was safe and that it could consistently produce reliable, useful results.

Sones realized from the outset that for reasons of both safety and efficacy he would need a catheter that was suitable for the new job. The coronary arteries and their openings are narrower and harder to get to than the openings through which dye was injected into the aorta, so a catheter with a finer, more flexible tip was necessary. Moreover, it would have to be more manipulable than catheters then in use to be successfully maneuvered into the openings of these arteries. So Sones designed such a catheter, which was maufactured by the United States Catheter and Instrument Company (USCI). By April 1959 it was ready for use.

Sones also experimented with 11", 9", and 8" image intensifiers, and 16mm as well as 35mm motion-picture cameras, finally settling on the

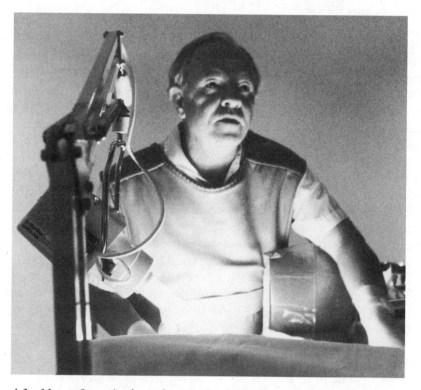

4.1. Mason Sones in the catheterization laboratory at the Cleveland Clinic, c. 1979 (Courtesy of Yu Kwan Lee, Cleveland Clinic Archives).

combination of a 5″ intensifier, which could amplify light 1,200 to 3,000 times and did not scatter X rays as much as the larger intensifiers, and a 35mm camera. This combination provided clear pictures with a minimum of X-ray exposure for the patient. He also established that 2 to 5 cc of dye—either 90 percent Hypaque or 85 percent Cardiographin—were enough to assure good, readable images.

Sones and Shirey began doing angiograms on a routine basis, even though by any reasonable standard the procedure was entirely experimental. Varying accounts of how they carried out their work exist, and some points, including the precise chronology, cannot be verified, but based on interviews with Earl Shirey, Royston, Lewis, William Proudfit, William Sheldon, and others who were at the Cleveland Clinic at the time and who worked with Sones, here is essentially what happened.

Sones told Carlton Ernstene, chairman of the Department of Medicine, that he had accidentally done coronary angiography and that he intended to experiment with patients until he could selectively and clearly image their coronary arteries. There was limited use for the information at that time because coronary artery bypass surgery had not been invented yet, but Sones worried that a large number of errors were being made in diagnosing angina pectoris and coronary insufficiency. He was among other things concerned that patients were being mistakenly diagnosed as having coronary artery disease, which meant that they needlessly were required to take drugs and limit their activity.

Ernstene gave him a go-ahead but insisted that Sones experiment with dogs first, which he did, using smaller amounts of dye injected at lower pressures than were typically used when dye was injected into the aorta. All three dogs died, which might or might not have had anything to do with the dye injections. Lots of dogs were lost in the labs in those days as a result of bad anesthesia, among other things. But Sones apparently did not try to find out what had gone wrong. He was both impatient and confident that he was right, so instead of trying more dogs he went right back to experimenting on humans.

Sones told Shirey that the first thing they were going to do was learn how to manipulate the catheter. "We're studying young people with valve disease, twenty-five, thirty, thirty-five years of age or less, and maybe a congenital defect," Shirey recalls Sones saying. "After we've solved their problem, after we've taken pictures based on our clinical impression of what the problem was, a leaky valve, whatever, then let's take about five minutes and just manipulate the catheter and see if we can learn how to get the catheter in there."[53]

"That would never go today," Shirey said softly. "You'd have to go to fifteen or twenty committees to do that. But in those days [people said]:

Let's just keep this quiet. Let's just take about five more minutes of fluoroscopy. It doesn't hurt the patient. And let's just learn how to do this.' "
In describing the learning curve, Shirey said that "Everybody sort of came
up with their own way. We knew that if we turned a catheter clockwise,
it would turn this way; if you turned it counterclockwise, it would go that
way. You sort of just tried different things and you found, 'Hey, this seems
to work.' "[54]

Shirey also said that he and Sones studied the anatomies of hearts taken
from patients who had died. To the best of his recollection, no permission
was granted by the dying person or his or her family for this use of the
organ. He said he thought that both medicine and the public benefited
from the freedom researchers had at the time to experiment without bureaucratic constraints, as long as no one was hurt.

Sones and Shirey's subjects for their four-year experiment were "everybody who comes for a catheterization," no matter whether the reason was
to diagnose valve disease, heart failure, congential defects, or anything else.
When asked whether the patients gave permission for the procedure to be
done, Lewis laughed and said, "No, no."[55]

Although Sones did not publish for years, word got around quickly
about the new procedure he was doing and, as might be expected, the
more conventional-minded practitioners didn't much like it and were often
vocal about it. One day Lewis, who had left Sones's lab by then, ran into
Shirey who told him this story, which illustrates how personal the opposition got:

"Mason . . . came into the lab, bustling away, taking off his shirt, and
he said, 'Earl, you gotta catheterize me.' Shirey asked him, 'Why, Mason?'
And Sones said, 'I was talking at a medical meeting and some sonofabitch
said I was doing something crooked and criminal and he said, 'You haven't
done it on yourself.' 'Nobody's gonna tell me that again.' "[56]

Sones got up on the table then and there and Shirey went ahead with
the catheterization, beginning with an injection into the right coronary
artery. The dye caused a small spasm, which subsided. Then Shirey injected
the left anterior descending artery without a problem. He checked the
pictures and told Sones that his coronaries were normal. Geraldine Sones
said her husband didn't tell her about the procedure until after it was over.
"He just decided to show everybody that he could be all right with it,"
she said.[57]

Shirey said their greatest fear while doing the first thousand angiograms
was that patients would go into ventricular fibrillation and die. The first
death of this kind happened when Sones was away. Shirey had injected dye
into the right coronary artery of a patient he suspected had coronary artery
disease, and the heart began to fibrillate. He quickly opened the patient's
chest and applied the paddles of an AC defibrillator, hoping to shock the

heart back into a normal rhythm. But it was no good. The patient, who had been informed of the experimental nature of the procedure, died. "I felt very bad having the first one," Shirey said. But when Sones got back, he made little of it. "Let's just go on," he told Shirey.[58]

About a month later, a doctor named Mike Criley, who was interested in the photographic aspects of arteriography, was visiting the clinic to watch Sones in action. While Sones was doing a coronary angiogram, Criley told him about a physician named William Kouwenhoeven, who had induced ventricular fibrillation in dogs and then massaged their chests, which would drive enough blood to the brain to keep the dogs alive for a short time. While Criley was describing the experimental procedure, Sones's patient's heart began to fibrillate. Sones reflexively asked for a scalpel, but Criley said, "Why don't you get on his chest?"

Sones jumped up on the table and began to frantically massage the patient's chest, at which point the patient woke up and screamed, "Get off my chest! You're trying to kill me!" "Mason hadn't done this before," Shirey said, "and I'm sure the [patient's] sternum hurt like hell." When Sones let up, the patient immediately lost consciousness. They called a surgeon, who opened an incision and defibrillated the man's ventricle by applying the paddles of an AC defibrillator. His heart began to beat, but he died two weeks later of a blood clot in the lung. Not long afterward a direct-current defibrillator was invented that could return the heartbeat to normal when applied externally to the chest.

During the almost four years before Sones decided that he had collected enough data to publish, a steady stream of cardiologists came to Cleveland to watch the procedure and make up their own minds. Here and there, others began to do coronary angiography, but Sones's basement lab remained the mecca. A major test came in the fall of 1962, when the American Heart Association's annual meeting was to be held in Cleveland. This meant that dozens of cardiologists would visit the clinic to observe the pioneers at work.

At that time, Sones and Shirey were experimenting with different contrast agents. They were trying alternatives to Hypaque and Cardiographin, one of which seemed to produce fibrillation more often than the others. But it had not been used enough times to rule out chance as the reason the fibrillation rate was higher. Shirey suggested that while the AHA meeting was on they should use only Hypaque and Cardiographin. But Sones, in his usual bull-in-the-china-shop fashion, said, "No way. I'm just going to do exactly what we would do if they weren't coming." At this point Earl Shirey's voice dropped to a whisper as he described what happened:

He [Sones] had a roomful of visitors and he was using one of these new contrast agents. I think he studied three patients and two of them fibrillated.

They went out of there and said, "Those people at the Cleveland Clinic are crazy. They're butchers. They're crazy people."[59]

The year 1962 was a crucial one for Mason Sones and for the treatment of coronary artery disease. In July Sones and Shirey finally published "Cine Coronary Arteriography," their report of studies done on 1,020 patients.[60] It was also the year René Favaloro came to the Cleveland Clinic and began haunting Sones's laboratory in search of better ways to get oxygenated blood to the heart muscle surgically. And it was the year when Sones performed coronary angiography on two patients who had had Vineberg operations.

A skeptical medical community thought Vineberg's claims of success for his operation were at best extravagant. And Sones was among the biggest skeptics. Sones didn't like Vineberg and his hard-sell tactics and thought his idea was "nutty." Sones wanted to know how you could dig a tunnel in the heart without doing more harm than good.[61] At a medical meeting, the combative Sones challenged Vineberg publicly to send him some patients for arteriography so he could study them and once and for all show that Vineberg's operation did not work. Vineberg accepted the challenge.

When he got back to Cleveland from the meeting, Sones told Elaine Clayton, "You're gonna get a call from Vineberg. He's gonna send two patients." In January 1962 Clayton got the call, the first patient came to the clinic, and Sones did the study. When it was completed, Clayton remembers a furious Sones stomping back from the lab muttering, "That goddamn bastard, he's done it."[62] The second patient was studied in March, with similar results.[63]

Soon thereafter, Cleveland Clinic surgeons began doing Vineberg's procedure. They and others continued doing it into the early 1970s, well after bypass surgery had become a routine operation. Yet even today, at the end of the twentieth century, there is still controversy over the operation's effectiveness because the tiny collateral vessels stimulated by the implantation were difficult to see in the shadowy, angiographic images. David Sabiston, who did the first coronary artery bypass operation, also in 1962, rejected Sones's angiographic evidence, saying that no one ever demonstrated "any real flow" going through the connections between the internal mammary artery and the bed of tiny arterioles in the heart muscle.[64]

5

Accidents and Innovations

As a young surgeon working under Alfred Blalock at Johns Hopkins, David Sabiston tried Arthur Vineberg's implantation operation on pigs and dogs, with poor results. But many other surgeons and cardiologists insisted that it worked, especially when the internal mammary artery was implanted in the most oxygen-deprived areas of heart muscle. As evidence that the operation worked, René Favaloro, who perfected bypass surgery, cited a case in which he accidentally severed an implanted artery during a reoperation he was performing, resulting in a massive heart attack and the death of the patient. What better proof could you want? he asked.[1]

There are patients living today whose angiograms show blood flow to the heart muscle through an implanted internal mammary artery. Rosalind Talisman, for example, had a Vineberg implant done by Favaloro at the Cleveland Clinic when she was fifty-two years old in 1969. Since then she has had two bypass operations, the last one done in 1992 by Bruce Lytle, also of the Cleveland Clinic, who discovered the implant done by Favaloro during a last-minute angiogram that he ordered because there seemed to be something odd about Mrs. Talisman's coronary anatomy.[2]

In 1997 Mrs. Talisman was a spry eighty-year-old, a living testament to the work of Mason Sones, Arthur Vineberg, René Favaloro, Floyd Loop (who did her middle bypass operation and who now heads the Cleveland Clinic), and Bruce Lytle. She is active in Mended Hearts, a national organization of survivors of bypass surgery, and is a regular visitor to Cleveland Clinic patients awaiting bypass surgery.

Back in January 1962, when Mason Sones showed that Arthur Vineberg's operation could bring fresh red blood to the heart, there was no other way to do it. Three months later, however, Sabiston used a length of saphenous vein from a patient's leg to bypass a blocked right coronary artery, much as Alexis Carrel had done with a piece of carotid artery on a dog half a century earlier. But the patient died of a stroke three days later.

An autopsy showed that the stroke was caused by a blood clot that formed where the saphenous vein was sutured to the patient's aorta and

was then "swept into the cerebral circulation." For fear of this happening
again, Sabiston did not repeat the operation until after Favaloro, a cabinetmaker's son from La Plata, Argentina, showed in 1967 that it could be
done safely. And he did not publish a report on it until more than a decade
after his first attempt.[3]

Favaloro had been practicing general surgery in Jacinto Arauz, a small
town in the rural grasslands west of La Pampa Province. He and his brother
had gone there in 1950, opting for a country practice largely because they
felt they would be freer than in Buenos Aires under the dictatorship of
Juan Domingo Perón. They turned a big, old house into a twenty-three-
bed clinic and did anything that could be "defined as general surgery."

They also subscribed to a range of medical journals from abroad. Favaloro read articles by Robert Gross, Alfred Blalock, and C. Walton Lillehei, among others, describing heart surgery Favaloro did not know was

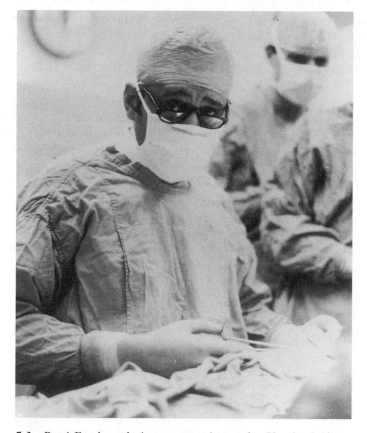

5.1. René Favaloro during an operation at the Cleveland Clinic,
c. 1971 (Courtesy of Cleveland Clinic Archives).

possible. Next to what these men were doing, he thought, the accomplishments of a country doctor in rural Argentina were pretty humble. "I could
not help thinking to myself," he wrote years later, " 'This is not the place
for you, it never was. You are capable of bigger things and you are wasting
your time.' "[4]

In February 1962, driven by his new ambition to be a heart surgeon,
Favaloro and his wife, Toni, boarded an airplane for the first time in their
lives and flew to New York. After an overnight stay near Idlewild [now
Kennedy] International Airport, they flew to Cleveland. The newly arrived
couple hailed a cab and asked the driver where they could stay near the
Cleveland Clinic, which, although they didn't know it, was in a bleak,
crime-ridden neighborhood. The driver dropped them off at a tired-
looking but respectable hotel called the Bolton Square. They checked in,
and a couple of hours later Favaloro walked four blocks to the office of
George Crile, Jr., the clinic's chief executive.

His timing could not have been better. Specialized units for the care of
coronary patients were spreading rapidly in the United States in the early
1960s, and results were beginning to come in from the Framingham Heart
Study, in which the residents of a Massachusetts town were being continuously followed to assess the importance of a wide range of suspected risk
factors for heart disease.

The tall, olive-skinned Favaloro showed up at the Cleveland Clinic without an appointment or even a phone call. He handed Crile's secretary a
letter of introduction from his mentor in Argentina. Crile saw Favaloro
after a brief wait and listened patiently as his Argentine visitor explained
in brushed-up high-school English that he had come to Cleveland to learn
to be a heart surgeon. Instead of turning him away, as he might easily
have done, Crile passed him on to Donald Effler, the clinic's chief of thoracic and cardiovascular surgery.

Effler asked Favaloro if he had taken the exam required for working as
a resident in the United States, and Favaloro told him he'd never even
heard of it. This ruled out a real job, at least for the time being, so Effler
took a low-risk option and offered to let Favaloro be an unpaid observer
while he studied for the exam. Favaloro accepted, came to work daily, and
began, unassumingly, an unpredictably brilliant surgical career.

When Favaloro arrived in 1962, the Department of Thoracic and Cardiovascular Surgery at the Cleveland Clinic consisted of two senior surgeons, Effler and Laurence Groves, both patrician WASPs, and two residents, Niall Scully from Hawaii, and Alfonso Parisi, a Canadian, who like
Favaloro was of Sicilian descent. They were doing a lot of lung surgery,
operations on the esophagus, and cardiac procedures such as blue-baby
operations. Although David Sabiston had already done the first coronary

artery bypass operation on a human being, no one at the clinic knew about it.

Within weeks, Favaloro was helping out in the operating room, mainly as a scrub nurse, inserting Foley catheters in patients to measure urine flow, washing their chests with surgical soap, and so forth. It didn't take him long to discover B-10. Soon after coming to the clinic he began joining groups of visitors watching Mason Sones and Earl Shirey do coronary angiograms and then, on his own, he started going to the archives to study angiographic films.

One day Favaloro asked Elaine Clayton to introduce him to Sones because he had been having trouble interpreting two films. Sones viewed them with him and answered his questions, thereby beginning a long, productive, and, given Sones's prickly nature, remarkably uncontentious relationship. Despite their profoundly different backgrounds, they became close friends, perhaps partly because they were both totally consumed by

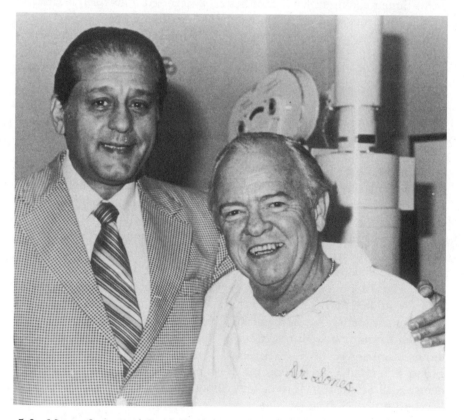

5.2. Mason Sones and René Favaloro at the Cleveland Clinic during a visit by Favaloro, c. 1982 (Courtesy of Cleveland Clinic Archives).

medicine. But Geraldine Sones believed it was more than that—that there was real "love" between the two men. "When Mason was terminal," she said, "René came to see him and he sat in the apartment in tears, broken up totally."[5]

During his first year at the clinic, Favaloro habitually went to the basement when he finished surgical rounds, often studying Sones's films until nine or ten at night. He wasn't entirely without a social life, though. In the beginning, the Favaloros saw a few couples of Sicilian or Argentine background, including Parisi and his wife, Adeline, who was also of Sicilian descent; Vicente Profeta, an Italo-Argentine electrician at the clinic and his wife, Maria; and some of their working-class friends, with whom the Favaloros would occasionally have traditional Argentine barbecues. But mostly he worked, as a result of which his network of friends expanded in time to include a number of physicians on the clinic staff.

In September Favaloro passed his residency exam and became a junior fellow, which gave him a small salary and the right to do what he had already been doing by then—assist in and perform actual surgery. He also sat in on consultations where he observed with dismay the terse, blunt way clinic surgeons told patients about their illness, without any effort to soften the blow, even if the disease was cancer. The coldness offended his Latin sensibilities and was contrary to his practice as a country doctor.

Favaloro took to revisiting some of these patients before surgery to comfort them and explain more about their disease, often making simple sketches for them of the planned operation. Years later, during a course Favaloro was giving in Miami, a former patient of his sent him sketches of his operation as a keepsake with a note of thanks for having kept him alive long enough to celebrate his golden wedding anniversary. And Rosalind Talisman, Favaloro's patient in 1969 who remembers him with warmth, said he "always held my hand while he was talking to me."[6]

A year after coming to Cleveland, Favaloro used his two-week vacation to travel to Boston to watch Dwight Harken, who advanced cardiac surgery in the battlefield hospitals of World War I,[7] and Robert Gross perform surgery. Later Favaloro went to the Mayo Clinic to watch John Kirklin operate and to see Mayo's less-traumatic heart-lung machine—using a membrane oxygenator—that Kirklin and his colleagues had developed.

Then, in 1964, when he was chief resident at the clinic, Favaloro was sent to Houston to evaluate a heart-lung machine with a new type of disposable bubble oxygenator being used by Denton Cooley. The clinic's oxygenator had to be cleaned after every use, which meant that it could be used for only two operations a day. Favaloro came home impressed with Cooley's exceptional skill and speed in doing valve operations and other heart surgery, but he said that angiography in Houston was poor and as a result Cooley knew relatively little about coronary artery disease. He was also impressed with the oxygenator, which bubbled air through the blood, and when he returned to the Cleveland Clinic, surgeons there began using the new device.

Favaloro was now doing just about every kind of surgery done by Effler and Groves. This included Vineberg operations, which they had been goaded into doing by Sones, who proselytized for the procedure he once scoffed at after he proved to his own satisfaction that it worked.[8] As a result, he was getting experience removing one end of internal mammary arteries from the wall of the chest, a technique that was considered difficult at the time but that was a precursor to today's standard surgical procedure for coronary artery disease, an internal mammary artery graft to either the left anterior descending coronary artery, the right coronary artery, or both.[9]

With this experience under his belt, Favaloro returned to Argentina in 1965, planning to rejoin his extended family and share what he had learned with his colleagues at home. But as hidebound as the American medical establishment was, it was nothing compared to the Argentine bureaucracy. Within months he headed back to Cleveland and accepted a job at the clinic at $18,000 a year.

But there was one more hurdle to clear before Favaloro, now forty-three, could become a full-fledged surgeon on the clinic staff. He was in a kind of legal limbo because he still had to pass a four-day state licensing examination testing medical school knowledge, most of which had little relevance to his surgical practice of the past two decades. Ohio only let U.S. citizens take the exam, so Favaloro had to take it in a state with which Ohio had reciprocity. Meanwhile, a fiction needed to be maintained. All of his operations were listed in the clinic's official records as having been done by Effler and Favaloro or Groves and Favaloro, even though neither of the senior surgeons actually participated.

During this period Favaloro performed the first successful pulmonary embolectomy ever done at the Cleveland Clinic. This was the same operation whose difficulty inspired John Gibbon to invent the heart-lung machine. Without a heart-lung machine, Favaloro's removal of numerous small clots from the patient's pulmonary artery almost certainly would not have been attempted, or if it had been, it almost certainly would have failed.

Knowing that the exam could be tricky, Favaloro decided to take it in both Virginia and New York, so that if he failed on the first try he would have a second chance. After taking the exam in Virginia he told Effler that he thought he might have failed. But he felt more confident after taking it in New York. He needn't have worried, however. The results were announced six weeks later, and he had passed both. He was formally appointed a staff surgeon at the beginning of 1966, four years after having arrived unannounced from rural Argentina.

Favaloro's workload was mainly cardiac operations, including Vineberg procedures. It occurred to him that in some of the worst cases it might be possible to implant both internal mammary arteries to provide even more oxygen to the heart muscle than could be accomplished with a single implant. Sones told him that the chest wall couldn't stand the loss of blood from both arteries, but Favaloro reviewed the anatomy over and over again, finally concluding that Sones was wrong.

Favaloro's first case, very carefully selected, was a good candidate for a standard single implant, but Favaloro persuaded the referring cardiologist to let him try the new procedure. It was successful. Ten months later, an angiogram showed that both mammary arteries were connected to the majority of the branches of the left coronary system. Favaloro did thirty-eight double Vinebergs with zero operative mortality. He developed instruments to perform these highly traumatic operations, stressing to his assistants that "the heart must be treated gently, caressing it as though it were a woman."[10]

But the Vineberg operation, single or double, left a great deal to be desired. Even when the operation appeared to work, it took months before it did any good—that is, until new channels opened, allowing blood to perfuse the heart muscle. And the worst disease, obstruction of the left main coronary artery, remained virtually untreatable. Every time a patient with left-main disease was scheduled for surgery, the renal transplant team, in a ritual at once ghoulish and benevolent, gathered in hopes of harvesting the kidneys for one of their own anxiously waiting patients.

Although at the time Favaloro knew nothing of at least three earlier human surgical experiments using saphenous vein grafts in the coronary circulation,[11] and one using an internal mammary artery graft,[12] and very little about the animal experiments done by the Canadian surgeon Gordon Murray, among others, he was familiar with the use of saphenous veins to repair peripheral and renal arteries.

If it worked in the peripheral circulation, Favaloro wondered, why not in the coronaries? He discussed the idea with Sones, who said he thought it was worth trying. A South African cardiologist at the clinic, David Ferguson, identified a suitable patient in May 1967. She was a fifty-one-year-old woman with a blocked right coronary artery that could be easily seen on an angiogram.

With no fanfare, Favaloro cut out the section of artery containing the blockage and sewed a section of vein taken moments earlier from the woman's leg in its place. Eight days later Sones did another angiogram on the patient, who seemed to be recovering normally. Sones ran the film in his office for Favaloro, William Sheldon, and a couple of other colleagues, and to their delight it showed that this "interposed" graft was wide open. Favaloro remembers an elated Sones "waving his arms about and congratulating me."[13]

In their fifteenth operation, Favaloro and his colleagues Effler and Groves tried a technically simpler procedure. Instead of excising the blockage and interposing the vein graft in the coronary artery, they connected one end of the graft to the front wall of the aorta and the other to the clogged artery beyond the blockage, thereby bypassing the source of the trouble.

This simple mechanical solution to insufficient blood supply to the heart muscle was essentially the same operation done by David Sabiston in a planned procedure in 1962. A team including Edward Garrett, Edward Dennis, and Michael DeBakey did it as an improvisation in 1964 when the target artery was too fragile to permit the planned reaming out of the vessel known as endarterectomy. In this case the patient recovered. But neither repeated the operation—that is, not until after Favaloro and the Cleveland Clinic team recognized its importance and kept on doing it.

Despite skepticism from leading cardiologists such as Eugene Braunwald and Willis Hurst, soon everybody was doing it, beginning with Dudley Johnson at Marquette University in Milwaukee, who might have been the first to connect a coronary artery directly to the aorta. Within a decade, thousands of bypass operations were being done a year, and today the annual number worldwide is about 900,000, about 350,000 of which are done in the United States. In 1970 René Favaloro returned to Argentina. This time he stayed to establish and run his own cardiovascular surgery center in Buenos Aires.

From the perspective of the end of the twentieth century, there is a remarkable matter-of-factness about the birth of bypass surgery. It seemed right to a creative surgeon, who bounced it off an inventive cardiologist, who agreed. So they tried it on a human patient without the benefit of having done a single animal experiment. They knew Alexis Carrel had done bypass surgery on a dog almost sixty years earlier, but with a piece of carotid artery, not a vein, and that Carrel had interposed vein grafts in the peripheral arteries of animals but not in the more delicate coronaries.

Although bypass surgery was eventually shown in three large clinical trials to be effective for some but not all coronary artery disease, it was not unusual then, nor is it unusual now, for new surgical procedures to skip a step, such as animal experiments, or clinical trials, both of which are legally mandated for fundamentally new drugs or medical devices.

Innovative surgery is often improvised on the operating table in an effort to save a patient who is fading fast, as was the case with Edward Garrett's saphenous vein bypass operation in 1964. Or it is tried when there is no known treatment and death within a short time is considered certain. Or, as was the case with Favaloro and coronary artery bypass grafting, a surgeon gets a bright idea and acts on it. In each case, if the operation works, it is tried again. And if it doesn't work but looks promising, it is tried again, following Cutler's dictum that "mortality figures alone should not deter further investigation."

Of course, surgeons sometimes conduct extensive animal experiments before trying out their radical operations on human patients. Claude Beck did for the Beck I and Beck II operations, and so did Arthur Vineberg for the internal mammary artery implant. Vineberg wrote in 1982 that there must be "laboratory proof for a new revascularization surgical procedure before its use in the treatment of human coronary artery disease. The same is true when surgical techniques that have been shown to be of benefit in the laboratory and in the treatment of human coronary artery disease are modified. Such modifications should not be used until they are laboratory-proven."[14]

On the other hand, in his brief 1992 book *The Challenging Dream of Heart Surgery,* Favaloro argued that animal trials are sometimes indicated and sometimes not. He wrote: "It is evident that in medicine animal experimentation is of great importance, but it is not always obligatory. In our own case, the bypass [operation] resulted from intensive work on hundreds of patients affected by coronary disease and meticulous analysis of every patient."[15]

Although some animal rights activists disagree, there is a consensus among mainstream bioethicists and biomedical scientists that animal experimentation is the only way to conduct certain kinds of critically important medical research without causing excessive harm to human subjects. Animal experiments may not be necessary in all cases, but what principles should guide surgeons who must decide when animal experimentation is "obligatory" and when it isn't?

And what about the specific case here, inventing coronary bypass surgery? Vineberg is clear: Animal experiments must precede surgery on humans. But Favaloro said he did not consider animal experimentation obligatory. He gives two reasons: (1) the extensive experience he and his colleagues had in surgically treating coronary artery disease, and (2) the careful follow-up they conducted of the treated cases.

The Cleveland Clinic's experience in treating coronary artery disease surgically mostly involved implanting one or two internal mammary arteries into the heart muscle in the hope of forming connections to the native circulation and thereby bringing needed blood to the muscle. Other techniques tried were endarterectomy, which consists of opening a blockage by forcing a stiff catheter through the artery, and so-called patch grafts, in which an artery is opened, the blockage is partly removed, and then the vessel is repaired by sewing over the opening a piece of tissue taken from, for example, the pericardium, the membrane in which the heart is suspended.

Unlike bypass surgery, none of these methods involved clamping the aorta, or connecting a vein segment to the aorta and to a coronary artery. The clinic's experience, therefore, was inadequate to predict, among other things, the likelihood of causing a stroke by clamping the aorta, or the likelihood that the vein graft would close, causing a heart attack. And even the most careful follow-up studies of the older procedures were irrelevant to assessing these potentially traumatic effects of the new operation.

Experience is a necessary basis for innovation in surgery, but it is not a sufficient one. It provides deep, detailed knowledge of variations in anatomy and of the organic processes of physiology that cannot be obtained in any other way, and it sharpens surgical skill. But it does not enable surgeons to anticipate the consequences of new procedures, nor is it the source of the insight from which they spring.

Absent a "stroke of luck," which is the way John Kirklin characterized the Garrett operation,[16] surgeons need the same qualities artists rely on to create original works: courage, intuition, and imagination. With these attributes, both artists and surgeons can creatively apply the lessons learned from experience, revising them as needed.

Just as an artist's creative act illuminates previously obscure relationships, so a surgeon's innovative act illuminates previously unrecognized ways of treating disease. Afterward, other, less creative surgeons see the new procedure's potential and learn to do it themselves. "We knew instinctively," Cleveland Clinic surgeon Paul Taylor said of Favaloro's bypass procedure, "that this was a better operation."[17] But without Favaloro's imaginative leap the collective instinct Taylor mentioned would have lain dormant for nobody knows how much longer.

Of course, Sabiston had the courage and the creativity to do it. But neither he nor his colleagues at Johns Hopkins had the courage to repeat it, very likely because his patient died. Garrett's patient, on the other hand, lived. Still, apparently neither he nor either of his great surgical colleagues in Houston saw its potential: not Michael DeBakey and not Denton Cooley.[18]

Moreover, for years after Favaloro showed that it could be done, bypass surgery was criticized by leaders in the medical community. Favaloro believes that an inability to interpret angiograms was responsible for some of the initial skepticism.[19] Another possible reason, rarely aired outside physicians' circles, was the threat to cardiologists' status and livelihoods. Bypass grafting had the potential to turn a medical disease into a surgical disease. And this was not just any ailment. It was the nation's biggest killer—half a million Americans annually; and it cost the nation an estimated $90.9 billion in 1997.[20]

Henry Zimmerman, who broke a major taboo when he became the first researcher to catheterize the left side of the human heart, wrote in the *American Heart Journal* in May 1969, exactly two years after Favaloro's first vein graft operation, that "the surgical management of coronary artery disease is in almost total chaos" and that "there are no valid objective studies to show the merit of" bypass surgery.[21]

And in 1971, Braunwald, then chairman of the Department of Medicine at the University of California, San Diego, quite properly called for prospective, randomized clinical trials to answer a long series of questions about bypass surgery, including whether it extended life.[22] Three such trials, comparing bypass surgery to drug therapy, were carried out.

Veterans Administration Cooperative Study*

Between 1972 and 1974 a total of 686 patients with stable angina were randomized—332 to bypass surgery and 354 to drug therapy—at 13 Veterans Administration hospitals scattered around the country. To no one's surprise, the preliminary results of the VA trial, reported in the September 22, 1977, issue of *the New England Journal of Medicine*, demonstrated that bypass surgery provided better, longer relief from angina than drugs. But at three years they did not show a survival benefit.[23] The take-home message seemed to be that if you let the surgeons saw open your chest, the payoff was nothing more than a marginally better quality of life for a limited period of time.

To make matters worse, an editorial by Braunwald, who by then had moved to Harvard and was on his way to becoming the dean of American cardiology, noted that "it would be difficult for the surgical results to be substantially better than those of medical treatment, so far as longevity is concerned, simply because the medically treated group exhibited a cumulative survival of 87 percent at thirty-six months, a mortality rate approximating only 4 percent per year!"[24]

Note the exclamation point at the end of Braunwald's sentence. By the

---

*See Appendix A for an account of how clinical trials are designed, conducted, and reported to the profession.

standards of the bland academic journalese in which such articles are normally written, this punctuational excess thrusts like a dagger into the heart of the surgical camp.

However, the pace of publication in academic medicine at the time was—and often today is—glacial, so it was not until July 1978 that a large-bore response to Braunwald's editorial appeared. It was written by Floyd Loop, a renowned cardiac surgeon who now is chairman of the Cleveland Clinic Foundation, and two of the clinic's most respected cardiologists, William Proudfit and William Sheldon. That is to say, it came directly from the heart of the surgical camp, even though two of its authors were cardiologists. It was published by *The American Journal of Cardiology*, not a surgical journal. It leveled many criticisms at the VA study and at Braunwald's acceptance of the study's principal finding that, excluding the 13 percent of patients with left main coronary artery disease,[25] bypass surgery does not increase longevity.

The most telling criticism of the VA study was that, based on risk-adjusted mortality data, much of the surgery in the trial was second-rate and was therefore not useful for judging the operation itself. The thirty-day mortality rate for the entire trial was 5.8 percent, high considering that about two-thirds of the patients were relatively low-risk. The mortality range among the 13 hospitals, all of which were doing a low volume of bypass surgery, was 2 percent at the best and just over 12 percent at the worst. Loop, Proudfit, and Sheldon offered for comparison a thirty-day mortality rate for 1,400 consecutive patients at the Cleveland Clinic in 1973—the middle year of the VA study—of 0.6 percent. Since the clinic took all comers it is unlikely that the VA study population was sicker than the clinic's comparison group.

Using the same time frame and patient samples, the comparative figures for heart attacks is 18 percent in the VA study and 4 percent at the Cleveland Clinic. And at three years, 87 percent of the Cleveland Clinic patients had open grafts compared with 69 percent of the VA patients, and 95 percent of the Cleveland Clinic patients were alive, compared with 88 percent of the VA patients.

Loop and his colleagues also took issue with Braunwald's contention that since lots of hospitals in the United States at the time had mortality rates similar to the VA average, the study should not be discounted. "Why should we judge a mode of therapy on the basis of mediocre performance?" they ask. "A high operative mortality rate, high perioperative infarction [heart attack] rate, and low rate of graft patency [openness] are manifestations of technique. Demonstration of the utility of an operation to prolong life requires nearly ideal surgical results. The clinical trial is designed to study the operation, not the surgeon."

Loop et al. criticized the VA trial on many other grounds, including inconsistent data, statistical errors, inappropriate comparison of the relatively low-risk patient population of the VA study with a broad cross section of patients with coronary artery disease, and a failure to discuss surgery's beneficial effects on quality of life and a patient's ability to return to work.

These are on the whole substantive concerns, but the two big questions are: Did the VA study really prove that bypass surgery provides no survival benefit (Not at seven years? Not at eleven years?) compared to drug treatment? And did the VA trial provide any other important information?

The obvious answer to the first question, which will be discussed later in the context of the results of the two other large clinical trials comparing bypass surgery with drug treatment, is no. But the answer to the second question—whether the trial provided any other important information?—is a resounding yes.

Patients with disease of the left main coronary artery showed a highly significant survival benefit from bypass surgery. Surgical treatment of patients with three or more blocked arteries and a poorly functioning left ventricle showed a trend toward benefit that, while not statistically significant, bore watching. This information was immediately useful to surgeons and cardiologists who had the wit to extract it from the study. Additionally, the patients treated with drugs alone in the VA study, especially those with two- and three-vessel disease and good left ventricular function who did as well as the surgical patients, provided a baseline against which surgical success could be measured in the future.[26]

Coronary Artery Surgery Study

By the summer of 1975 another large, multicenter study, this time comparing bypass surgery combined with drug therapy to drug therapy alone, was getting under way. This trial was sponsored by the National Heart, Lung, and Blood Institute, and its twin goals were to find out whether bypass surgery increased longevity in patients with coronary artery disease and whether it decreased the number of nonfatal heart attacks they suffered. It was called the Coronary Artery Surgery Study (CASS), and the participating centers (fifteen in a registry and 11 in the randomized trial) included the elite of academic medicine: Harvard, Yale, Stanford, Duke, and the Mayo Clinic.

When results were finally published in 1983, they did not settle the debate over bypass surgery; they stoked the fires. Once again a controlled, randomized clinical trial, this time with low operative mortality, had failed to show that the very traumatic operation known as coronary bypass surgery extended life. And this time it also failed to show that patients treated surgically suffered fewer heart attacks.[27]

Predictably, like the VA study, CASS came under withering fire from surgery's heavy artillery. And, like the VA study, it was vulnerable. Perhaps the most damaging blow was struck by the nation's best-known heart surgeon, Michael DeBakey, and his colleague Gerald M. Lawrie, both of Baylor College of Medicine in Houston, Texas. DeBakey and Lawrie's main point was that the 780 CASS patients weren't very sick or very old, therefore they could be expected "to have an extremely good prognosis," with or without surgery.[28]

This is important because by the mid-1980s it was already apparent that the patients who benefited most from surgery were the sickest, the ones at greatest risk. It would be misleading, DeBakey and Lawrie argued, to extrapolate the results of CASS to the high-risk patients who were the best candidates for bypass surgery.

The Baylor surgeons also took a close look at what CASS had to say about subsets, as critics are wont to do when the main findings of a trial don't come out the way they want. DeBakey and Lawrie focused on the small group of patients whose ejection fraction—the percentage of blood in the left ventricle that is pumped into circulation with each heartbeat— was relatively low. These patients showed a higher survival rate with surgery, but the number of patients was too small to yield a statistically significant result. The CASS investigators themselves recommended follow up of this subset of patients,[29] which was done, and subsequent studies confirmed that indeed they did survive longer with surgery than if they were treated only with drugs.[30]

There is one other criticism of CASS that is bound to make anyone unfamiliar with clinical trials wonder how the CASS researchers could have done what DeBakey and Lawrie said they did. This is because the normal way of doing things is counterintuitive. Clinical trials are usually conducted according to a principle called "intention to treat." A patient assigned to one group, such as surgery or drug treatment, at the beginning of a trial, even if later switched to the other group because of a change in or a reassessment of their condition, is counted in the trial results as having had only the treatment to which he or she was originally assigned.

This is done to eliminate the ability of investigators to manipulate trial results by inappropriately switching patients from one group to another in midtrial. What's important here is that in CASS an unusually high percentage of patients—38 percent—crossed over from drug treatment to surgery. Many of the patients who crossed over had disease in three coronary arteries.

Because the percentage of patients with three-vessel disease who crossed over to surgery from drug treatment was high, and because the number of patients in the drug-treatment group with three-vessel disease was small to begin with, DeBakey and Lawrie argued that this "seriously affects the statistical validity of the study." They added, "[A]s the authors of the CASS report themselves indicated, 'Because of the small sample size, a large improvement in survival due to immediate surgical intervention cannot be excluded as a possibility.' "[31]

When the CASS investigators began reporting their results, bypass surgery had been around for more than fifteen years and was being done at an ever-increasing rate, mounting into the hundreds of thousands annually. But the cardiology community was still deeply divided over whether this highly invasive procedure was really anything more than a very expensive pain reliever.

European Coronary Surgery Study

The European Coronary Surgery Study, in which 767 men were randomized between 1973 and 1976, showed a statistically significant survival benefit for bypass surgery over drug therapy at five years.[32] Moreover, the benefit, while smaller, was still statistically significant at twelve years.[33] Here at last was a result the surgeons could be happy about. Moreover, in the twelve-year follow-up report, the authors offered a possible methodological explanation for the diminished difference in survival rates between five and twelve years. This is what they wrote:

> Hypothetically, the large number of coronary bypass operations performed on patients in the medically [drug] treated group (n=136) might have improved late survival in this group, whereas the survival rate in the surgically treated group might have declined with time as a result of the progression of disease affecting both grafts and native coronary arteries.[34]

Despite the appropriately cautious use of the word "hypothetically," this paragraph makes points that even the most rigidly original-intent-oriented statisticians—the Nino Scalias of clinical trials—cannot easily ignore. Between five and twelve years, because of worsening symptoms, 136 subjects—about 36 percent of the patients in the drug-treatment group—had bypass surgery. For a clinician to ignore the possibility that this fact contributed to the narrowing of the difference in survival rates between the two groups would be irresponsible.

The second clause in the sentence refers to "progression of disease affecting both grafts and native coronary arteries." This distinction is important because saphenous veins taken from the patient's leg were the state-of-the-art graft of the 1970s, and they clogged 20 to 30 percent of the time within a few years. Therefore it is not entirely illogical to attribute deaths resulting from such blockages to failure of the surgery. But by the 1980s the state-of-the-art graft was an internal mammary artery, and late blockage rates were on the order of 5 percent. As for blockages in native coronary arteries, no one was claiming that a bypass operation cured coronary artery disease. The claim was only that it could relieve angina symptoms for years and perhaps extend life by bypassing existing blockages.

Finally, the twelve-year report by the investigators of the European Coronary Surgery Study concluded that the main reason why it found an overall survival benefit for surgery and why the VA study and CASS did not is that there were important differences in the subjects randomized in the three trials. Because of the complexity of the comparisons involved, the claim that these differences, mainly in severity of illness, significantly affected the results may be difficult to prove statistically, but it makes good sense.

Twenty years of clinical experience with bypass surgery, as well as subset results and meta-analysis [combined analysis of the data from several studies][35] of the trials themselves, support the position that a trial studying patients suffering from mild disease should show little or no relative survival benefit for surgery, whereas a trial studying the sickest patients should show considerable relative survival benefit.[36] And in fact, patients from all three trials with diseased left main coronary arteries, or with three or more diseased vessels and weak left ventricles, have been shown to survive significantly longer with bypass surgery than with drug therapy.[37]

As late as 1977, a decade after Favaloro's groundbreaking surgery, Braunwald pointed out that it had not been proved that bypass surgery offered patients a survival benefit and that it was expensive and might siphon off funds from other possibly more needed areas of medical care.[38] Zimmerman and Braunwald did not care to rely on instinct. They wanted scientific proof.

Others, of course, rose to the defense of bypass operations,[39] and eventually the controversy led to the mounting of the trials discussed above, an unprecedented response for a surgical procedure, although not one that slowed the pace of its use. Over fifteen to twenty years, partly because of data generated by these trials and partly because of the evolution of the operation and increasing success rates, the supporters of bypass surgery prevailed. Their instincts, it turned out, were more right than wrong. Sabiston, Garrett, DeBakey, Cooley, Zimmerman, Braunwald, and other skeptics were not fools. They raised the right questions. Their skepticism was absolutely appropriate. In the end, it just proved unjustified.

There is a narrow sense, however, in which the skeptics were right. Bypass surgery did explode into practice before its benefits were adequately demonstrated, before its risks were well enough understood, and before patient selection was sufficiently refined. But the clinical trials, while not proving that bypass surgery extended life in all or even most cases, also did not support the claim made by the opponents of the operation—that compared to drug therapy, bypass surgery, except in very limited circumstances, did not extend life at all. Time has shown that with increased knowledge and improved technique, for perhaps tens of thousands of patients annually, bypass surgery has increased their longevity as well as improved their quality of life.

Advances such as the use of internal mammary artery grafts, improved oxygenators and less-traumatic blood-plastic interfaces in heart-lung machines, better means of protecting the heart during surgery, innovative blood conservation methods, better anesthesia techniques, and better postoperative care have all improved survival rates, although not necessarily nonfatal heart-attack rates for surgical patients.

Robert Califf and his colleagues at Duke University reported in 1989 that "surgical results have improved significantly" since enrollment was completed for the CASS and European trials. According to an analysis of data on 5,809 patients treated with bypass surgery at Duke, they wrote, survival benefits "are now larger than the results of these trials would predict."[40]

The development in the late 1970s of balloon angioplasty to open blocked arteries and of stenting in the late 1980s to keep them from closing brought to about 800,000 in 1995 the number of procedures designed to bring more blood to the heart muscle. This raises the following question: Why were more than twice as many procedures—angioplasties, placing of stents, and bypass operations—done in 1995 for coronary artery disease than there were in 1986, even though the incidence of the disease has declined about 1 percent a year for the last thirty years?[41]

Part of the answer is the truism that a new procedure that makes physiological sense and shows even a marginal benefit will be used by those trained to use it. To a man with a hammer, everything looks like a nail. But there is more to it than that. Cardiologists and cardiac surgeons were finally beginning to understand, for example, that women—especially postmenopausal women—suffered from coronary artery disease, so they were treated surgically or with angioplasty and, more and more frequently, angioplasty and stents.

As they got better at bypass surgery, the surgeons also concluded that they could operate with high success rates on patients in their seventies and eighties, even though some of them had other diseases, such as diabetes, that made surgery more difficult. And they did many more operations on patients who already had had bypass surgery once, or even twice, some because the job was not completed the first time, some because of graft closure, and some because of progression of the underlying disease.

Some needless bypass surgery was being done, and undoubtedly still is.[42] The reasons are several: poor clinical judgment; inadequate data on which to make patient specific diagnoses; cowboy syndrome, in which, as Laurence Groves put it, "It got to be a kind of a game to see how many vessels we could graft";[43] diagnostic errors, or some other form of mistake; and, rarely, greed. To use a worst-case example, the Cleveland Clinic's Proudfit said, "We've studied a number of patients here who've had bypass surgery who didn't have coronary disease."[44]

There is no indication at all that the spread of bypass surgery was slowed because of the trials or warnings from opinion leaders such as Braunwald, who declared in his 1977 editorial in *the New England Journal of Medicine* that the rapid growth of the procedure was an "insidious problem" because "an industry is being built around this operation. This rapidly growing enterprise," he wrote, "is developing a momentum and constituency of its own. . . ." that eventually may lead to bypass surgery on "many hundreds of thousands. . . . This course would escalate the annual national cost into many billions of dollars, which in turn could result in a radical redistribution of medical-care resources."[45]

Here is America's most respected cardiologist warning in one of the nation's most prestigious medical journals that rushing headlong into mass use of the bypass operation was potentially courting disaster. Many if not most cardiologists were as skeptical as Braunwald. Yet it seems to have made little if any difference. Why?

There is no single, simple answer. Several factors were involved, a number of which have already been touched on. For one thing, whether it extended life or not, the operation had already been shown to eliminate angina in large numbers of patients for many years. For most of these people, this was enough to justify the trauma of surgery, especially in a high-volume, high-quality center where operative mortality was low and patients suffered few nonfatal heart attacks or strokes. Then, of course, for persons with severe disease and limited life expectancy, something, even if unproved, was better than nothing. And bypass surgery offered hope. So to some degree, the takeoff of the operation was consumer-driven.

But there were other important drivers, not the least of which was that bypass surgery was a cash cow for surgeons and hospitals alike. And, as it turned out, it proved lucrative for cardiologists, too, because advances in bypass surgery begat advances in diagnostic technology, which made new tests for coronary artery disease available, each of which could be billed for separately.

For a relatively small investment a community hospital could hire a cardiac surgery team, equip a couple of operating rooms with heart-lung machines and the necessary monitoring equipment, and open shop to offer an operation that generally took two and a half to five hours and at the time cost about $12,500 (today it is more like $40,000, about $5,000 of which is the surgeon's fee).

Of course, as noted earlier, the operation was also driven by the surgeons' belief in it and desire to do it. And neither technique nor technology stood still. The more the surgeons did it, the better most got at it. They learned to suture smaller and smaller arteries, and arteries that were more difficult to reach, to graft fragile vessels, such as those of diabetics, and to use the almost atherosclerosisproof internal mammary artery as their graft of choice.

6

Surgeons

Bypass surgery works. The operation is done successfully, without mortality or morbidity, about 95 percent of the time. The VA, CASS, and European trials helped identify the patients who benefit the most from it. But the VA trial unintentionally made another point: The key variable in surgery is the surgeon.

What does it take to be a heart surgeon? Not just any heart surgeon, but the one I would like to do my bypass should I need one? What are the character traits and physical gifts of the men and the women who perform these operations, who direct a team of anesthesiologists and perfusionists, surgical assistants and nurses, who saw bone and cut flesh, who fondle and stroke living hearts in search of buried arteries, who dissect delicate vessels from the chest wall, who sew with thread as fine as human hair, who know that a slip of the hand, or a split-second mental lapse, can be the difference between life and death?

John Kirklin and Paul Taylor, both now retired, are vastly different in temperament and style, but they were surgeons I would have trusted. Each performed more than ten thousand heart operations. The following sketches from their lives illustrate some of the qualities, attitudes, and skills that, it seems to me, are common to first-rate surgeons.

One brilliantly sunny Saturday morning in the early autumn of 1938, a hundred or so neatly dressed Harvard medical students sat waiting for a class to begin in the steeply pitched amphitheater of the old Peter Bent Brigham Hospital. A slender first-year student, wavy hair combed in bangs over his forehead giving him a slightly pixieish look, was among them. His name was John Kirklin, and he had recently graduated *summa cum laude* from the University of Minnesota. He wasn't particularly looking forward to the lecture, which was on wound healing, a subject he thought at the time was uninteresing.

When Robert E. Gross walked onto the stage, however, concerns about a dull lecture on a dull subject evaporated. Kirklin was starstruck. Gross was in his midthirties, tall, dark-haired, and dark-eyed, with regular features, and dressed in a well-tailored navy blue suit, crisp white shirt, and fashionable tie. Every hair was in place. He stopped for a moment and surveyed the room. Then he stepped to the lectern, still not having spoken, and focused on the fresh faces.

This young professor, who captivated his audience by his elegant, self-assured presence, just a year earlier had ventured into the virtually unexplored territory of cardiac surgery. He had closed a patent ductus arteriosus, a relatively rare defect in newborns that results when a normal channel in the fetal heart, which is meant to close by itself before birth, fails to do so. This failure results in the recirculation of arterial blood through the lungs, which in turn leads to numerous complications, some of which are likely to be fatal, especially in late adolescence or early adulthood. The procedure Gross pioneered was done with the infant's heart beating.

Recollecting the events of almost sixty years before, Kirklin, his hair thinner, and gray rather than brown, but still combed in a fringe across his forehead, reflected that Gross that day, not for what he said, but for who he was, "made a hundred Harvard medical students decide to be cardiac surgeons. I was one of them."[1]

While Kirklin, at eighty, no longer performs surgery, he studies it. His peers consider him to have been one of the best of all cardiac surgeons. He is soft-spoken, courtly, deliberate, intellectual, circumspect, and diffident. But when he detects inattention, sloppy speech, or careless thought, he can be curt or even acerbic. He speaks carefully, sometimes plainly, sometimes with academic precision, sometimes with biblical overtones, often pausing to ponder a word's nuance, or even enunciating it to try out its sound. One must listen to his sentences, weighing their meaning, attending to their occasionally complex structures.

In the quotation above, for example, Kirklin did not say, nor did he mean, that the hundred Harvard medical students in the Brigham amphitheater became cardiac surgeons, but rather that at that moment, in that amphitheater, the presence of Robert E. Gross compelled them to decide, if only for a moment, to become cardiac surgeons, a decision all the more remarkable because at the time there was no such discrete surgical specialty. And more relevantly, he did not say, nor did he mean, that his own decision to become a cardiac surgeon rested solely on Gross's compelling presence. Kirklin is not given to such simplicities.

"There's no single reason anybody ever does anything," he said, explaining his own decision to become a cardiac surgeon as "some sort of combination of opportunity, drive, desire, balancing the problems of living with the problems of training, all those things."[2] Then he thought back to his childhood at the Mayo Clinic, where his father was a radiologist, and delivered what sounded suspiciously like, if not a single reason, then a precipitating cause for becoming a heart surgeon. He remembered a man named Arleigh Barnes, who was chief of cardiology at Mayo and who used to go fishing for muskies in northern Wisconsin with his father. Because of Barnes, Kirklin said, "[I] knew a little bit about cardiac surgery, and I knew nobody could do it. Barnes said it's gonna happen, it's gonna be exciting, it's gonna change totally the practice of cardiology. Sounded good to me."[3]

About eighteen years after John Kirklin came under the spell of Robert Gross, around Christmas, a hulking high school football player from Shaker Heights, Ohio, named Paul Taylor was invited to the Cleveland Clinic by Donald Effler, the head of thoracic surgery there. Surgery was nothing new to Taylor. He had spent three summers working as a scrub technician in operating rooms at the clinic. He had also worked in a dog lab, where his duties included collecting blood drained from cattle slaughtered for kosher meat, which, according to Jewish dietary laws, must be bloodless. The blood was used to prime the pump of the lab's heart-lung machine.

That school vacation Taylor watched Laurence Groves, a patrician-looking, technically brilliant, ambidextrous surgeon, close a patent ductus arteriosus. The operation by Groves, who had watched Robert Gross operate when he was a student at Harvard, was the first cardiac surgery Taylor had ever seen. It transported him, much as the words of Arleigh Barnes and the charisma of Gross had transported John Kirklin.

"I was lost in it," Taylor said, "totally consumed in it. I virtually went off to college with the idea, I didn't want to be a physician, but I wanted to be a surgeon, probably a heart surgeon, which is just ridiculous. I mean, how would you know that?"[4] In 1957, the year Taylor went to college, that was a fair question because there was *still* no such thing as a heart surgeon. The specialty as such would not exist for more than a decade.

Like John Kirklin, Paul Taylor followed through and became a highly respected cardiac surgeon. Unlike John Kirklin, he is not soft-spoken, courtly, deliberate, intellectual (at least not in an obviously self-aware way), circumspect, or diffident. He is acerbic, outspoken, anti-intellectual in some of his views about surgery, hard-edged, and loud. His language is muscular and direct, tending toward mechanical metaphors. For example, "The heart is an engine. You can't lose all the fuel lines."

Taylor's operating room is a theater for his stand-up act of often irreverent, sometimes obscene one-liners and political commentaries delivered in a booming voice, sometimes against a background of boogie-woogie piano, which he plays as well as appreciates.

Yet, despite their substantial differences, Kirklin and Taylor share a culture—share certain rituals that help define the culture—that can be observed in any heart surgeon's operating room. The music might vary from Mozart to Jelly Roll Morton, but with rare exceptions there is music. And the tone and subject matter of the conversation can vary almost as much as the music, but there is usually conversation.

Take, for example, one day in October 1996, in Taylor's operating room at the Cleveland Clinic. The patient is a sixty-four-year-old diabetic male from Morgantown, West Virginia. Taylor is planning to use both internal mammary arteries to bypass blockages in his left anterior descending and circumflex arteries. This is not everyday surgery, but neither is it rare. Taylor has done it many times.

The operation entails detaching one end of each of the two internal mammary arteries, easily accessible vessels that feed blood to the chest wall, and hooking them up to two important coronary arteries on the left side of the heart. The ends of the internal mammary arteries will be sewn into the left anterior descending and circumflex arteries downstream from fat-and-fiber blockages that are preventing blood from irrigating two segments of the heart muscle. If all goes well, blood from the internal mammary arteries will then course through the coronary arteries and nourish the heart muscle where needed. The chest, as Favaloro demonstrated, will do fine because it receives enough blood even if both mammaries are rerouted.

Before Taylor comes into the operating room, the preliminaries are taken care of. The patient's chest is sawn in half in a few seconds. His ribs are wrenched apart by steel retractors. The lungs naturally deflate when air enters the chest cavity. They are then stitched to the chest wall to keep them out of the way. Plastic lines from the heart-lung machine are attached. Dark, venous blood will be pumped from the right atrium into the machine instead of the lungs; it will be cooled to about 82 degrees Fahrenheit to lower the body's temperature thereby slowing the metabolism of the tissues; purified, oxygenated, and, now crimson, returned to the circulatory system through the aorta.

The opening in the patient's chest is about a foot square and looks eerily empty. The fibrous pericardial sac has been slit open. The heart is slick and still beating. Gauze "sponges" strategically placed in the open chest soak up small amounts of blood. One of Taylor's assistants dissects the mammary arteries off the chest wall and trims off fat and other tissue.

The mood seems relaxed. The team—assisting surgeons, nurses, anesthetists, and heart-lung machine technicians—chat amiably like people who work regularly together and are comfortable doing it. There is something reassuringly blue-collar about the atmosphere, a sense of being among the working class of the age of technology. The surgeons especially are, in a manner of speaking, master craftsmen of the space age—high-tech carpenters, plumbers, and electricians rolled into one.

The physical environment, with its flickering TV monitors, yards of plastic tubing, consoles, roller pumps, membrane oxygenator, trays of stainless steel instruments, and the exposed operating field displaying a rack of ribs on either side of the heart, suggests a butcher shop sharing space with a computer lab.

Then, momentarily unnoticed by the rest of the team, Taylor, a masked presence in blue surgical scrubs, enters the operating room. Once the nurses and surgical assistants see him, work continues, but conversation stops. Taylor is powerfully built; well over six feet tall and well over two hundred pounds. A nurse quickly passes him a towel to dry his dripping hands and then helps him into translucent rubber gloves, which give his hands a soft, white, feminine look. He begins to talk. For the next two hours his deep, loud, resonant voice dominates the operating room.

Dr. Sukesh Chigarapalli-Reddy, an Indian surgeon who has assisted Taylor dozens of times, gets the brunt of his running diatribe this day. He is criticized first for not changing a set of surgical loupes quickly enough and then for not trimming one of the internal mammary arteries carefully enough. Taylor, who is giving orders to the technicians and the other assistant surgeon about anesthesia, cardioplegia, and the heart-lung machine, which has been turned on, shifts gears and lets fly a blast of invective at Bill and Hillary Clinton, him for being "sleazy," her for "screwing up medicine," and both for just being "liberal."

There is a momentary break during which I ask him a question about the components of the cardioplegia solution, the chemical cocktail used to stop the heart's contractions so it can be manipulated safely and operated on with greater precision. "As long as there's enough potassium in it," he says offhandedly, "the rest might as well be V-8 juice."

Taylor is now handling the patient's heart in the detached fashion of experienced surgeons, looking for the arteries he will bypass, cradling the still, bloodless organ in his left hand, probing it with his right index finger. He is now talking about the difficulty of the operation, the fragility of the patient's arteries resulting from his diabetes, the calcification of the vessels, the diffuse disease, and that the arteries are buried deep in muscle. He finds the circumflex, a lateral branch of the left main coronary artery, fairly easily and completes the hookup quickly, using a separate suture and tiny curved needle for each stitch. This is a technique called interrupted suturing that is considered old-fashioned by most cardiac surgeons but is still used by some at the Cleveland Clinic who believe it yields a tighter, longer-lasting connection.

Now Taylor begins hunting for the left anterior descending, the long artery that runs from top to bottom down the left side of the heart and nourishes the majority of the left ventricle, the main pumping chamber. He runs his finger along the surface of the heart, hunting for the vessel, which is no more than three millimeters in diameter. His touch is sensitive but not delicate. The flaccid heart does not require delicacy. He can't find it, and says, "Shit, at my age I don't want to do three of these a day anymore."

At last, after about twenty minutes of probing, he thinks he has it. "You think this is it?" he asks Chigarapalli-Reddy. The Indian doctor's reply is softly spoken and hard to understand. "Don't mumble," Taylor says. "You can mumble in India because everybody mumbles there. But you can't mumble here." Taylor has a gift of being simultaneously jocular and serious. His political incorrectness is on the whole well tolerated by the surgical team, which may be the only choice in this most autocratic of environments.

He is now silent as he continues to feel along the front surface of the patient's heart. Finally, in a tone reflecting the surgeon's creed—usually right, but never in doubt—he announces that he's found the LAD, the vessel he must bypass. He carefully dissects the artery out of the muscle, makes a quick, tiny incision, there's a spurt of blood, a clamp is placed, and he begins to suture again. Now he's talking with relish about a planned trip to the Cayman Islands for skeet shooting and the joys of handmade bamboo fly rods. When the sewing is done he instructs his assistants to close and leaves as unobtrusively as he arrived.

What was it that John Kirklin responded to in "the man" Robert E. Gross? What was it that affected Paul Taylor so profoundly when he watched Laurence Groves close a patent ductus arteriosus? What, more generally, are the characteristics surgeons have in common, whether they are upper-middle-class midwestern WASPS like Kirklin and Taylor; New York Jews like Greg Ribakove, who is a leading heart surgeon at NYU; second-generation Sicilians from West Virginia like Paul Corso; or ex-hippies from North Dakota like Bruce Lytle, who wears corduroy and leather and rides his Harley Hog to work at the Cleveland Clinic?

Why are these men surgeons especially, not just physicians? Surgery, after all, is something other than just a specialty of medicine. It pursues its palliative and curative goals by means associated with the infliction of pain and death. Its instruments are carpenters' tools—saws, drills, and clamps. The professional forebears of its practitioners are medieval barbers. Somewhere inside most of us, although we honor surgeons and pay them more than their medical colleagues, we believe that what they do is barbarous and wherever possible must eventually be replaced by more humane forms of treatment. So what is it then that leads men and women to choose surgery as their life's work? Why heart surgery? And what sets surgeons apart from other physicians who choose less aggressive, more contemplative medical specialties?

John Kirklin, who has a gift for precise, comprehensive characterizations and biting irony, offered this appraisal: "I think surgeons, generally, are more decisive. I think surgeons are generally more driven; driven to consummate whatever it is they are doing, a sense of urgency, maybe; a more tangible, achievable goal rather than a vague, more distant goal. Surgeons generally tend to be people who find it easy, and rewarding, to do manual things, carpentry, surgery, whatever. In the [nonsurgical] medical world there are lots of people who are completely content not to be able to tie their shoes very well."[5]

Kirklin's vision is complex. It captures more than just decisiveness, drive, urgency, tangible goals, and manual dexterity. There is an intellectual component. He himself is interested in the gross and micro workings of the human body; in physiology and microbiology. And he is by nature a problem-solver, which has put him at the forefront of a new approach to medicine that emphasizes better collection and analysis of data. As a resident, Kirklin filled notebooks with descriptions of the operations he would do once it was possible to work inside the heart. And as a young staff surgeon at the Mayo Clinic he successfully led a small group of men bent on improving John Gibbon's revolutionary but still crude heart-lung machine.

"I don't have much faith in committees," Kirklin said, alluding to the Mayo experience with what may have been a surgeon's tendency to view the world from the perspective of a soloist. But, he added, "I have a lot of faith in a small number of individuals working intimately together"[6]— the surgeon as conductor, the surgical team his chamber orchestra.

For Kirklin, unraveling the complexity of modern surgery is a multifaceted intellectual activity to which engineers and statisticians as well as surgeons may make important contributions. On the other hand, Paul Taylor, who is as different in style from Kirklin as Jackson Pollock was from, say, Piet Mondrian, articulates a view of surgery that both overlaps with and diverges from Kirklin's.

"I think that surgeons are extremely aggressive, decisive people," Taylor said. "I think that often . . . they are very athletic types. [But] Effler always said, 'Don't be too smart. You'll outthink yourself.' " Indeed, in a review of three years of bypass surgery at the Cleveland Clinic, Donald Effler wrote: "Coronary artery procedures that are unduly complex" are more likely to fail. He argued for bypass surgery that is "both simple and safe."[7] "When things are difficult, or too complex," Taylor said, "they may not work out as well. Everybody wants to do something to somebody. Sometimes you don't need to do anything."[8]

It is evident from their comments that neither Kirklin nor Taylor is addressing the overly broad question of what makes a surgeon, but rather a more restricted question: What makes a *very good* surgeon? What are the mental and physical qualities, the character traits, that make them very good? And are these qualities common to all very good surgeons?

To begin with, everyone would like to think that wherever they go for surgery, from large urban academic medical centers to small rural community hospitals, at a minimum they will find surgeons with "good hands." But will they? Laurence Groves said tartly during an interview in October 1996 that "I've seen a lot of motor morons in the operating room."[9] And Groves's Cleveland Clinic colleague Leonard A. R. Golding said, "There are some guys I wouldn't send a sick dog to."[10]

Groves and Golding may have higher standards than most, and their choice of words might have been a bit overheated, and judgments about manual dexterity and hand-eye coordination are somewhat subjective, but few of Groves's and Golding's colleagues would disagree that differences in mortality and morbidity rates, corrected for the difficulty of the particular surgeon's caseload, are frequently due to variations in technical skill. In other words, some people die in the operating room, or have nonfatal heart attacks or strokes, simply because the surgeon lacks the fine-motor capacity needed to do the job.

Another quality self-evidently common to all very good surgeons is an exceptional ability to concentrate for extended periods of time. It is evident from spending many hours with John Kirklin and Paul Taylor that both men are extraordinarily focused; their minds do not drift; they concentrate until a line of thought, or a surgical procedure, is completed, however long that takes. The same is true of Michael Mack, Jorge Garcia, Paul Corso, John Stevens, Bruce Lytle, Valavanur Subramanian, Greg Ribakove—of all the very good surgeons interviewed—and observed doing surgery—for this book.

In the operating room their concentration is sustained by whatever ritual it takes to keep them relaxed. In Taylor's case, it is his bombast, the sound of his own voice, the rhythmic intricacies of James P. Johnson's stride piano; in Ribakove's, it is ironic New York kibitzing, light rock, and DJ patter. Each surgeon's operating room seems to have its own style.

This background is created to provide an aura of normality in what is in fact a singular and somewhat peculiar setting. Its purpose is to sustain the necessary level of concentration in as relaxed an environment as possible for whatever time it takes for the surgeon and for the support team to complete their demanding and often delicate work.

So far the qualities described—manual skill and concentration—might well be those of a master cabinetmaker. And that, to a degree, is the way many cardiologists—only half in jest—subtly demean surgery and assert the superiority of their own discipline.

These practitioners view themselves as working in an intellectual tradition, as thoughtful interpreters of hard-to-detect symptoms identified through the use of highly developed clinical skills and sophisticated diagnostic equipment. While many of them admire surgeons, it is often with the genuine but qualified admiration of artists for artisans, not quite with the all-embracing admiration fine artists and intellectuals reserve for those they consider their equals.* Indeed, a few nonsurgeons, such as Stephen Oesterle, Massachusetts General Hospital's outspoken, sometimes hyperbolic director of interventional cardiology, dismiss "all surgeons [as] idiots."[11]

However, after several hours of conversation with John Kirklin, it is hard to give much credit to a view of "very good" surgeons that excludes or even minimizes the role of intellect and judgment. And the same can be said of the other surgeons interviewed for this book, Paul Taylor included, despite his posture of abhorring complexity. Even Oesterle, if pressed, will agree that not every surgeons is an idiot.

The best surgeons, after all, design, participate in, interpret, and publish the results of complicated, multicenter clinical trials; they compile large databases, carefully analyze the data, and apply it to individual patients; they have invented better ways to preserve a patient's blood and reuse it during an operation, thereby avoiding transfusions; they have devised means of protecting the heart while it is being repaired, of reducing damage to blood cells during cardiopulmonary bypass, of lessening other kinds of trauma during surgery, and so on. To be a very good surgeon, therefore, intellect and good judgment are clearly part of the package.

Manual dexterity, exceptional powers of concentration, and intellect are all qualities common to very good surgeons, but when I asked surgeons themselves what characteristic most set them apart from other physicians, almost to a man they said "decisiveness." It is not clear whether those destined to be very good surgeons typically bring this character trait to the operating table as interns and residents, or develop it in training. But, like fledgling fighter pilots, if they do not have it or quickly develop it, they

---

*In fairness, surgeons are no more charitable toward nonsurgical medical practitioners than nonsurgeons are toward them: To wit, Groves's caustic comment "I know an awful lot of respected internists in town whose patients do fine, unless they get sick." Moreover, there are surgeons who sometimes refer to their nonsurgical colleagues as FLEAs, which stands for fucking little esoteric assholes.

will either wash out or be second-rate in a profession where second-rate is unacceptable.

A surgeon must have a quick hand and a prepared mind because an open chest, like an enemy fighter, is not an object of tranquil contemplation, it is an occasion for action. A patient whose coronary arteries are filled with surprises does not need a surgeon who will in due time write a brilliant paper about it; he needs a surgeon who will on the spot improvise a workable solution. A very good surgeon must react reflexively to the unexpected, not rarely but often, because given the relatively primitive although rapidly improving state of cardiac diagnostic techniques, the unexpected is still a common occurrence.

There is a handful of additional qualities that very good surgeons almost certainly must have. These include stamina, because surgeons work long hours on their feet under continuous mental strain; intense short-term goal orientation, because once a surgeon starts something he must finish it, except in those rare cases where he is confronted by an unexpected situation such as exceptionally diffuse disease or contorted coronary anatomy that he can only make worse; and perhaps an unquenchable enthusiasm for the work, a sense of excitement that in John Kirklin's words "keeps your adrenaline level continually a little elevated."[12]

Of course, no discussion of what it means to be a heart surgeon can be complete without confronting death. Heart surgeons face it every day. Successful heart surgery is often the only thing that stands between a patient and death. If a cardiac surgeon's performance is imperfect, or at times, even if it is perfect, some patients will die under his knife. For very good heart surgeons like Taylor and Kirklin, who take the toughest cases, the lifetime operative mortality rate—including operations done in the early days of open-chest surgery—may be 3 to 5 percent. That's more than one death a month, year in and year out.

What kind of a psychological toll does that much death take? Is it the reason why so many surgeons maintain a cool demeanor, seem detached or even callous? Kirklin says the coolness is "usually a cover-up . . . the playing out of the realization that it could have ended differently,"[13] with survival instead of death, or vice versa.

His implicit question is how could any surgeon accept the responsibility, stand the emotional roller coaster, without a well-prepared defense? No doubt Kirklin is right about the psychological barriers some or even most surgeons erect. But, almost certainly, such barriers, at least for some, in time become permanent; they constitute a new reality. It becomes correct to say that these surgeons are cool to death, or detached, or even callous.

Yet, René Favaloro believes it is his fault every time one of his patients dies in surgery or before leaving the hospital. He has almost no emotional tolerance for the death of his patients. For him, the issue is not having caused the death because of an incorrect judgment, or a technical error, but rather having failed to prevent it. Favaloro once told a resident that "Deaths related to surgery would be *his* [my italics] deaths, and he would carry them on his shoulders for the rest of his life."[14]

Favaloro dreams of something that transcends surgical perfection, because surgical perfection alone cannot guarantee zero mortality. Most people do not think of surgeons as dreamers. They think of them, by and large, as surgeons think of themselves—as pragmatic, concrete, and focused on the immediate. And that is what they are, except that the best surgeons, like the best writers or painters, musicians or molecular biologists, tend to be somewhat less bound by stereotypes, by old paradigms, than average professionals; they let their imaginations range a bit more freely; they very likely are more willing to challenge conventions, as Alexis Carrel and John Gibbon did before Favaloro.

But in the end even the very best surgeons and cardiologists must make treatment choices for—and more and more with—their patients based on incomplete evidence. This is because the results of clinical trials and other kinds of studies frequently offer only general guidance applicable to large populations, not clear-cut, patient-specific answers. The case of Lewis Hollander in chapter 8 illustrates how difficult it can be to choose.

Moreover, the choices are no longer limited to standard bypass surgery of the kind developed by René Favaloro and performed by Kirklin and Taylor. Today bypass surgery is also done through small incisions in the chest and on a beating heart; angioplasty is an alternative to bypass surgery in many cases, and so are stents, tiny metal scaffolds permanently inserted into arteries to keep them open. These new treatments are the result of collaborations between inventive cardiologists and cardiac surgeons, engineers, and entrepreneurs. Their cooperative ventures have brought to market a whole range of new treatments. They have also raised a new set of ethical questions.

7

Smart Operators

As a premed undergraduate at Stanford University in the late 1970s, Wes Sterman was assigned a faculty adviser who was in the process of founding a company. The adviser's name was Bill New, and he had invented a photoelectric device that now can be found in almost all operating rooms and intensive-care units. It is called an oximeter, and it uses a photoelectric cell to measure the oxygen saturation of the blood without puncturing the patient's skin. Sterman found New fascinating, even brilliant, and came to view him as a mentor.

When New, a professor of anesthesiology, suggested to Sterman that he try to remain at Stanford for his medical education so he could audit courses at the business school, he took the advice. Sterman applied and was accepted into the Class of 1986.

For Sterman, a medical student already flush with entrepreneurial ambitions, it was an ideal setting. Stanford, after all, had been midwife and wet nurse to dozens of Silicon Valley start-up companies. Moreover, while its average medical-school salaries were low by national standards, it more than made up for this by giving faculty members time off to consult for medical-device companies. In this environment designed to nurture invention and entrepreneurship, Sterman not only met the demands of first-year studies at one of the country's most rigorous medical schools but also started a company of his own.

He was struck by the fact that he and his fellow students were paying the school bookstore a lot of money for their instruments—stethoscopes, ophthalmoscopes, otoscopes, etc. He speculated correctly that if he could go directly to the manufacturers with a block of guaranteed sales, he would be able to buy the same equipment for less than the bookstore paid. He put together a group of about eighty students, bought the instruments from 3M at a sharp discount, and sold them for exactly what he paid. His profit, apart from experience and the gratitude of his fellow students, was on the float. He held the money for sixty to ninety days, earning what he could with it.

As Sterman progressed through medical school toward a surgical internship, his company, called MedSurge, flourished. Before he graduated he was selling supplies to medical students at the University of California's campuses at Davis, San Diego, San Francisco, and Los Angeles, to nursing and chiropractic students, and to residents, fellows, and some faculty members. With this experience and medical school behind him, Sterman entered the Stanford business school full-time and completed an M.B.A.

In early 1987, instead of pursuing and internship, Sterman, then twenty-eight years old, went to work for a venture capital firm as their specialist in biotechnology, biopharmaceuticals, medical-device technology, and health-care services. It was a perfect opportunity for him to get an overview of the industry and to learn about dealmaking. While working at the firm, called Menlo Ventures, he started a company called Endovascular Technologies (ET). Menlo put up the money to get it started. At ET Sterman, who was impressed by the reduction of surgical trauma resulting from the use of a laparoscope in gallbladder surgery, developed a less-invasive means of treating abdominal aortic aneurysms, a dangerous ballooning and weakening of the main artery supplying blood to the lower half of the body.

Instead of opening the abdomen to get to the deeply situated aorta and repair it with a Dacron tube, Sterman devised a means of inserting the tube through an artery that runs near the surface of the leg. To do this the tube had to be made collapsible, and a way had to be found to hold it in place without sutures. This was accomplished by a kind of lattice of metal hooks that replicate the action of suture needles, but the hooks themselves remain in place instead of sutures.

The hooks are made of elgiloy, a metal used in making space shuttle tiles and that has excellent antifatigue and anticorrosion characteristics. Eventually the blood vessel grows a new lining right over the hooks. This procedure reduces trauma and length of hospital stay and cuts operating time from four hours to half an hour. The company was sold to Guidant Corporation and the device is undergoing clinical trials required for FDA approval.

The venture capital job and running a small company like Endovascular Technologies were formative experiences for Sterman. They provided the practical business know-how he needed to go with his M.D. and M.B.A. degrees. But they were not a perfect fit for his interests. Almost from the beginning of medical school Sterman was attracted to the challenges of treating a sick heart. As a medical student, he found cardiac physiology, cardiac anatomy, and cardiac surgery the most interesting and exciting areas of medicine. He also believed that diseases of the heart were "qualitatively more important than [diseases of] any other organ."[1]

As an entrepreneur, Sterman's focus remains on the heart, but his angle of vision and vocabulary shift into business mode. He talks about the extra sexiness of devices, biopharmaceuticals (drugs made from living organisms), and medical services (such as cardiac surgery, angioplasty, and stenting) in the cardiovascular area, pointing out that the companies that compete in this market tend to have "the highest valuations, the highest gross margins." In addition, he notes, cardiac surgeons are among the most highly paid surgeons, and the procedures are often the most expensive procedures, the most dangerous and complicated. "There are," he says, "a lot of characteristics that all add up to a potentially good business opportunity."[2]

Sterman sees nothing fundamentally wrong with viewing disease as a business opportunity. Indeed, he sees this approach as socially productive despite the inherent conflict of interest between maximizing profits and benefiting patients. He would surely agree with Robert Petersdorf, ex-president of the Association of American Medical Colleges, who said, "[M]ost biomedical research [is] ultimately aimed at bettering the life of patients, and the industry that aid[s] and abet[s] this goal [is] acting in the public good."[3] Cancer surgeon Steven Rosenberg has pointed out, however, that "The increasing involvement of for-profit . . . companies in medical research has provided new sources of funding, but with this involvement has come an emphasis on the ethical and operational rules of business rather than on those of science."[4]

Sterman is not terribly concerned about the short-term risks encountered when for competitive reasons a new device is rushed to market too quickly. While acknowledging that some patients might be treated inappropriately—a circumstance that historically has caused a large but unknown number of deaths—he argues that in the long run the scrutiny of the clinical community and regulatory bodies such as the FDA protects patients adequately.

Moreover, even though he can't prove it, he believes that the trade-off between lives saved and lives lost by getting devices to market quickly provides a net benefit to the public. Petersdorf, however, also made a subtler point. He said that "the culture of the biomedical enterprise was changing from a primary emphasis on scholarship to a focus on entrepreneurial success."[5] Although he did not say so explicitly, he implied that this shift in emphasis would entail some unknown cost to the public.

Given his interest in cardiovascular medicine, when Sterman began to look around for new business opportunities it was natural that he turned to John Stevens, his medical-school classmate from Salt Lake City who was pursuing a career as an academic cardiac surgeon. The two intelligent and energetic young men were natural collaborators. Although Stevens elected to pursue an academic career, he was interested in business and was among Sterman's few medical school friends who encouraged him to pursue an M.B.A.

Over a period of about six months in 1991 they batted around ideas, finally concluding that they could succeed at something no one else had ever tried—coronary bypass and valve surgery done without splitting the patient's chest. One of the things they liked most about the idea was that nobody had tried it, and most surgeons thought it was impossible. They saw these as ideal conditions for starting a new company.

They would learn the lessons of laparoscopic gallbladder surgery, arthroscopic knee surgery and other minimally invasive procedures and apply them to the heart. Sterman had already taken a step in this direction with his minimally invasive treatment for abdominal aortic aneurysms. The business opportunity seemed enormous, possibly billions of dollars a year.

Devices, which generally depend on relatively cheap, straightforward engineering for their development, could be brought to market quickly and inexpensively compared to drugs, which depend on expensive, complex cellular and molecular science. What's more, without the trauma of a foot-long incision, the main reason for most lengthy postsurgical hospitalization, patients could go home in a couple of days and return to work and other normal activities in a week or two. This would be attractive to third-party payers because it would reduce costly hospital stays. And it also would be attractive to private employers and the federal government because it would result in less productivity loss than standard bypass surgery, which usually requires a five- to ten-day hospital stay and up to twelve weeks of recovery time.[6]

In late 1991 Sterman and Stevens quietly set up Stanford Surgical Technologies, which later became Heartport Corporation. They began with a quick $3 million cash infusion from just two carefully chosen venture capital firms, Sierra Ventures and Kleiner, Perkins, Caufield, & Byers. The two friends did not want word of what they were doing to spread in the venture-capital community.

They resisted the temptation to present any of their early work on the techniques of minimally invasive heart surgery at medical meetings and even held off from using their name of choice, Heartport, because it revealed too much about what they were doing. Sterman had been burned before when word got out about his aortic aneurysm procedure, and a number of companies with similar technologies popped up like mushrooms to compete with ET.

One of Stanford Surgical's first employees was a young toolmaker named Chuck Taylor. While Sterman, a straight-arrow businessman's son from Los Angeles, was speeding along a twin track at Stanford, Taylor, who seemed destined by birth for the straight and narrow academic path, was in the process of rejecting it.

Taylor grew up in New Haven, Connecticut, the son of the provost of Yale University. He attended Phillips Academy in Andover Massachusetts, the American International School in Zurich, Switzerland, and graduated from the Putney School in Putney, Vermont. From early childhood, however, what delighted him most was making things, working with his hands. He built model airplanes, and by the time he was in prep school he was on his way to becoming a cabinetmaker. He built looms, a guitar, and one summer, at his family's country property in western Massachusetts, together with his father he built a barn.

While working on the barn, Taylor met a man who had been a blacksmith. The idea of making things from forged metal excited him so much that when he graduated from prep school he found a blacksmith in Connecticut to work with. This was not an Old West shop that made horseshoes and the like. They made finely detailed reproduction ironwork for early American buildings, using a technique similar to that still used in making forged, stainless-steel surgical instruments.

After his apprenticeship with the blacksmith, Taylor entered Brown University. While a freshman there he took a machine-shop course at the nearby Rhode Island School of Design. He couldn't get enough of it. After a year he quit college to work in a machine shop full-time. He learned to be a toolmaker and how to make delicate jewelry chains. Once he felt he had learned the trade, Taylor decided he would practice it in the journeyman tradition by going on the road as an itinerant machinist. His idea was to travel from place to place picking up jobs, work as long as he liked, and then move on. But it didn't take long for him to discover that employers really weren't interested in having someone come to work for a week or two or three and then be gone.

Taylor settled instead for a small machine shop in Conway, Massachusetts, which he operated for a couple of years. During this time he got married and he and his wife, Ravenna, moved south from New England to rural Arkansas. He set up a shop deep in the country near a town named Fifty-six and did whatever jobs he could get. "I ended up repairing a lot of sewing machines, bulldozers, road graders, farm equipment," he said. "I made machines for people; I made a potter's wheel for a guy, set up a welding shop to mass-produce satellite dishes."[7]

By his thirtieth birthday Taylor had been in rural Arkansas for seven years. He still enjoyed working with his hands, but some of the fizz had gone out of it. He was eager to do something more sophisticated, but that still involved making things. So he and Ravenna moved to California. They headed straight for Silicon Valley, where high-tech companies sprout as easily as asparagus does in the Central Valley. He got a job making tools and machinery for a company that manufactured electronic maps for cars. The year was 1985. The company was a little ahead of its time.

Taylor was next hired by Advanced Cardiovascular Systems, the grand-daddy of all medical device companies in Silicon Valley. John Simpson, its founder, had built a better medical mousetrap, an angioplasty catheter over a guidewire that could be more accurately maneuvered than the original wireless variety. In the tradition of Silicon Valley, Simpson sold the company, got rich, started up another company, and then another. Simpson hired Taylor because he could make machines, and they needed machines to manufacture prototypes of their catheters.

For the next five and a half years Taylor built machinery and developed new technology and products, not all of which had obvious applications. Then he ran a little "skunk works" for a consortium of medical-device companies that produced interesting items such as a three-dimensional printing process to make microparts in preassembled form. Six months later, Taylor left this job to work for what was to become Heartport.

But Taylor didn't stay. He had entrepreneurial dreams of his own and left after a year and a half to pursue them. Like so many Silicon Valley inventor-entrepreneurs, he started a company in his garage. Like Sterman, Taylor was well aware of the advantages of surgical procedures done through small incisions. He, too, saw a business opportunity. He believed there was a market for sewing machines that surgeons could use in all kinds of minimally invasive surgery. But he thought the real future was in surgery done through tiny portlike incisions, with the surgeon sewing while look-ing at a television picture of the structures being sutured, not through surgical loupes at the actual structures.

This was precisely what Heartport's founders had in mind for cardiac surgery. Taylor's initial focus, however, was on gallbladder surgery because, at the time, this was the most common minimally invasive operation. Tay-lor believed that one day there would be a market for his sewing machines in heart surgery, too, but a medical-device industry investor named Jack Lasersohn persuaded him that Heartport was going about it in the wrong way.

Lasersohn convinced Taylor that suturing tiny coronary arteries under indirect vision would be too difficult for most surgeons and also that the operation would require the patient to spend too much time on the heart-lung machine, a source of trauma to blood cells and possible complications such as stroke and postsurgical cognitive deficits. He also told Taylor some-thing he had not known: Open-chest bypass surgery had been done many times on a beating heart, which meant the risks of the heart-lung machine were avoided.

But Lasersohn said there were two problems: Sterman and Stevens had convinced the investment community that opening the chest was a terrible thing to do to a patient, and beating-heart surgery was too difficult to do through a small incision. If a company was going to successfully promote beating-heart surgery, Lasersohn believed, this impression had to be neutralized. Taylor, however, looked at it differently. He saw a technical challenge: devising a way to do minimally invasive beating-heart surgery. This was the kind of problem he was good at solving.

He began working with Mark Ratcliffe, a cardiac surgeon at San Francisco Veterans Hospital, and familiarizing himself with the literature on beating-heart coronary artery surgery. It turned out it had a long history, going back at least to 1964 in the Soviet Union. In recent years it has been done mostly in Argentina, Brazil, and, less frequently, in the United States. It was done often in Argentina and Brazil mainly because it is much cheaper to do heart surgery without a heart-lung machine than with one. Indeed, many hospitals in poorer countries do not even own one of the $250,000 devices.

It is done in the United States mainly because some surgeons believe that avoiding potentially devastating short-term complications such as strokes, which in a small number of cases are caused by the heart-lung machine, is a good trade-off for the possibility of a less-precise incision, which can be caused by sewing on a moving heart and which can result in a poorer long-term result. When oxygen bubbles into the blood, cells are damaged, which leads to several problems: White cells become less effective in preventing infection; inflammatory substances are released; and platelets are damaged, which can cause bleeding. Tiny clots also can form around oxygen bubbles, causing strokes.

Ratcliffe was skeptical about beating-heart surgery. He told Taylor, "I'm just not convinced that I can sew a good anastamosis [juncture] while the heart is bouncing up and down."[8] Taylor's response was to begin working on a device to stabilize the coronary artery being sewn so it would move less than the underlying heart muscle. He tested his prototypes in Ratcliffe's animal laboratory, unaware that a group in the Netherlands was working toward the same goal.[9] He also began working on a business plan, which he knew he needed to attract start-up capital.

Taylor also wanted to go to South America to observe the surgeons who had the most experience with the operation, Federico Benetti[10] in Argentina and Enio Buffolo[11] in Brazil. But he didn't have the money to do it. He was living on his fast-diminishing savings and was close to being forced to take a job and give up on beating-heart surgery altogether.

Then one day Taylor's phone rang. It was a woman named Judie Vivian, who runs ProMedica International, a company that organizes educational activities for surgeons. Vivian told Taylor that Federico Benetti was looking for someone to help him make instruments for a procedure he had just developed—minimally invasive bypass surgery on a beating heart. The call was a shot of adrenaline for Taylor. He immediately phoned Benetti, who agreed to come to San Francisco and discuss working with him. "He probably would have worked with anybody," Taylor said in retrospect. "He was eager to have anybody pay attention."[12]

Benetti began doing beating-heart bypass operations in an open chest in May 1978. He was working in a poor clinic in Buenos Aires, and the combined cost of using a heart-lung machine and dealing with the strokes and other problems it sometimes caused made the off-pump, beating-heart approach attractive. Not quite sixteen years later, on January 25, 1994, with no fanfare at all, he tried the operation through a small incision for the first time. The patient was an eighty-four-year-old woman who was still alive in September 1997.

It was only with his third patient, however, in June 1994, that it dawned on Benetti that he was doing something radically new. To avoid problems with the clinic adminstration, he operated on this patient at 10:00 P.M., when the building was nearly deserted. After the surgery, which took forty-five minutes, the patient walked from the operating room to the intensive-care unit. He was discharged thirty-six hours later.[13]

In June 1995 Benetti flew to the United States to talk about forming a company and to demonstrate his operation for Taylor; Rich Ferrari, a Silicon Valley businessman with medical device experience; Ratcliffe; and a handful of others. The patient was a pig, and the operation was done in an animal lab at the University of California, San Francisco. Ratcliffe assisted Benetti. Taylor remembers the excitement:

> He [Benetti] made a little hole in the pig about two inches square and went in and did an IMA [internal mammary artery] to LAD [left anterior descending artery] graft and Mark Ratcliffe said, "It's not the greatest-looking anastamosis I've ever seen, but, hey, it's flowing, the pig's alive, and it didn't take long and the pig had a little hole in him like this and he'd had a bypass graft."[14]

From that moment on, things happened very quickly. Taylor signed an agreement with Benetti. Ferrari came on as temporary CEO. Potential investors were shown a videotape of Benetti doing the operation on a human, they were impressed, and with the proviso that Ferrari would become the full-time CEO, they put up about $5 million to begin making devices to stabilize the arteries being sutured and instruments to remove the mammary artery from the chest wall through the small incision and to cut and sew. This happened in September 1995, and by April 1996 Cardio-Thoracic Systems (CTS) had gone public and was poised to take on Heartport, which had gone public at about the same time.

By early 1997, CTS already had made major inroads among surgeons and Wall Street analysts. This was partly because of Heartport's stealth strategy in the public relations arena. Mostly, though, it was because open-chest beating-heart surgery had been around for a long time and the "key-hole" version didn't require any sophisticated new technology. One financial analyst observed that Heartport still hadn't "convince[d] clinicians and investors of the true potential of the arrested heart [on-pump] approach."[15]

Meanwhile, there was plenty of skepticism about both operations among leading surgeons, which was reminiscent of the skepticism that greeted standard bypass surgery thirty years before. Bruce Lytle, a motorcycle-riding cardiac surgeon at the Cleveland Clinic, summed up his and his colleagues' wait-and-see attitude with a terse line from Bruce Springsteen's "Thunder Road": "The door's open but the ride it ain't free."[16]

A more prolix establishment view came from the Council on Cardio-Thoracic and Vascular Surgery of the American Heart Association: "Despite tremendous enthusiasm on the part of patients, industry and the press, [the] widespread adoption [of minimally invasive heart surgery] cannot be endorsed until suitable data have accumulated and a conscientious critique can be done."[17]

Sterman, who owns 13 percent of Heartport's stock, and Stevens, who owns 10 percent, remained confident, however. By this time they had plenty of money in the bank from venture capitalists; a somewhat inflated market valuation of about $800 million, compared to CTS's $250 million, multiple patents, most importantly for their improved version of catheter-based technology to hook up the patient to the heart-lung machine; and about 250 employees, including various kinds of engineers, lawyers, and clinicians, as well as sales, marketing, and promotional professionals. They also had a four-year lead on the field—which at this point was only CTS and Heartport—and, they believed, a less-traumatic way of doing all but the most complex bypass operations.

But before long big, rich companies such as Baxter Healthcare Corp., Johnson & Johnson, and Boston Scientific were moving fast to join the fray. U.S. Surgical was ready with a beating-heart kit to compete with CTS's, and Medtronic was about to begin marketing a $10,000 reusable Dutch stabilizer for beating-heart surgery. This device is known as the Octopus because of the suction pods that hold it in place. It was no longer shaping up as a two-way battle with a winner and a loser, but as a free-for-all for shares in what might or might not turn out to be a major surgical market.

Sterman and Stevens, who had looked at beating-heart surgical techniques early on, concluded that suturing precise enough to obtain optimum long-term results could only be done on a stopped heart that was emptied of blood and fully manipulable. This conclusion was questionable, however, for operations involving only one or two arteries on the front of the heart. Beating-heart surgery of this kind had been done for years with good results, but in an open chest.

In triple- and quadruple-vessel cases, however, even though surgeons in Argentina and Brazil, including Benetti, had done a few, the Heartport founders seemed on stronger ground with the contention that only with their method's ability to stop and empty the heart was it possible to bypass any number of vessels, irrespective of where they were, through a small incision. And valve surgery, which is done inside the heart—the coronary arteries are on the heart's surface—can be done only on a stopped heart.

Sterman and Stevens also believed that despite its technical challenges, most surgeons would quickly become comfortable doing the operation because it retained the familiar heart-lung machine and arrested heart. Moreover, the heart would be stopped with a standard cardioplegia solution and the patient would be hooked up to the heart-lung machine by a catheter-based system inserted through the groin, a method similar to one that had been used in the past.

Since the operation had to be marketed to surgeons before it could be marketed to the public, it was important that as much as possible seem familiar, especially because along with the similarities to standard bypass, there were some radical differences. For example, the surgery would be done with specially designed long instruments through small ports, and visualization would be indirect, using scopes and a television screen.

The key to the Heartport system is to get the patient on the heart-lung machine without opening the chest and then to stop the heart from beating. During standard open-chest bypass surgery the hookup is relatively straightforward. The right atrium and the aorta, to which the pump must be connected by plastic tubes, are fully exposed and easy to reach. This is not the case in keyhole surgery.

Using the Heartport method, the tubes that drain deoxygenated blood from the venous system and return oxygenated blood to the arterial system are connected to the right atrium and the aorta by a catheter that is inserted through the femoral vein and artery in the groin. A balloon is also inserted into the aorta by catheter. When the balloon is inflated, it keeps blood from backing up into the heart during surgery. Once the tubes are in place, the pump is turned on, the balloon is inflated, and cardioplegia is delivered to protect and stop the heart.

The surgeon then begins working in a cavity not much larger than the heart itself. Sterman argues that the small size of the opening, formed by soft-tissue retractors that pull apart the sides of the incision, makes it all the more important that the heart be motionless.

Sterman and Stevens knew what they wanted to do, but the technological barriers were formidable. A complex catheter thin enough to slip up the femoral artery to the heart, but capable of handling multiple tasks, had to be devised. It would have to hook up the patient's arterial and venous systems to the heart-lung machine; deliver a balloon to the aorta and inflate the balloon; deflate the heart and empty it of blood; cool the heart, stop it, and protect it.

Optical systems had to be designed and ways had to be found to place scopes so the operating field could be clearly visualized, new instruments had to be made, and, perhaps most difficult of all, it had to be demonstrated that any good heart surgeon could master the operation. Similar technologies were being used for operating on other organ systems, but the relentlessly pulsing, life-sustaining heart posed much greater difficulties.

Heartport developed its system of catheters within catheters over a period of about two and a half years, discovering only at the end of the process that an Australian named Will Peters had patented an almost identical system. They overcame this obstacle by buying the patent and hiring Peters. Although femoral-access bypass had been done before, it had never been done in combination with delivery of a balloon clamp and cardioplegia.

Sterman argues that the balloon is much gentler than the external clamp used in open-chest surgery, which crushes the tubular aorta flat. He also contends that the four causes of stroke associated with the heart-lung machine[18] are eliminated in the Heartport approach.[19]

The Heartport system of catheters, cannulas, balloon clamp, and specialized long-handled instruments won FDA approval in 1996 but may face patent challenges. A similar Dutch product is being brought to market in the United States by Medtronic, and another system is being developed by Baxter.

While one team of engineers and clinicians at Heartport was developing the catheter-based system of hooking up the patient to the heart-lung machine, others were working on the surgical side, figuring out how to do valve operations and coronary bypass operations through ports. Since for coronary surgery the plan was for surgeons to view the tiny arteries on a television screen while operating, the optical systems had to be both flexible and of very high quality; and since the heart would have to be manipulated through the ports with unfamiliar instruments rather than the standard tools, of which surgeons' fingers were perhaps the most important, new instruments would have to be designed and made. And then, of course, heart surgeons would have to learn to work in a new way.

As the prototype instruments came out of the engineering shop, Stevens and his colleagues, including Greg Ribakove, an NYU surgeon who was spending a year at Stanford, tested them on dogs, sometimes on arteries less than one millimeter in diameter (a human coronary artery is rarely less than two millimeters, or eight hundreths of an inch in diameter). By 1995, with FDA approval, Heartport began testing the procedure in the United States on human patients. Simultaneously, human trials were conducted in England and Germany. By 1996 the Heartport operation was being done at New York University, Duke in Durham, North Carolina, Brigham and Women's Hospital in Boston, Barnes Hospital in St. Louis, Johns Hopkins in Baltimore, and at about five other major centers.

Things were going well, but something fundamental in the Heartport approach had to be changed. Doing the surgery through minute ports while viewing imperfect images on a TV screen turned out to be too hard, at least for the present. As a result, the Heartport-trained surgeons began doing the operation under direct vision through a three- to four-inch incision, just like the one used in the beating-heart operation.

Meanwhile, minimally invasive heart surgery had become the hottest topic at the major cardiology and cardiac surgery meetings. Wall Street was hyperbolic. Smith, Barney reported that minimally invasive cardiac surgery will "revolutionize the way cardiac surgery is performed [and] it will likely be the focal point for cardiovascular product development for years to come."[20] And Alex. Brown & Sons, Inc., said, "With an estimated $4.0 billion market potential, it could eventually become the largest medical device market known."[21]

The mass media were also beginning to report the story and casting it, predictably, as a fierce competition for market share. Financial analysts were trying to figure out which companies would succeed and which would fail. If anyone was thinking that maybe none would succeed, they weren't getting much ink or airtime. It was widely assumed that the surgical community would accept minimally invasive bypass surgery and that a consensus would eventually form about the appropriate uses of the on-pump and off-pump versions.[22] But this hadn't happened yet, and by early 1998 the ardor for on-pump minimally invasive surgery—and for Heartport stock—had cooled substantially. And by July 1999 Heartport's market capitalization had dropped from a maximum of about $800 million to $50 million.

But analysts still had to speculate what the market for each procedure would be in the long run. This calculation depended on the answers to questions such as these: Would beating-heart surgery always be limited to the arteries on the front of the heart? Would it draw many patients, as the inventor and Stanford surgeon Tom Fogarty believes it will, from the large number now getting angioplasty or stents?[23] How significant a factor would the lower cost of beating-heart surgery be? How good would the long-term results of beating-heart surgery be? Would improvements in heart-lung machine technology neutralize concern about complications linked to its use? Is arrested-heart, less-invasive surgery significantly safer because a case can quickly be converted to open-chest surgery if necessary? And would computer-assisted surgery eventually dominate the minimally invasive surgery marketplace? The answers to these questions would largely determine where investors would put their money.

Heartport gained some support among surgeons at first, but CTS attracted more. A few early converts at Washington [D.C.] Hospital Center had done hundreds of beating-heart operations by 1995, but with an open chest.[24] They recognized that older and sicker patients were especially vulnerable to complications as a result of being put on the heart-lung machine, so in the late 1980s they decided that when they could, they would operate on these patients without it. Their mortality rate in a cohort of 220 carefully selected patients was 1.4 percent, compared to a mortality rate of 3.1 percent for all bypass surgery done in 1995.[25] At about the same time, however, a group at Loma Linda University in California was less selective and had poor results.[26]

When the Washington Hospital Center group heard that Federico Benetti was doing minimally invasive beating-heart surgery, they invited him there. They were impressed with his numbers, and under his watchful eye they tried the operation. The patient went home in forty-eight hours and was back at work in a week. After Benetti left, they did six operations in quick succession.

One of the surgeons was Paul Corso. He said, "The first patient was about ready to walk off the operating table. All six patients did very well. They did get out in a couple of days. They did go back to work in a week. And stress tests were negative. Some were recathed [had angiograms] and they looked good."[27] This took place in June 1996, one year after Benetti operated on the pig.

The Washington Hospital Center surgeons were operating on beating hearts without stabilizers, in Corso's words, "using a few tricks. I can use little Silastic tapes that I can put under the vessel to sort of hold it up gently; a little stitch over here to hold it gently, just little things to cut down on the movement of the vessel."[28] These "little things" also include the use of drugs such as adenosine or esmolol to slow the heart rate to about forty beats a minute so that the surgeons can stitch between beats.

Corso, who owns a small amount of CTS stock, and his colleagues were successful without the $2,000 disposable CTS kit, whose most important elements are a simple, forklike stabilizer, an access platform to which it is attached, and special instruments to remove the internal mammary artery and ease access to multiple vessels. But they were receptive when asked to teach the company's technique to other surgeons and help standardize the procedure. Others also signed on with CTS as training centers, including St. Vincent's Hospital in Indianapolis; the University Medical Center in Hanover, Germany; and the two largest health-care chains in the United States, Columbia/HCA and Tenet. Columbia and Tenet hospitals also have done the Heartport operation. CTS estimates that 600 hospitals use its kits. Heartport says its system is used at more than 100 hospitals.

By mid-1999, however, Heartport, whose market value had plummeted mainly because surgeons found its procedure too hard to do, had begun marketing a kit to do beating-heart operations in an open chest. The company was under new management and Sterman and Stevens had receded into the background. This was clearly an attempt to get back into the running, but the field was now crowded with big-name players. Heartport or its clones may make a comeback because the on-pump operation is well suited to treating multivessel disease and it can be used for valve surgery. But there are surgeons such as Fogarty, the iconoclastic CTS board member, and Corso who believe that ways may be found to do beating-heart surgery on more vessels than is currently possible. Corso is both vague and careful in discussing the possibility of multivessel operations on a beating heart, emphasizing that at this point he is not "out to sell that." But he does say this much: "We're doing some other techniques to work on some other vessels, different innovations. We're sort of walking our way up. There may be a way of doing a different movement of the heart to do one of the branches of the right [coronary artery] through the small incision. There is an ability on certain patients to get some of the more lateral vessels through the same incision if you pull the pericardium this way and use the stabilizer in a different way."[29] And CTS's Rich Ferrari adds that "We're working toward more multiple-vessel orientations; some greater anatomical reach in the system."[30]

There are other even more visionary surgeons, engineers, and entrepreneurs who are already conducting human trials on port-access robotic operations in which the operator views a computer-generated, three-dimensional virtual image of a moving heart that appears bloodless and motionless, and eliminates all but the essential structures from the surgeon's view. The surgeon is able to guide from a control panel instruments that are synchronized by a computer to the target artery's actual movement.

The instruments are inserted into the chest through two one-centimeter incisions. A scope with a tiny camera is inserted through a third such incision. In one of the two systems being tested this scope is voice-controlled by the surgeon. In both systems a relatively gross movement of the surgeon's hand yields a very fine movement of the instrument. Costs are high, but so is the cost, for example, of magnetic resonance imaging (MRI), which is widely used in the United States.

Another important consideration is that the market for minimally invasive surgery is not solely in the population where surgical patients are usually found—the one defined by blockages in more than one artery. It may be that many candidates will be drawn from the large group of patients with one-vessel or two-vessel disease who today are routinely treated with angioplasty or stents. The reason for this is that the rate at which arteries reclog after surgery on an important single vessel such as the left anterior descending coronary artery is about 5 percent over fifteen or twenty years. The reclogging rate for angioplasty on this vessel is as high as 40 percent, and for stents, 20 percent or more, with almost all of the reblockage occurring in the first six months. This means expensive repeat procedures.

If angioplasty is done twice, the overall cost will roughly equal that for one bypass operation. As our medical system, including Medicare, moves toward capitation, under which hospitals will be paid a fixed sum annually for each patient they treat, there will be strong financial incentives to avoid such repeats. In an effort to find the optimum means of preventing vessels from reclogging, hybrid operations that combine beating-heart bypass surgery and stenting are also being tried.

No one knows for sure where—or how big—the major market will be in ten years' time, or how it will be divided up among Heartport, CTS, U.S. Surgical, Baxter, Johnson & Johnson, Medtronic, and others. Both Heartport and CTS might well be gobbled up by one of the device-industry giants such as those named above. Partly for this reason, the majority of heart surgeons are still cautiously watching from the sidelines, waiting to see more results, assessing as best they can how hard these new procedures are to do.

A 1997 article in *Circulation*, a journal of the American Heart Association, quotes a number of surgeons warning their colleagues in the interest of safety to go slow and not to overreach. John J. Collins, Jr., a professor of surgery at Harvard, characterized beating-heart surgery as "converting an operation that should be totally safe into a hair-raising adventure," and Bruce Lytle of the Cleveland Clinic said of minimally invasive surgery generally, "I don't think that people know whether over time the operation will turn out to be safe enough."[31]

Some thoughtful surgeons worry about the fast pace even when the operation is being performed only by the best and most experienced among them. "What scares me about any new technique or device," Paul Corso said, "is that we or Wall Street might sell a procedure that we're not ready to sell. We think we're doing it well. But are there some problems that need to be addressed? Or are there some truths that need to be demonstrated? Absolutely. And I tell every patient that."[32]

Does every surgeon tell every patient that the procedure he is offering them is experimental or, using the euphemism of choice, innovative? Probably not. Most surgeons become committed to a procedure as soon as they are convinced it works and they can do it successfully. Their satisfaction in doing it comes from both their success rate and the degree of difficulty of the operation. Because they are competitive by nature, the harder it is, the better they like it. Because they are decisive by nature, commitment to the new procedure—that is, belief in its safety and efficacy—comes quickly. So why worry the patient?

The opposite, of course, is also true: Those surgeons who can't do a procedure comfortably resist its introduction at their institution for fear that they will lose patients to those who can do it. Such surgeons may also warn patients that the procedure is unsafe.

Although Heartport and CTS are both based in California, and Heartport's system was first tested at Stanford, and minimally invasive beating-heart surgery was first done in Argentina, the most interesting and perhaps the most illuminating place to compare the two procedures is New York. A competition, although the surgeons reject this characterization, occurred in the late '90's between a group at New York University Hospital and an India-born Lone Ranger at Lenox Hill Hospital. The NYU surgeons, led by Aubrey Galloway, had done Heartport's on-pump operation more than any other surgical group anywhere in the world. At Lenox Hill, Valavanur Subramanian had done more minimally invasive beating-heart operations than anyone.

Subramanian is slim, dark, quick, brusque, and supremely confident. His style in the operating room is cool, efficient, and all business. There is none of the monologue, music, or radio chatter that goes on throughout surgery when, for example, Paul Taylor or Greg Ribakove are operating; there is more palpable tension. Many of his fellow cardiac surgeons consider him arrogant and dislike him, but they acknowledge that he is a highly focused, first-rate technician.

Whatever his colleagues think of him, Subramanian's reputation is now linked, for better or for worse, to the success of off-pump surgery, and he proselytizes for it tirelessly and effectively. It is also, at least for the moment, linked directly to the success of CTS, in which he is a stockholder. His short-term patency rate—the rate at which bypassed arteries remain open within thirty days of surgery—was a relatively poor 89 percent before he began using the CTS stabilizers, retractors, and instruments, and a much better 96 percent after he began using them.

Greg Ribakove, who holds what he characterizes as a minor financial interest in Heartport, and Aubrey Galloway are on the whole less controversial among surgeons than Subramanian. Galloway is the director of research at NYU and author of the chapter on heart surgery in a major textbook.[33] Ribakove is a University of Chicago-trained New Yorker who is also interested in research. Both do beating-heart surgery in the cases where they think it is indicated, and they are no longer as committed to on-pump minimally invasive surgery as Subramanian is to the beating-heart version. Both Ribakove and Galloway are persuaded that the trade-off between imperfect suturing and pump-related complications favors doing on-pump surgery in most cases. Galloway argues that if the pump runs are kept below three to four hours, complications are rare.[34]

The availability of the competing surgical treatments poses a dilemma for New York City cardiologists and some of their patients who are candidates for minimally invasive surgery.[35] For such patients, a diligent cardiologist has to do the following; read the limited literature on both procedures (there have been no head-to-head trials); factor in what is known about risks associated with the heart-lung machine and imperfectly sewn bypass grafts; consider the skill of the surgeons and the over-all quality of the cardiac-surgery programs at the institutions doing each procedure; try to share this rather vague, uncertain information with anxious and often ill-informed patients; give them an adequate account of the standard bypass and angioplasty options with their trade-offs; and finally, help the patient choose a treatment. If this is difficult for the cardiologist, imagine how hard it must be for these patients, who are suffering from a potentially lethal disease.

Wes Sterman, John Stevens, and Greg Ribakove, and Rich Ferrari, Chuck Taylor, and Valavanur Subramanian are interested parties who have one or more reasons for wanting to influence the choice patients make in consultation with their cardiologists. It was undoubtedly with this in mind that some of them shared their valuable time with me and with reporters from the *New York Times*, the *Wall Street Journal, Newsweek,* and other mass media outlets. It is why Sterman and Ferrari cultivate the Wall Street analysts who handicap the medical device business.

Eugene Braunwald did not have minimally invasive surgery in mind when he warned twenty years ago that "an industry is being built around" bypass surgery. Nor did he necessarily foresee Wall Street's influence on the direction of bypass surgery. But today he looks prescient nonetheless. And his concern that bypass surgery would develop "a momentum and a constituency of its own" has proved accurate. Other thoughtful surgeons, such as Michael Mack of Dallas, have expressed serious concern about the extent to which stock prices and market share are driving their profession.[36]

The commodification of a surgical procedure generates a variety of moral problems, some of which Braunwald has hinted at. For example, when two new companies with similar products compete for the same set of patients, the pressure to get to market first provides an incentive for cutting corners and fudging data. If the company is publicly owned, the rationale for cutting and fudging would likely be a duty to shareholders: Being second can have disastrous financial consequences.

Treating an operation as a product also sets up potential conflicts of interest for physicians in a position to benefit financially if one procedure wins greater market share than another. It is not yet certain how these two types of surgery will develop in the next few years, but here are two plausible scenarios that illustrate the kinds of conflicts that might arise.

Cardio-Thoracic Systems or U.S. Surgical shows a reasonable probability that surgeons using its stabilizers can suture mammary arteries to coronary arteries as precisely as surgeons operating on a fully stopped heart using a heart-lung machine. Moreover, beating-heart surgeons figure out how to consistently bypass three major arteries with long-term results equal to those achieved with open-chest bypass surgery. And finally, there is mounting evidence that the heart-lung machine is causing substantial cognitive loss in many of the patients over seventy[37] who now commonly undergo bypass surgery. If you are John Stevens, cardiac surgeon, Heartport cofounder and major stockholder, what do you offer patients over seventy who under these new parameters are viable candidates for beating-heart surgery?[38]

Or, alternatively, at three years the rate at which bypassed coronary arteries are remaining open after beating-heart surgery is down to about 88 percent compared with 97 percent for on-pump surgery. And there is now persuasive although not definitive evidence that advances made in the heart-lung machine and its tubing have reduced the rate of complications in on-pump surgery to about the same as the complication rate with beating-heart surgery. What do you offer your patients if you're Valavanur Subramanian?

These are, of course, hypothetical situations that might never occur. Still, they could. It is impossible to know in what proportions men like Fogarty and Stevens, Subramanian and Ribakove are motivated by ambition, money, or desire for fame, the satisfaction of problem-solving, defensiveness about their clinical judgment, or the duty and the desire to give their patients the very best care they possibly can. But it would be ostrichlike to say that the presence of money in the mix, in the form of equity or other financial arrangements, is not a potentially significant factor. In the beginning it is a positive force, a powerful incentive for developing a new therapeutic agent, device, or technology, and developing it quickly. Down the line, however, the glitter of profits can blind physicians, not only to the new treatment's weaknesses, but also to the strengths of competing treatments.

How important, for example, were financial considerations to the physicians who continued to promote use of the antiarrythmia drug Tambocor for mildly symptomatic or asymptomatic patients after it should have been clear that it was killing more of them than it was saving?[39] Or to what extent, if any, did stock options or holdings in Genentech, or paid consultancies, influence choices made by steering committee members and clinical-trial investigators testing the company's clot-busting drug tPA (at a first-dose cost of more than $2,000) against its competitor streptokinase (at an initial cost of less than $200)?[40] Does the fact that twenty-three out of twenty-four physicians who wrote articles in support of calcium channel blockers "had financial relationships with manufacturers of those drugs" suggest undue commercial influence on researchers?[41]

Or consider the case of Maurice Buchbinder, an interventional cardiologist at the University of California, San Diego, who served as principal investigator of a multicenter clinical trial to evaluate an artery-opening device called a Rotablator. The catheter-based, 190,000rpm, diamond-coated burr is manufactured by a company in which, at the time, Buchbinder owned stock and held stock options valued jointly in the neighborhood of $10 million. Did his financial interest influence the way he ran the trial? Buchbinder says no. Were the normal safeguards built into the clinical trial process adequate to prevent manipulation of any kind? Buchbinder says they were. Moreover, he says he sees no conflict of interest inherent in the situation. Indeed, he says there are no such things as conflicts of interest, there are only dualities of interest.[42]

An FDA audit of the research found several deficiencies, notably a failure to do follow-up examinations on 280 patients and inappropriate use of the device on severely ill patients. As a result of the audit, Buchbinder was banned by the university for an indefinite period from doing research on human subjects. At the time of the trial, the University of California cardiologist also served as the unsalaried medical director of the Rotablator company, Heart Technology, Inc.[43]

Of course, a physician's honest intellectual commitment can also distort judgment and influence choices. It is possible to fall blindly in love with a hypothesis. In the clinical research community the word is that "It's okay to sleep with a hypothesis, but you should never marry one." The plot gets even thicker if an investigator has staked his academic reputation on the truth of his research. William Boyd captured the essence of this kind of deeply emotional commitment in his novel *Brazzaville Beach.* When Hope Clearwater, a young researcher, discovers that a quarter century of work by the world's leading primatologist is wrong, the eminent researcher tries to suppress her findings and to beat her to death with a stick.[44]

But is intellectual commitment likely to bias research outcomes as much as a nontrivial financial interest? This, to me at least, seems like a question without a definitive answer, although the larger the amount, the greater the strain on my belief in anyone's power to resist. Individuals vary in their ability to withstand pecuniary temptation just as they do in their ability to be objective when testing a treatment to which they have an intellectual commitment. But there is a fundamental difference: Financial conflicts of interest can be avoided. Intellectual commitments, because they develop organically out of the research itself, cannot.

When it comes to research, the medical ethicist Baruch Brody points out, the main risk of financial conflicts of interest is not outright fraud— that is, faking data—even though minor falsifications can determine whether an important result is statistically significant. It is rather the subtler problem that arises when investigators, either consciously or unconsciously, make "inappropriate decisions about the design and conduct of clinical trials."[45]

Biased decision-making on matters such as who will be enrolled or not enrolled in the trial, how the hypothesis to be tested is framed, or what will count as a good result can affect the outcome as much as out-and-out fraud, and it is probably far more common. For example, the difference between choosing a clinical outcome such as the death or heart attack rate to test a treatment's effectiveness, and choosing a surrogate outcome such as high blood pressure, can be highly significant, since high blood pressure may or may not cause heart attacks or death.

Bioethicists such as Brody and physicians such as Roger Porter have been quick to point out the conflict that exists when a clinical researcher has a financial stake in study results or treatment choices such as which drug, device, or procedure to use. "The worst scenario," Porter wrote, "occurs when the scientist has direct financial interest in the outcome."[46] But the NIH allows research institutions to set their own conflict-of-interest standards, overlooking the fact that the institutions themselves derive income from the grants, which itself creates conflicts of interest. In 1998 the FDA announced new rules that go into effect in 1999 that require only disclosure of proprietary interests such as patents and equity of more than $50,000, and only to the agency, not to the public.

By and large, leaders in the medical profession have gone only halfway in recommending an appropriate response to conflicts of interest. Often, rather than an outright policy banning stock ownership by investigators, they recommend disclosure of relevant holdings to sponsoring agencies and in journal publications,[47] or a ban with a time limit.[48] But once the drug or the device is approved for use, it is not clear how this disclosure or ban, whose term has usually expired by then, will curb any tendency to inappropriately prescribe or promote it in the clinical researcher's medical practice. This is especially problematical because unless the physician's stock ownership becomes a mass-media sensation, few patients will ever hear of it.

8

A Momentous Decision

Just before 7:00 A.M. on February 2, 1998, Lewis Hollander,[1] a sixty-four-year-old Washington, D.C., lawyer, was lying in a hospital bed, mildly sedated. His sister, brother-in-law, and nephew were at his side. They were talking softly. Hollander was about to be wheeled into an operating room to undergo coronary bypass surgery. The operation was going to be performed unconventionally—without the use of a heart-lung machine. His heart would beat throughout the surgery. The tiny arteries to be bypassed would be moving targets.

Hollander was Paul Corso's first case of the day. The tall, loose-limbed surgeon, dressed in light-blue scrubs, was on his way from a locker room to the pre-op area to say a reassuring word to his patient. Corso is good at relaxing people. His manner is direct, concerned, and self-confident. He moves with the athletic grace of an expert skier, which he is. He has a high forehead, dark brown eyes, and a brushlike mustache whose tips turn slightly upward. The overall effect is vaguely evocative of nineteenth-century Sicilian nobility.

Corso's father arrived in West Virginia from Sicily as a child. He grew up to be a railroad fireman and then an engineer. His mother, who is of Scotch-Irish background, was the head nurse in a forty-bed hospital in Charlestown, which is in the state's panhandle region, not far from Washington. Corso came to the Washington [D.C.] Hospital Center, where he is chief of cardiac surgery, because he saw in it the potential for a hybrid career in clinical practice and research. Time has proved him right. Since the late 1980s, he and his colleagues have pioneered surgery on a beating heart without the use of a heart-lung machine.

Corso walked into the pre-op waiting area at exactly 7:00 A.M., took Hollander's hand, and squeezed it. He said a few reassuring words and then slipped down the hall for a last quick look at the angiographic film of the blockages he was about to bypass. Satisfied that everything was as he remembered it, he headed toward the large, tiled operating room where Hollander was now stretched out naked on a narrow, leather-covered table.

A nurse tuned the radio to a classic rock station. An anesthesiologist was holding a plastic mask over the patient's mouth and nose and instructing him to take deep breaths. Electrocardiogram leads were attached to his chest and earlobes. The readouts could be seen on monitors behind the patient's head. When he was fully anesthetized, a clear plastic breathing tube about three-quarters of an inch in diameter was inserted into his windpipe and a long, narrow tube, perhaps one-quarter inch in diameter, was threaded down into his stomach to keep it empty. Another quarter-inch tube was placed in his esophagus to monitor his temperature and heart rate.

While the tubes were being put in place, a nurse wheeled a steel cart covered with sterile instruments up to the foot of the operating table. A surgical assistant put a Foley catheter into Hollander's penis to evacuate urine, and a nurse quickly shaved the front of his body and swabbed it with iodine antiseptic roughly the color of shellac. Hollander was totally vulnerable—naked, anesthetized, and intubated.

Hollander's body was quickly covered with a special green drape with a clear plastic area that adhered to his chest, keeping the skin stable and clean. Other drapes were hung until it was no longer possible to tell that there was a human patient on the table. I had seen a videotape a week earlier of experimental surgery on a calf, and this could as easily have been the domestic animal. The drapes not only keep the area sterile, they also help distance the surgeon from the patient's humanity and from the primitive, even brutal—albeit salutary—thing he is about to do.

Corso took a knife from a nurse and unceremoniously made a seven-inch cut down the middle of Hollander's chest, exposing his breastbone. Blood oozed through the slit plastic and was blotted away by a nurse. Corso said "Saw, please," and was handed what looked like one of those multipurpose electric tools advertised on television. He placed the small, oscillating blade on the top of Hollander's breastbone just below the neck and ran the blade straight down, slicing through the entire structure in perhaps three seconds.

He then used a slim, yellow-handled instrument called an electrobistoury to cauterize the inner walls of the split bone. This work was accompanied by wisps of smoke and the smell of seared bits of flesh and bone. Assistants sucked out excess blood through plastic tubes or sopped it up with surgical sponges.

The conversation around the table was unrelated to the surgery. It could as easily have been taking place in an auto repair shop. The surgeon assisting Corso said he'd just sold his motorcycle and bought a BMW automobile. Corso dryly accused him of becoming a "yuppie."

The assisting surgeon mounted a stainless steel rod in a ring on the side of the operating table. On the ring he hung a crosspiece, from which were suspended two heavy steel forks with curved prongs. The assistant then hooked the prongs around one side of Hollander's inch-thick sternum and turned a small handle on the device, ratcheting the bony frame several inches upward, thereby giving Corso access to his patient's chest wall. This was necessary because Corso was going to remove one end of Hollander's left internal mammary artery (LIMA) from the wall and attach it to both clogged arteries beyond where they were blocked.

The blood that normally flows through the LIMA, a multibranched vessel that runs north-to-south along the chest wall from just below the clavicle to just above the abdomen, would be redirected to Hollander's heart muscle. Since structures fed by the LIMA—the chest wall, the diaphragm, and the organs between the lungs such as the heart, trachea, and esophagus—get enough blood from other vessels, the internal mammary artery can be diverted safely.

Corso sat on a stool looking into Hollander's chest through a hole that was now about seven inches long and four inches wide. He was wearing glasses to which were attached 3.5-power loupes, much like the ones jewelers use to examine gems. Richie Valens was singing "La Bamba" on the radio.

Using the electrobistoury, Corso delicately cut away tissue and removed the artery in its fatty covering from the chest wall. Once this was done he let his assistant complete the job of trimming away the fat and other tissue while he went off to make phone calls. The assistant also opened the pericardium, exposing the pulsing organ.

A quarter-million-dollar heart-lung machine stood to the side of the operating table. But Corso did not plan to use it unless there was an unforeseen emergency. The patient's heart would continue to pump at a normal rate during the operation, supplying his body with blood without any mechanical assistance.

Corso has a strong preference for operating without a heart-lung machine whenever possible because he believes there is a lower risk of strokes, heart attacks, and other complications when the machine is not used. He also believes he can sew as precisely with the heart beating as when it is stopped. Not everyone agrees. A report to the 1997 meeting of the American Association of Thoracic Surgeons concluded that "beating-heart bypass produces results intermediate between conventional bypass (best) and angioplasty (worst)."[2] But Corso's own mortality and morbidity record appears to justify his self-confidence.

When Corso returned to the operating room, Hollander's left internal mammary artery was almost completely trimmed. The surface of his healthy-looking, roughly three-quarter-pound heart, covered by a thin layer of yellow fat with purple and red blotches in places, filled much of the opening in his chest.

"Time to do some sewing," Corso said.

Most of the talking that had accompanied the surgery until this point stopped, and the nurses and assistants came up close to watch. Fats Domino was singing "Blueberry Hill." Corso quickly stitched the flaps of pericardium to the chest wall to get them out of the way. He then tied off the first artery he was going to bypass—a diagonal branch of the left anterior descending coronary artery (LAD), which is the main artery running down the left side of the front of the heart—so it wouldn't bleed while he was sewing.

The old-fashioned-looking stainless steel retractor that had lifted Hollander's breastbone had been removed and a different one was put in place. It was made by CardioThoracic Systems, Chuck Taylor's Company. The retractor is plastic and is part of a simple, disposable kit. It opens a cavity about eight inches by six inches and serves as a platform for a movable plastic arm with a two-pronged, forklike instrument at its end that raises the coronary artery slightly and keeps it relatively still while it is being sutured. It does this by forcing the prongs down on either side of the artery, thereby pushing up the tiny vessel just enough to give the surgeon good access.

Corso picked up the mammary artery between his thumb and forefinger and sliced off the last of the fat, much like an electrician trimming insulation from wire. The vessel is about three millimeters in circumference and pale beige in color. He exposed a length of several inches because this single mammary artery was about to be attached to both blocked coronary arteries. After tying off the diagonal artery with a Silastic cord, he laid the trimmed section of the mammary artery across it, made small incisions in both vessels, and with a long needleholder and tiny curved needles, sewed the sides of the two arteries together. This took about eight minutes.

Corso then removed the little piece of Silastic that had been closing off the diagonal branch and tied it around the LAD. He then sewed the end of the mammary artery to the side of the LAD. This also took roughly eight minutes. Corso's work ended as it had begun, without ceremony and few words.

"That's it," he said. "It looks good."

Corso walked across the room and sat down. It was 10:25 A.M. The entire operation had taken about two hours. But it wasn't quite over. An assistant was putting Hollander's sternum back together with steel wires heavy enough to set off alarms in airports, and then sewing his skin to

complete the closing of his chest. Moments later all the tubes were removed and the anesthesiologist was talking gently to the patient, who
showed some eye movement but no other response.

Less than a minute later, however, a dazed-looking Hollander sat halfway up, as if he wanted to get off the table. Instead, not surprisingly, he
expelled a high-pitched wail of pain, and his head dropped back down.
Four days later, however, he was recuperating comfortably at home. And
two months after that, he was out playing golf again.

The perilous journey that ended so successfully in Paul Corso's operating
room had begun on a golf course. Lewis Hollander was vacationing at the
luxurious Homestead resort in Virginia in August 1997. He had been
feeling a bit under the weather and after a round of golf he felt generally
achey, especially in his right arm. He chalked up his discomfort to a touch
of the flu. However, when the achiness continued after he returned home,
he decided to see his doctor. His daughter was getting married later in the
month, and he wanted to be sure he would be well for the wedding. He
asked his family physician, Dr. James Ramey, whether he thought the
symptoms might be heart-related, but Ramey assured him it was the flu
and that he would be fine.[3]

And indeed within days he felt much better. He went to the wedding,
played some more golf, and for a while everything was okay. Then the
pains started up again. Friends suggested he take a test for Lyme disease.
He did, and it was negative. In early October he went to see Ramey again,
and again Ramey found nothing. This time, however, he suggested a
shoulder X ray if the pain didn't go away. When it persisted during walks
and on the golf course, Hollander returned to Ramey. It was now early
December.

This time Hollander's son Art pressed him to get a stress test. Ramey
asked a cardiologist in his practice to give him the test, which Ramey said
he was sure he would pass with flying colors. But at the highest heart rate
he achieved on the treadmill—150 beats a minute—there were signs of
inadequate blood flow to the heart muscle.

The cardiologist said it could easily be a false positive but recommended
a thallium stress test, in which the patient is given trace amounts of a
radioactive isotope that accumulates quickly in the cells of the heart muscle. This test provides an assessment of the blood flow reaching the muscle
and of its condition. Mr. Hollander agreed, and the test was done at
Georgetown University Hospital, where it was covered under his health
plan.

This time the result was definitive. It showed a severe blockage in the
left anterior descending coronary artery and possibly additional blockages.

It was beginning to look like an invasive procedure such as angioplasty would have to be done to remove the obstructions and restore adequate blood flow to the heart muscle.

The predictable next step was an angiogram, the invasive test in which dye is squirted into the coronary arteries and X-ray pictures are taken that show where they are narrowed. Hollander was not happy about the idea of an angiogram, which requires an incision in the groin and carries with it small risks of death, stroke, or heart attack. He remembered reading an American Medical Association report indicating that this test was overused.

Hollander was also worried that, in general, things were moving too fast. He asked his doctors whether they couldn't first try additional non-invasive tests such as an echocardiogram, which provides information about the motion of the wall of the heart, among other things, or a heart scan (electron-beam computed tomography) to measure calcium content, which is associated with arterial blockages, or perhaps even treat him with drugs.

The answer was that given the results of the thallium stress test, it was unlikely that these other tests would be useful. Stuart Seides, an interventional cardiologist to whom Hollander was referred by Ramey, persuaded him that only an angiogram would provide the kind of information needed to complete his diagnosis and decide on a course of treatment.

Seides told Hollander that based on the thallium stress test he thought he might be a candidate for angioplasty, a treatment in which a catheter is used to insert a balloon into an obstructed artery where it is inflated, crushing the plaque causing the blockage against the arterial wall. This widens the channel through which blood flows to the heart muscle. But Seides was careful to tell Hollander that until he saw the results of the angiogram he could not be sure that Hollander would not need bypass surgery.

The angiogram was done in early January at Washington Hospital Center, the capital's preeminent facility for heart care. The procedure was performed under local anesthetic and took fewer than twenty minutes. As soon as the lights dimmed in the equipment-filled catheterization laboratory, an unusually clear picture filled the screen of a TV monitor suspended from above.

It showed a beautiful, lacy network of "collaterals," tiny, dormant vessels that had opened to replace some of the lost flow from the blocked LAD. The collaterals might have prevented Hollander from having a heart attack in the short run. But they could not provide enough flow to adequately replace a major vessel for the long haul. The angiogram also showed a blockage in a diagonal artery branching from the LAD.

The angiographic result meant that Hollander was about to get more bad news. First he had been told he had no heart problem. Then he was told he had a heart problem, but he probably would not need surgery. Now he was going to be told he did need surgery. The position and lengths of the blockages were such that Seides thought angioplasty would be too difficult to do successfully.

Seides did think, however, that Hollander was a good candidate for an operation known as a MIDCAB, which stands for minimally invasive direct coronary artery bypass. This operation is done through a three-inch incision on a beating heart and does not involve splitting the sternum. Seides gave Hollander the news and said he would see if Paul Corso was available for a surgical consultation.

Corso was in the hospital and met Seides a few minutes later. Together they reviewed the angiographic film. Corso's best judgment was that because of the location of the blockage in the diagonal artery, the surgery should be done in an open chest. This was still another negative change for Hollander to deal with. The operation would require sawing through his breastbone.

Thomas J. Ryan, a cardiologist at Boston University, once said that in coronary artery disease, "in contrast to all other diseases about which I [know] something, the severity of symptoms [does] not necessarily correlate with the severity of disease."[4] This was true in Hollander's case. Ryan might also have expressed some skepticism about the ability of diagnostic tests to identify appropriate treatments.

Hollander was now in a semiprivate room, and Corso went to see him. He introduced himself over the blare of *Sanford and Son* from the TV on the other side of the curtain and sat down on the end of the bed. He began to explain what the angiogram showed and why he thought surgery in general, and beating-heart, open-chest surgery in particular, was a better choice for Hollander than angioplasty.

Corso told Hollander that with a catheter-based treatment such as angioplasty there was a 40 percent chance that the blockage would recur within six months and that there was some risk. He said the same was true with stenting, a procedure involving the permanent placement of a tiny metal scaffold inside an artery to keep it open. Surgery, he said, is more traumatic, but the long-term results are significantly better, adding that with the operation he proposed to do there was a 90 to 95 percent chance that the arteries would be open in five years and that the chances were good that they would stay open for far longer than that.

He went on to explain that not all bypass surgery is the same. Using his index finger on Hollander's chest, he traced the small incision under the left nipple used for the MIDCAB and explained how it was done. But he quickly added that working through a "keyhole" incision would compromise his ability to bypass the diagonal branch. "The other option," Corso said, "is to do a standard incision from here to here." Again he ran his finger along Hollander's chest, this time vertically along the sternum, but less than its full length. He added that the operation would be done without a heart-lung machine.

"We're able to do that with some instruments that we have and then we bypass the major arteries and it's done," Corso said. "Now, it's still an operation; you still can have a heart attack; or there's a tiny chance that you won't survive. But you've got a 99 percent chance that you'll do fine, without a heart attack, without dying, without a stroke."

Corso went on to say that the risk was smaller without the heart-lung machine. If it were neccesary to use the machine, he said, the overall risk of complications or death would be about 3 percent. But the beauty of not using the machine, he told Hollander, is that you "recover quicker, feel better quicker." He also told Hollander about an operation through a small incision in which the heart-lung machine could be used, but that he thought that was inadvisable because it would be too difficult to bypass the blockage in the diagonal artery without fully exposing the heart. Finally, he said that drug treatment was a poor alternative because on drugs he would have to limit his physical activity and would be more vulnerable to a heart attack than he would be after surgery.

This was a lot to deal with for a man who had just had an angiogram, a scary procedure for many people under the best of circumstances, and who was expecting to be told that angioplasty would take care of his problem. Now he was being told that he needed a major operation—coronary bypass surgery—and that if he accepted Corso's advice, it would involve splitting his breastbone wide open and doing the operation unconventionally—that is, without using a heart-lung machine.

He was also being told that there were alternative kinds of surgery that could be done without sawing through his sternum from top to bottom, including one done through a small incision using a heart-lung machine with his heart stopped. But these methods, according to Corso's judgment, were not the best options for him. What about angioplasty, Hollander wondered, or stents? Should they be eliminated from consideration because Seides and Corso said they were bad options? Were drugs out as an alternative to surgery because they said so? Corso, after all, made his living doing surgery.

Hollander was still somewhat sedated from the angiogram. But he said nonetheless that his head was clear enough to follow everything that Corso had told him. He asked Corso why he favored an open-chest, beating-heart operation over a small-incision operation using a heart-lung machine. Corso explained again that the small incision limited access to the heart, which in his case was likely to make it difficult or impossible to bypass the diagonal artery without using the heart-lung machine.

Adherents of the small-incision, "on-pump" operation say they can rotate the heart to get access to blocked branches such as Hollander's and that additional risk associated with the heart-lung machine in such an operation is in the range of minuscule to zero. But Corso and his colleagues at Washington Hospital Center, like a significant minority of heart surgeons, believe that the risk of complications such as heart attacks and strokes associated with the machine are somewhat greater than this and that they should be avoided whenever possible.

Hollander then asked whether both operations involved breaking a rib. Corso said that the operation he was proposing did not, but on this point there was a lack of clarity in his explanation. "We actually split the sternum and wire it back together," he said. "There's no break or anything." Hollander, however, did not seem confused by Corso's implicit distinction between breaking a rib and splitting the breastbone, or sternum.

Just then Hollander's son walked into the room. "I guess you didn't get the news you were expecting, big guy," he said. Hollander asked Corso if he would mind summarizing for his son what he had said so far. Corso did so. Father and son then asked several questions about recovery time and how long it would take to return to normal activities after the different operations. Corso told them that Hollander might be in the hospital a day or so longer with the open-chest surgery, but otherwise there would be little difference.

Art Hollander then began to question Corso knowledgeably about his experience. "How many of these procedures have you done?" he asked.

"Probably about 350," Corso said. "I do about 500 heart operations a year."

"Is there someone who's done more?"

"Not to my knowledge."

"I'm just trying to gather information," Art Hollander said, aware that his questioning sounded a little too aggressive, too much like an interrogation.

"My ego's not involved here," Corso replied calmly.

Corso then laid out the comparative risks when cases considered suitable for beating-heart surgery are done with and without a heart-lung machine. The statistics for death, heart attack, and stroke—based on his own clinical experience and that of a handful of other surgeons who do significant amounts of beating-heart bypass surgery—were marginally better across the board when the machine was not used.

Art Hollander then praised the reputation of Washington Hospital Center but persisted in his questioning. He asked Corso where else in the world this operation could be done well. Corso advised him to stay in the United States. He said there were hospitals in Indianapolis and Minneapolis with good results but with fewer cases than Washington Hospital Center.

"You've done the most?" Art Hollander asked.

"Yes," Corso said.

"He doesn't need to go to Hopkins or Mayo?"

"I would not suggest Hopkins or Mayo," Corso said.

The conversation then turned to second opinions. Corso suggested they talk to both Seides and their family doctor. He also recommended a surgeon and a cardiologist at a nearby northern Virginia hospital.

Art Hollander then asked how it was possible that a couple of days before the angiogram, his father had been able to walk eighteen holes of golf without pain. Corso explained that the collateral flow probably was getting just enough blood to the heart muscle to prevent pain. Art asked whether the operation had to be done immediately and whether angioplasty, by a top operator, was really not an option. Corso said surgery did not have to be done immediately, and while there might be someone out there who would do angioplasty, he did not recommend it because of the length and location of the blockage, and the artery involved.

Corso sat on the end of the bed for a while longer, patiently answering questions. Then, aware that they were going over ground that already had been thoroughly covered, he said:

"You know, if you want to talk to another cardiologist here, someone who does a lot of angioplasty, to get his impressions, I'd do it. Stuart Seides could set you up and introduce you to one of the guys here. I want to give you options. Nobody wants to go through an operation. But if you make the decision, you want to be as comfortable with a lousy decision as you can be."

Art Hollander, indeed, still wanted more information. He asked Corso when he would have the surgery done if it were his heart, and what his schedule was like over the next few weeks. Corso answered the first part of the question by saying it was a matter of personality. "If it were my heart and I had nothing to do tomorrow that would affect my family or my income, I'd get it done tomorrow. But I'm not telling you that it's medically necessary." He added that except for a weekend trip to New Orleans, he was available and could fit Lewis Hollander into his schedule.

Over the next fifteen minutes Corso provided additional information for the Hollanders. He explained that since Washington Hospital Center had only nine years' experience doing bypass surgery in which the heart-lung machine was not used, he could not project twenty-year results with certainty. But at seven years, he said, the results were better for patients operated on without the machine than with it.

Corso also emphasized to the Hollanders that bypass surgery does not cure coronary artery disease; that it creates conduits around existing blockages but does nothing to prevent new blockages from occurring. Corso told Hollander that he would recommend lifestyle changes after surgery, including cholesterol-lowering by either diet or drugs, and an aspirin a day for the rest of his life.

Corso then said, "Why don't I let you talk it over with whomever you want so that you will have a good understanding (1) that it's the right decision, (2) that it's here that it should be done, and (3) that it's me who should do it." He got up from the bed, not abruptly, but with body language indicating that he had said all he could usefully say, shook hands with Lewis and Art Hollander, and left the room.

Father and son talked a bit longer and decided that they would decide nothing immediately. The decision was too important. They still knew too little, and what they knew was confusing. They needed time to think, to talk things over with Hollander's wife, Jane. The one thing they agreed they should do quickly was to get at least one more professional opinion and possibly two. This they did over the next week.

Ramey sent Lewis Hollander to Bernard Gersh, the chief of cardiology at Georgetown University Medical Center. Gersh reviewed the angiographic film and concurred with Seides and Corso that surgery was the correct treatment. He also said that Corso was a good surgeon and that Washington Hospital Center was a high-quality institution. But he added that he had a preference in Hollander's case for a small-incision operation using the heart-lung machine. As it happens, a surgeon who does this operation had joined the Georgetown center's surgical staff six months earlier. Gersh said he did not believe that the arteries could be sutured together as precisely on a beating heart as they could if the heart were stopped and that an imperfect sewing job could mean trouble in a few years' time.

Gersh's advice prompted Hollander to speak to Seides again. Seides said that he thought Hollander should decide what to do based on the following order of priorities: (1) the odds that his arteries would remain open for the longest time; (2) the procedure that would require the least time on the heart-lung machine, with the ideal being no time; (3) the procedure that would cause the least physical trauma.

A week later Hollander went to Fairfax Hospital in nearby northern Virginia, which is generally considered second only to the Washington Hospital Center for heart surgery in the Washington area. He consulted a surgeon there named Robert Albus, who agreed that surgery was the right way to go. Albus said he did not believe, however, that the operation should be done through a small incision or on a beating heart. He recommended standard bypass surgery with an open chest using the heart-lung machine.

Hollander had also collected literature on bypass surgery, including booklets on treatments for heart disease prepared by Yale-New Haven Hospital and the Mayo Clinic. But they were of little use because while they described standard bypass surgery, which is still done in about 98 percent of all surgical cases, they mentioned beating-heart and small-incision operations only in passing. They also lacked the detail to help with a choice of the kind he had to make.

He and Jane then consulted with a neighbor named Joseph Giordano, a surgeon at George Washington University Hospital who operated on President Ronald Reagan after he was shot. He said Corso's treatment plan sounded good to him. They also talked to one of Hollander's college classmates, who is chief of cardiology at Newton-Wellesley Hospital near Boston. He, too, said he thought it was wise to avoid the heart-lung machine. At this point Hollander concluded that it was time to stop gathering information and decide.

There was a sense, Hollander realized, in which he was a lucky man. He is educated, intelligent, sophisticated, and insured. He had access to numerous centers where bypass surgery and angioplasty were done well. Indeed, had he chosen to, he could have gone anywhere he wanted for surgery, angioplasty, or other therapy. Moreover, he did not require emergency treatment, which meant there was time for careful decision-making. Nevertheless, he faced a difficult, stressful choice.

Hollander is a rational man—not the kind of patient who goes shopping for a doctor who will give him the treatment he prefers rather than the one he needs. He was persuaded by Seides, Corso, Gersh, Giordano, and others that he needed surgery, and he was prepared to have it. His wife and son supported him in this choice. But how was he to choose among the various forms of surgery being offered to him?

Should he have an operation with his chest split open while his heart continued to beat, which Gersh said might compromise the long-term result? Or would he be better off to have an operation through a small incision using a heart-lung machine and a potassium solution to protect his heart and stop it from beating? The heart-lung machine, he had been told, raised his risk of stroke and could cause some short-term cognitive deficit. Or should he have standard bypass surgery, the tried-and-true kind done by most cardiac surgeons most of the time in an open chest and also using a heart-lung machine?

With his wife and son's concurrence, he chose beating-heart open-chest surgery because in the end he trusted Corso and the statistics he cited. Although he made his decision as rationally as possible—that is, on the basis of competent professional advice—it would not have been irrational to seek still more advice elsewhere and perhaps to have made a choice other than surgery.

There are no clinical trials that suggest, for example, that someone with blockages such as Mr. Hollander's will live longer with surgery than with angioplasty or drug treatment. It is likely that surgery will provide a pain-free, active life without the need to take multiple medications for years longer than would be the case with angioplasty. But many entirely rational people are willing to pay the price of being less active, of having repeat angioplasty, or of taking drugs for the rest of their lives to avoid surgery.

Hollander is a vigorous man who loves golf. A choice to avoid surgery in his circumstances might have limited his physical activity, but it would not necessarily have done so. He probably could have found an aggressive interventional cardiologist who would have been willing and able—at some unknown increased risk—to treat him with angioplasty, or angioplasty and a stent, or two stents. There would have been about a 30 or 40 percent chance of his needing repeat angioplasty or bypass surgery, but there is a reasonable chance that he would have been able to play golf and avoid surgery.

It might even have been possible, had he shopped a bit more, to find a respectable cardiologist who would treat him with drugs for the foreseeable future. Surgery is more likely to provide a better quality of life for a longer period of time than angioplasty or drugs, but these choices are based on statistical probabilities, not certainties, and the differences can be marginal.

There are other considerations that Hollander might have taken into account. For example, did the physicians he consulted factor costs to third-party payers into their treatment recommendations? It may be unlikely that they did so in this case because surgery is the most expensive of the available options. But in an age of managed care, in which physicians often must justify their clinical decisions to insurance companies, in principle this is not an idle question. And neither is it an easy questions to answer. Most physicians try hard to put their patients' welfare first, but they are also sensitive to pressures to keep costs down and, unsurprisingly, they look after their own interests.

Did any of his physicians have conflicts of interest that might influence the treatments they recommended? It is not uncommon, for example, for diagnosing cardiologists who do angioplasty to recommend angioplasty for blockages that a noninterventional cardiologist would send to surgery or treat with drugs. (In Hollander's case, despite the fact that Stuart Seides does angioplasty, he recommended surgery.) In some cases the conflict may be intellectual. A cardiologist may be overcommitted to one form of treatment because he invented it, or pioneered its use. And sometimes it is overtly financial, as in cases where cardiologists or surgeons own large amounts of stock, or derive substantial income from drug or device manufacturers.

And what about mass media reports? Hollander's daughter Elizabeth, for example, came across an article in the July 28, 1997, issue of *U.S. News & World Report*. It quoted Corso's opinion that patients should worry less about the size of the incision than the risks of the heart-lung machine, and that the key variable in all of this is really the surgeon's skill. But it also cited the American Heart Association's refusal to endorse the procedure on the ground that it is still experimental.

Although the article is informative, as a decision-making aid it is hard to assess. For example, it quotes several surgeons, but they range from the very well known—Delos (Toby) Cosgrove of the Cleveland Clinic—to the relatively unknown—Mart McMullan of Jackson, Mississippi. Just how and why these individuals were chosen is unclear. Was the idea simply to show what opinions are out there in the surgical community? Were these surgeons selected without checking possible conflicts of interest or worrying about the relative expertise and experience of the surgeons quoted? How should readers who lack expert knowledge about cardiac surgery evaluate their comments?

Is it possible for someone like Lewis Hollander, who is intelligent, thorough, and has many resources, to learn enough in a few weeks to be a real participant—that is, an adequately informed participant—in one of the most important decisions of his life, a decision hundreds of thousands of less well-prepared Americans must make every year? Or does it all boil down to trust based on one physician being more likable than another, or more persuasive? Or is it even possible that the predictable differences between outcomes in many cases are so small that flipping a coin might be almost as rational as struggling to arrive at some version of a best choice?

These are the kinds of stomach-churning questions patients must answer every day. They must do so when they are under the stress of dealing with their disease physically and psychologically. And if they hope to answer the questions successfully, they must come to grips at least to some extent with a science and a profession they have not been taught to understand.

9

Angioplasty: A Balloon on a Snake

In January 1964, a radiologist known widely as "Crazy Charley" saved the gangrenous leg of an eighty-two-year-old woman who had refused amputation. He did it by pushing a series of stiff little polyethylene tubes through a blocked artery. This was the first time what is now called angioplasty had been done on a human. The technique, which almost immediately became known as "dottering" for its eccentric inventor, Charles Dotter, was primitive. It consisted of snaking a tiny guidewire through the artery and then slipping increasingly larger catheters over the guide to incrementally scrape away plaque and widen the vessel's channel.[1]

Dotter got the idea for angioplasty when he was performing routine angiography. He passed a catheter over a guidewire, accidentally opening a channel in a large artery in the patient's abdomen.[2] Recognizing the potential therapeutic benefit of what he had done, he experimented in cadavers by pushing bigger and bigger catheters over a piano-wire guide. It worked, and he began doing it on patients. The new technique caused frequent blood clots at the puncture sites through which the large catheters were inserted, and potentially clot-producing bits of broken plaque were regularly carried downstream in the artery. Nevertheless, despite the risks, a handful of European radiologists such as Eberhardt Zeitler were quick to grasp the technique's potential and adopt it.

But in the United States, where vascular surgeons had a proprietary lock on invasive procedures, Dotter met substantial resistance and attracted almost no followers. Some say that even his associate Melvin Judkins, a three-hundred-pound, vegetarian, tee-totaling Seventh-Day Adventist who assisted with the first procedure and who became a major contributor to the field of interventional cardiology, was not really convinced that dottering was the right way to go.[3]

An example of this resistance and Dotter's response to it occurred soon after he and Judkins did the landmark procedure. A vascular surgeon sent Dotter a request for an angiogram to confirm the existence of a blocked artery in a patient's left leg. The request form had the following message handwritten across it in large block letters: *"VISUALIZE BUT DO NOT TRY TO FIX!!!"*

Dotter did the angiogram, confirming a narrowing in the left femoral artery. But the film also showed a substantial amount of plaque in the right femoral artery. Taking a strict-constructionist approach to the surgeon's request, which addressed only the artery in the left leg, he dottered the artery in the right leg and gleefully dined out on the story. Predictably, his cavalier attitude did not endear Dotter to his surgical colleagues. Nor did it help advance the cause of angioplasty in the United States.

Dotter, like Mason Sones, was an abrasive, creative maverick. He invented devices in his kitchen, looked like a cartoon version of a mad scientist, and didn't care whom he offended. He also took chances that more prudent men would have avoided, such as risking prison by smuggling wire catheter guides to a colleague in Czechoslovakia, at the time a rigidly authoritarian Communist dictatorship that would have had no qualms about arresting an American smuggler, physician or otherwise.

Dotter was an ardent mountain climber who scaled sixty-seven peaks, including every one over fourteen thousand feet in the contiguous United States. He was a photographer and a car buff. And on at least one occasion, dressed in a tuxedo, he spent the better part of a formal evening repairing his host's TV set.

There is nothing whatsoever to suggest that he was not fully possessed of his faculties. He was probably called Crazy Charley mainly because of his manic grin and fierce eyes. Some cardiologists who knew him say his appearance might have affected the way he was treated, which, in turn, might have had some affect on the way he behaved. It is worth noting, however, that he was first called Crazy Charley by vascular surgeons who viewed him as a threat to their livelihoods.

As a physician, he combined the practical approach of a handyman with the offbeat imagination of an artist, which he was, too. A skillful drawing he made of a crossed pipe and wrench became his trademark. "If a plumber can do it for pipes," he used to say, "we [physicians] can do it for blood vessels."[4] Dotter was aware, of course, of the profound difference between plumbing crafted of inert metal and living vasculature. But despite the hyperbole, his analogy was not altogether inappropriate.

Drawing on his blend of pragmatism and creativity, he in effect reconceptualized the snake, a device designed to clear gunk from drainage systems, into something that could ream out blocked arteries. He also used the chemical streptokinase to dissolve blood clots the way Drāno dissolves hair balls, which makes him an early precursor of thrombolytic therapy as well as angioplasty.

Dotter was probably the first physician to insert a balloon-tipped catheter into a dog's circulatory system,[5] he was the first researcher since Alexis Carrel to experiment with supportive scaffolding inside arteries, and he developed a high-speed magazine for X-ray film that made possible sharper angiographic images. But when people asked him what he did for a living, he was cryptic and self-deprecating. His stock answer was, "Dilation is my bag."

Given Dotter's reputation as an oddball and his lack of a following in the United States, it is not surprising that it was one of his European admirers who made the next big leap. Like Dotter, this German-born physician was drawn to mountains and fast cars. He skied and drove his Porsche at high speed. He also flew his own plane, charmed women, and consumed Teutonic quantities of wurst and wine. And like Dotter, he invented new devices to unblock arteries on his kitchen table.

In addition, he had a trace of Felix Krull in his soul. He used his wits to enhance his comfort. On planes, for example, he sometimes would board without having shaved, looking disheveled, sniffing, and sneezing. This would inevitably drive away passengers in nearby seats, allowing him to stretch out and sleep.

Andreas Roland Gruentzig was born at the beginning of World War II in Dresden, a beautiful baroque and rococo city on the Elbe River in eastern Germany, which, in 1944, would be decimated by Allied bombs. However, in 1940 his parents moved to the small town of Rochlitz, about sixty miles away. In 1945, at the end of the war, Rochlitz was occupied by American troops, who set up their headquarters in the Gruentzig house. Andreas and his mother and brother were forced to move out. His father, a soldier in the Wehrmacht, never came home.

Postwar life was difficult, so Charlotta Gruentzig took her family to Argentina for two years. But she brought them back in 1952 because she believed her children would get a better education in East Germany. Andreas entered an elite *gymnasium* in Leipzig and prospered academically. But by 1957 he found the repressiveness of the Communist regime unbearable. He fled through Berlin to Heidelberg, West Germany, where he joined his brother, who had escaped earlier. His mother followed. Andreas graduated from medical school in Heidelberg in 1964.[6]

The peripatetic Gruentzig split his internship among three German hospitals and then began a series of fellowships in various places in Germany and England, and in various fields of medicine. He trained in epidemiology, internal medicine, peripheral vascular disease, radiology, and angiology. The signal event in his training, however, occurred when he accompanied his chief to Frankfurt to attend a meeting at which, Eberhardt Zeitler lectured on the Dotter method of peripheral angioplasty. Gruentzig was deeply impressed. It was a signal event for Gruentzig's boss, too. He was outraged that anyone would try to force catheters through diseased arteries, and he made it very clear that no one was ever going to do it in his hospital.[7]

In 1969, therefore, at age thirty, Gruentzig moved to University Hospital in Zurich, where the attitude toward Dotter's technique was a bit more open. Soon after his arrival he was allowed to visit Zeitler to observe him doing the Dotter procedure, and this time he was even more impressed. His chief then permitted him to invite Zeitler to Zurich to do it on a patient with a severe blockage in a femoral artery. Zeitler manipulated the catheters with Gruentzig's assistance while ten members of the radiology department watched.

At first everything seemed to be going well, but the patient suddenly felt excruciating pain. Plaque had broken loose and lodged at the joining of two arteries in the lower leg, completely cutting off blood flow. Although this was a fairly common occurrence in the first decade of peripheral angioplasty, it was a major setback. Nevertheless, he was allowed to continue to pursue the new technique at the sufferance of the chief of medicine, Walter Siegenthaler, and with some support from the chief of cardiovascular surgery, the renowned Swedish surgeon Ake Senning. Working on his lunch hours, Gruentzig accumulated a small series of cases.

In 1974, however, Gruentzig's career veered sharply. He switched his specialty from angiology and radiology to cardiology, an area of medicine that had interested him since his early days as an epidemiology fellow. This switch placed him perfectly to seek the answer to a question originally posed by Charles Dotter: If angioplasty can be done in the peripheral arteries, why not in the coronaries?

To put a solid object like a catheter inside a coronary artery would be revolutionary. In the mid-1970s injecting dye for angiograms still made many physicians nervous. And the coronary arteries were much smaller and more delicate than the peripheral arteries for which Dotter's ingenious but nonetheless crude method was devised. Scariest of all, of course, was that the consequence of loose plaque blocking blood flow to the heart muscle, as opposed to a toe, for example, could easily be death, not just severe pain or loss of a digit.

Visionaries like Dotter and Sones believed in the possibility of coronary angioplasty, perhaps even its inevitability, but had done nothing to solve the technical problems that prevented it from becoming a reality. It remained for Gruentzig to devise the more refined and gentler system that would make it possible.

Gruentzig probably was aware that balloon-tipped catheters had been used in urology as far back as the nineteenth century, and later in other

areas of medicine. And he might have known that in 1971 Cesare Gian-
turco was the first to use a balloon to open a blockage in a femoral artery.
But the procedure, while successful, was not repeated because the patient
died when her entry wound opened during the night.

Gruentzig himself had toyed with the idea of making a balloon-catheter
for dilating peripheral arteries as early as 1972, and by 1974 he had done
so. With this success behind him, he believed that it might be possible to
design a low-profile balloon-catheter that could squash plaque against the
walls of coronary arteries, thereby reopening a blocked channel. The catheters had to be very small and the balloons had to be not only thin and
strong but also firm enough to crush the plaque rather than mold around
it. Dotter never even tried to use his latex balloons for opening blocked
peripheral arteries because he believed, probably correctly, that they were
too fragile.

Gruentzig began working evenings at home with the help of his wife,
Michaela, a psychoanalyst; his assistant, Maria Schlumpf; and her husband,
Walter. They fabricated balloon-catheters from rubber tubing, thread, and
glue, but each time they tried one in an experimental animal, instead of
squashing the plaque, the too-compliant balloon simply conformed to the
lesion's shape. They needed a material that would become rigid under
pressure and not expand beyond a predetermined size. Gruentzig came up
with the idea of wrapping the balloon in silk mesh to contain its expansion.
He got the silk material from a shoelace factory. But he still needed something from which to make a very thin balloon.

At about this time he met a retired chemistry teacher who told him
about a relatively new synthetic material called polyvinyl chloride. It was
the answer to his prayers. Gruentzig worked with heat molding and compressed air and after hundreds of experiments created a thin-walled,
sausage-shaped balloon segment integral to the polyvinyl chloride tubing
that was small enough to fit into a coronary artery and rigid enough not
to need a silk-mesh wrapper. It would, among other things, avoid the large
entry wounds that plagued patients treated with the Dotter system.

The next step was to make a catheter on which the balloon could be
mounted that could monitor pressure in the artery and provide blood flow
to the heart while also providing a channel through which fluid could be
pumped to inflate the balloon. It took almost a year, but this hurdle was
surmounted, too. In January 1975 the twin-channeled catheter Gruentzig
devised was successfully used to open a blockage in an abdominal vessel
known as an iliac artery.

While continuing to dilate peripheral arteries, the Gruentzigs and the
Schlumpfs immediately began working on a balloon-catheter small enough
to fit into a canine coronary artery, which is even smaller than a human's.

By September they had it. Gruentzig constricted a dog's coronary artery with a silk thread, maneuvered the catheter into the artery, and inflated the balloon, which snapped the thread. The age of coronary angioplasty had begun, if only for dogs.

Two months later, the dapper Gruentzig, in shirt sleeves and an ascot, presented his dog experiments at a meeting of the American Heart Association in Miami Beach. His presentation caused a small stir among the thousands of cardiologists and cardiac surgeons attending the meeting, but in the main was viewed as just a curiosity. Most of the heart specialists held a view similar to that of Spencer King, a young Georgian who, based among other things on his own postmortem examinations, believed that plaque "was a crumbling, hard kind of material."

King said he was surprised that anyone would think an artery could be opened with a balloon without shattering plaque, a result that would cause blood clots leading to strokes, heart attacks, and death. He told Gruentzig flatly, "This will never work."[8] King is now director of the Andreas Gruentzig Cardiovascular Center at Emory University in Atlanta, president of the American College of Cardiology, and a leading apostle of angioplasty.

There were a few exceptions who, despite the general skepticism, were excited by what they heard and saw. Among them was Richard Myler, a

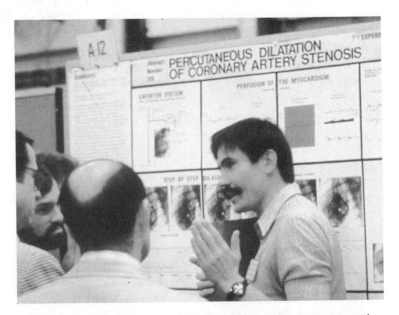

9.1. Andreas Gruentzig presents his work on canine coronary angioplasty at the American Heart Association meeting in Miami in November, 1976 (Courtesy of John Abele).

cardiologist practicing in Worcester, Massachusetts, who had attended a meeting in 1968 at which Dotter showed films of peripheral angioplasty and said he believed one day it would be possible to do coronary angioplasty. Myler says he remembers thinking, "Oh, my God, this is the future," and telling John Abele, a founding father of the medical device industry, "we need to begin working on this right away."[9]

In fact, Myler did just that. He quickly developed a metal, cagelike mechanism that when expanded shaved plaque off the arterial wall, trapped it, and carried it away. But he lacked a satisfactory means of directing it into the coronary arteries. When he left Massachusetts for San Francisco shortly thereafter, he dropped the project, but he remained interested in the general problem and discussed it periodically with Abele.

Several years later, in 1976, Myler went to the American Heart Association meeting knowing that Gruentzig would be there. He was aware of his attempts to extend angioplasty to the coronary arteries from Abele, who had visited Zurich in the fall of 1975 and had seen Gruentzig several times thereafter. "You guys have to meet," Abele told Myler, "because you're working on the same thing."[10]

After seeing and hearing Gruentzig's presentation in Miami, Myler was convinced that the balloon catheter would revolutionize the treatment of coronary artery disease. Myler wanted to go to Zurich immediately to see Gruentzig work, but family plans for Thanksgiving and other complications put off their next meeting until March 1977. They met in Nuremberg, West Germany, for the first course on peripheral angioplasty, which was run by Zeitler. Only about two dozen physicians attended. Dotter and Myler were the only Americans, and the only two who were not Zeitler's students.

At this meeting, Myler said, Gruentzig confided that he was frustrated by his superiors in Zurich, who tolerated his experiments with peripheral angioplasty on human subjects, and in the coronary arteries of dogs, but were adamantly opposed to his working in human coronaries. In response, Myler suggested that Gruentzig come to St. Mary's Hospital in San Francisco and that together they try coronary angioplasty in patients whose chests were already open in preparation for bypass surgery.

Myler reasoned that this would be a relatively safe way to start because even if something went wrong, like a piece of plaque breaking off and blocking an artery downstream, or the accidental damaging of the wall of an artery, they were already in the operating room, and the surgeons could handle the emergency. Gruentzig agreed. Myler found a skeptical but willing surgeon named Elias Hanna, and at the beginning of May, Gruentzig went to San Francisco.

In the first two weeks of May they did fifteen cases without a mishap.

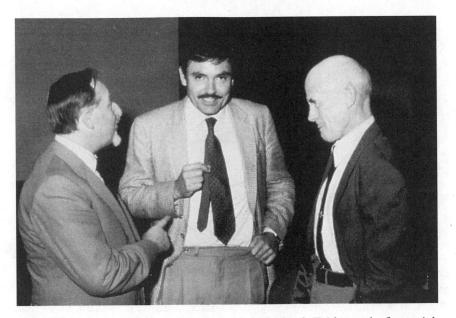

9.2. Charles Dotter, Andreas Gruentzig, and Eberhardt Zeitler, at the first peripheral angioplasty meeting in Nuremberg, Germany, March 1977 (Courtesy of Eberhardt Zeitler).

According to Myler, all of the patients agreed to the experimental procedure, which they were told was low-risk, would involve no pain, and would not increase their hospital stay, although they would have to have an additional angiogram.

The procedure consisted of inserting the catheter into a coronary artery through an incision already made for a planned bypass graft, advancing it through the blockage, and inflating the balloon to squash the plaque. Once the balloon was deflated and withdrawn, the artery was flushed out to check for plaque debris. None was ever found. Then the bypass graft was sutured in place. Postprocedure angiography showed that all of the arteries through which the balloon catheters had been passed had wider channels than before and had remained open.

Gruentzig and Myler immediately prepared an abstract, which they submitted to the American Heart Association. It was accepted, and they were invited to present their cases at the next meeting, in November. Gruentzig then went home to Switzerland.

The next steps were to learn how to maneuver hard-to-steer catheters into the tiny natural openings of the coronary arteries, and how to take blood-pressure measurements across the blockages. To accomplish these goals, Gruentzig came back to San Francisco, and he and Myler did some-

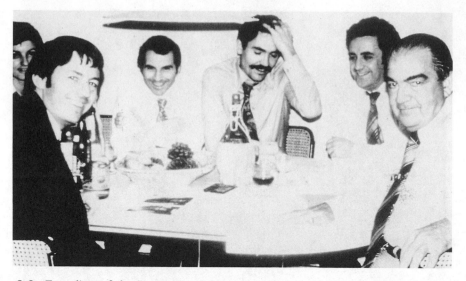

9.3. Founding of the International Dilatation Society: (clockwise) John Simpson, Maria Schlumpf, Lamberto Bentivoglio, Andreas Gruentzig, Richard Myler, and James Minor. The table they were sitting around was Gruentzig's workbench for developing his balloon catheter (Courtesy of Richard Myler).

thing very similar to what Mason Sones had done in 1958 after accidentally discovering selective coronary angiography: They practiced putting catheters into the orifices of coronary arterial branches during diagnostic angiograms. There was one difference, however: Myler said that, unlike Sones, they explained to their patients what they were doing and why they were doing it.

"It scared the hell out of us," Myler said. "We never hurt anybody. But we weren't going to help anybody. We were just trying to know if we could just manipulate the catheter into one branch or another. And we realized that we couldn't until we made guiding catheters with the tip pointed a little bit this way or a little bit that way. We put little tiny wires on the tip, one straight or one curved."[11]

Once he had achieved what he considered to be sufficient competence in manipulating the catheters, Gruentzig told Myler that he would like to do a real case, not in the open chest of a patient prepared for surgery, but through a small incision in the groin. Myler, however, still had concerns of what he referred to as "a medico-legal nature." It was relatively safe, he believed, to do the first human test in the operating room on a diseased patient who was going to have bypass surgery anyway, but the risk of doing it in a nonsurgical setting was unacceptable. Until the intraoperative cases, after all, the procedure had been done only on dogs whose arteries were normal and artificially constricted.

"Andreas," Myler recalls explaining somewhat elliptically, "about a mile and a half from our hospital is a fellow named Melvin Belli." Gruentzig looked blank and asked, "Who's Melvin Belli?" "The most famous malpractice lawyer in the world," Myler instructed him. "Richard," Gruentzig asked, "what is malpractice?"[12]

Malpractice was not a problem in Switzerland. When he returned to Zurich, Gruentzig began looking for the right patient. It would have to be someone with a single blockage that was relatively easy to attack. It would also have to be someone who would agree to be the subject of a dramatic medical experiment. The technique would be to thread a long catheter through a femoral artery in the groin up into the diseased coronary artery, inflate the balloon, crush the plaque, do it again if necessary, and get out. The procedure would be done under local anesthetic.

It took several months and there were a couple of false starts, but on September 15, 1977, with the help of a Zurich physician named Bernhard Meier, Gruentzig found a candidate named Adolph Backman, whose angiographically identified single blockage was easily reachable with the balloon catheter. He was ideal for the new procedure. The next day, this thirty-eight-year-old Swiss businessman became the first person to undergo an experimental intervention that most cardiologists at the time considered at best unsafe, at worst insane.

Gruentzig brought three balloons to the lab and promptly burst two while preparing for angioplasty in the patient's left anterior descending coronary artery. But once he began, the procedure, which required two fifteen-to-thirty-second balloon inflations, went smoothly and was a complete success. Gruentzig was very excited. He became extremely upset, however, when he learned that his patient had spoken to a newspaper reporter about the new treatment. A story in the lay press before publication in a peer-reviewed scientific journal would be a serious breach of protocol. To his relief, however, Gruentzig was able to persuade the journalist to hold his story for several months until he published a report in *Lancet,* a respected British medical journal.

Backman's willingness to undergo the procedure was courageous, but so was Gruentzig's willingness to do it. Gary Roubin, an eminent interventional cardiologist who has written on the history of interventional cardiology and who worked with Gruentzig at Emory, wrote: "To understand the resolve this must have taken, one must understand the prevailing thought at that time. Coronary angiography itself was still considered a relatively hazardous procedure. . . . The risk from plaque rupture and distal embolization and myocardial ischemia was quite unknown. . . . Andreas still had no support from his medical colleagues and if he failed, the personal consequences for his career would have been devastating."[13]

An angiogram a month later showed that Backman's artery was wide open. And when he was brought to Emory University for an angiogram ten years later, it was still wide open. And in 1997 "he performed a maximal bicycle ergometric test with normal results."[14]

In late 1977, only a few adventurous cardiologists, such as Myler, Martin Kaltenbach in Frankfurt, and Simon Stertzer in New York, were enthusiastic about percutaneous transluminal coronary angioplasty (PTCA), as Gruentzig called his new treatment. In October of that year, after doing another case in Zurich, Gruentzig did two cases in Kaltenbach's lab. But it would be almost six months before the first cases would be done in the United States.

In November, Gruentzig came to the annual American Heart Association meeting again to present the intraoperative work he and Myler had done. But by then, of course, the abstract they had written in May had been overtaken by events. Gruentzig had already done four coronary angioplasties, all successful, in which he had introduced the catheter into a femoral artery through a small incision in the patient's groin. The audience was small, perhaps fifty or sixty cardiologists and radiologists, and unaware that they were about to witness a historic event.

In the midst of delivering the abstract, with the room darkened, Gruentzig for the first time ever showed a professional gathering fluoroscopic film of coronary angioplasty. The effect was stunning. There was even applause, a rare reaction in the middle of a scientific presentation.

Among the cardiologists in the room was the profane, skeptical, but highly emotional Mason Sones. As Myler recalls it, Sones came up behind him, put his hands on his shoulders, and said: "I've got to meet your friend. It's a fucking dream come true." Not everyone at the meeting, however, was as impressed as Sones. And the national media showed no interest at all.

Myler returned to San Francisco the next day, happy with the results, but not overwhelmed. That evening Gruentzig called to say that he had been interviewed by a local reporter in Miami and that the reporter would be calling Myler, too. Myler was not pleased to hear this, because like Gruentzig's Swiss cases, their intraoperative cases had not yet been reported in a peer-reviewed journal. He asked Gruentzig what the name of the newspaper was. Gruentzig fumbled for it and finally came up with "the *National Enquirer.*" Myler groaned. But there was minimal fallout from the article.

Myler, who was becoming something of a transatlantic commuter, went to Switzerland again, in January, bringing with him this time a young, inventive, entrepreneurial cardiology fellow at Stanford named John Simpson, who had heard Gruentzig speak and who was thoroughly captivated. Simpson wanted to show Gruentzig a balloon-catheter he was working on that was easier to steer because it moved over a wire. But Gruentzig dismissed his idea with what Gary Roubin described as "a moment of infrequent but well-remembered arrogance."[15]

This incident, however, did not put a damper on the visit. One evening the three men, along with Maria Schlumpf, Gruentzig's young, beautiful assistant; Lamberto Bentivoglio, a Philadelphia cardiologist; and James Minor, a physician from Atlanta, sat in Gruentzig's dining room, drinking Chianti. When the last bottle was empty, in a spirit of wine-induced fellowship, they inscribed their names on the cork and formed what they decided to call the first International Dilatation Society. Gruentzig was declared president, Myler vice president, Minor treasurer, and Simpson, the youngest, keeper of the cork. They chipped in the equivalent of about $50 each, with Gruentzig paying Maria Schlumpf's share, and gave the money to Minor for safekeeping. Simpson can no longer find the cork, and, according to Myler, the money is missing, too.

A month later, Gruentzig's landmark publication appeared in the form of an extremely brief letter to *Lancet*. The text was fewer than 350 words, and it was accompanied by three frames from one patient's angiographic film and a small chart providing details of five cases. Gruentzig concluded the letter by writing modestly, "This technique, if it proves successful in long-term follow-up studies, may . . . provide another treatment for patients with angina pectoris."[16] His letter to the editor—no more than an abstract, really—signaled a major change in the direction of cardiology.

Traditionally, even when a new medical discovery looked promising, the discoverers had to overcome opposition, ridicule, or even scorn from their peers. As in the cases of Forssmann or Herrick or Gibbon, there was always a long struggle to win acceptance of their groundbreaking work. The Scottish physician Sir James Mackenzie, who died in 1925, lucidly described the form this conservatism typically took:

> When [a discovery] is first announced, people say that it is not true. Then, a little later, when its truth has been borne in on them, so that it can no longer be denied, they say it is not important. After that, if its importance becomes sufficiently obvious, they say that anyhow it is not new.[17]

But by the late twentieth century there was an unexpected and confounding factor in the equation, one Sir James could not have foreseen. The economic incentives for doing cutting-edge procedures such as angio-

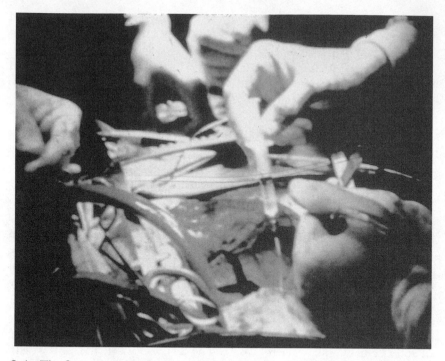

9.4. The first coronary agioplasty performed in May, 1977 by Andreas Gruentzig and Richard Myler in a patient about to undergo bypass surgery (Courtesy of Richard Myler).

plasty simply overwhelmed the medical establishment's innate conservatism. It still took a few years to overcome inertia, but once the potential rewards of doing angioplasty became obvious to everyone, cardiologists flocked to learn the procedure; new medical students flocked to become cardiologists; and physicians, in the spirit of entrepreneurialism, became inventors and businessmen.

Moreover, in part because traditional clinical skills, which remain the bedrock of care, were poorly rewarded by comparison with doing angioplasty and other interventions, competence in these skills declined, in some cases alarmingly. A 1997 study of 453 recent medical graduates, for example, showed that four out of five times they could not correctly identify the distinctive sounds of common heart abnormalities with a stethoscope.[18]

Until 1977, for all practical purposes, only surgeons treated coronary artery disease. Cardiologists diagnosed disease with increasingly sophisticated noninvasive tests and provided short-term relief with palliative drugs. Now, for the first time, cardiologists could move into the treatment arena not just with drugs, but also with an expensive procedure. This difference was important: Pharmaceutical companies got rich when physicians prescribed drugs; cardiologists would get rich from doing procedures.

Cardiologists would not only be able to compete with surgeons for patients but also would be able to charge fees approaching those charged by surgeons. Moreover, cardiologists now both diagnosed disease and treated it with angioplasty; this gave them the option of recommending a high-priced procedure they did themselves to patients whom previously they would have sent to a surgeon or treated with drugs.

It is unlikely that anyone in November 1977, including Gruentzig, understood that these largely economically motivated changes would occur. All that was obvious at the time was that for some patients he apparently had made available a less-invasive, less-traumatic alternative to bypass surgery. No one could tell yet how well it would stack up against surgery, against newer drugs that were just beginning to come on-line, or, for that matter, against doing nothing. But it had been done five times, the patients were all alive, and blood was flowing through their formerly blocked coronary arteries.

On March 1, 1978, less than a month after Gruentzig's publication in *Lancet,* Richard Myler on the West Coast and Simon Stertzer on the East Coast simultaneously became the first Americans to do percutaneous transluminal coronary angioplasty. Exactly how this timing came about, whether by chance or by design, is not clear. Myler vaguely remembers some coordination, possibly through Gruentzig, with whom he had regular contact, but Stertzer has no such recollection. In any event, both men were in effect anointed by Gruentzig, who taught them the procedure and supplied the catheters.

Stertzer had seen angioplasty for the first time shortly before this initial U.S. experience, when he visited Zurich to watch Gruentzig do several cases. A young cardiologist named William Grossman was there for the first time, too. Grossman was from one of the most prestigious of the Harvard-affiliated hospitals, Peter Bent Brigham. Both men were impressed with Gruentzig and with what they saw. Like Myler, they believed that angioplasty had a brilliant future.

Grossman returned to Boston and convinced the chief of cardiology at Peter Bent Brigham, Eugene Braunwald, to invite Gruentzig to Boston for a demonstration at their hospital under their auspices. Although neither of them can prove it, Myler and Stertzer, both of whom are intimate with the intrigues of major-league academic medicine, said they believed this was a power play by Harvard to claim angioplasty as its province.

Gruentzig was less impressed with Grossman, however, than Grossman was with him. Gruentzig was inclined to reject the invitation. But because it came from Braunwald, and Harvard, Siegenthaler prevailed on Gruentzig to accept. He flew to Boston but wasn't happy about it. In the catheterization laboratory Gruentzig found the usual skeptical audience, several surgeons among them, and a difficult case.

The patient was a woman in her mid-sixties with a heavily calcified blockage in her right coronary artery. In those early days of essentially unsteerable catheters without guidewires, and balloons that would burst under high pressure, the few people who had done angioplasty would usually turn down such cases. And if they did take them, they would stop in midcase if they were unable to get the catheter to slip easily through the blockage.

Gruentzig began the procedure by delicately maneuvering the catheter into the patient's right coronary artery, but even with insistent probing, he was unable to pass it through the blockage. He turned to Grossman and recommended that they stop and that the patient go to surgery. But Grossman said, "Let me try." Gruentzig said, "I don't think you can do it." But Grossman insisted. Gruentzig relented, saying, "Don't force it."

Grossman worked the catheter against the resistance of the blockage but could not cross it. At this point there is some disagreement about exactly what happened. Myler says Gruentzig told him the artery shut down and the patient had to be rushed to the operating room, where she underwent successful bypass surgery. Grossman says he does not believe that the artery closed, but agrees that the patient went to surgery and was successfully treated. In any event, the experience soured Gruentzig and, according to Stertzer, he vowed never to set foot in a Harvard hospital again.[19]

In early 1978 there were only four men in the world who had performed coronary angioplasty—Gruentzig, Kaltenbach, Myler and Stertzer. Myler, remembers asking himself, "What happens next?" He posed the question to Gruentzig, who came up with a daring answer—a live course in which qualified, interested, but probably highly skeptical radiologists and cardiologists would gather in a conference room to watch on television as he did a case in real time.

In its way, what Gruentzig was proposing was every bit as radical as coronary angioplasty itself. He had done only a handful of carefully selected cases, his equipment was primitive, yet he was willing to expose himself to the scrutiny of his peers under the most stressful possible conditions. No one had done anything quite like this before.

Without much enthusiasm, Siegenthaler permitted Gruentzig to offer his course in Zurich over Easter 1978, when there would be few researchers and staff around. He detailed a young surgeon to remain on duty in case of an emergency. Thirty-seven physicians attended, more than half of whom were Europeans, and more than half of whom were radiologists whose interest stemmed primarily from Gruentzig's earlier work with peripheral arteries.

The attendees gathered around a couple of small television screens. They watched Gruentzig operate on one screen, while on the other he showed the patient's angiographic film, freezing the frame from time to time and drawing on the screen with a grease crayon to show what he was doing. The patients did well, and the course was well received. Gruentzig would eventually offer fourteen such courses, four in Switzerland and ten in the United States.

The live course, often reaching large numbers of physicians by video, is now the standard way of teaching new procedures. Leading operators have grown comfortable with it, and the technology has advanced light-years since Gruentzig's first course. At the Transcatheter Cardiovascular Therapeutics meeting in Washington in September 1997, attended by more than six thousand interventional cardiologists, surgeons, and industry representatives, forty live cases were presented from hospitals in Washington; San Diego; Milan, Italy; and Toulouse, France. The audio and video satellite communications were interactive, permitting the operators to participate in a dialogue with the moderator and panelists at Washington's Convention Center.

The audience watched on four theater-size screens. One screen showed the operating room or catheterization laboratory, another showed angiographic film of the case in progress, another the moderator or panelist speaking, and the last flashed questions that each audience member answered by punching a numbered keypad at his or her seat. Thirty seconds later a tabulation of the answers showed on the screen in the form of a multicolored graph. In other words, an instant poll had been taken. The results were relayed to the operators in the United States and abroad by the moderator.

In 1978, not only was the communications technology primitive, so was the angioplasty technology. Perhaps two-thirds or more of cases that can be done routinely today were either initially rejected by the early angioplasters or were called off in midprocedure. This was usually necessary either because it was impossible to get the catheter's tip into the target artery, or because the operators couldn't get the tip beyond the blockage so that the balloon could be expanded to squash the plaque.

Over the next couple of years Gruentzig and others made improvements, especially in the guiding catheters, which are slightly larger than the balloon catheters that are threaded through them. They experimented with a variety of materials until they came up with a triple-layered catheter with many of the qualities they were looking for, such as torque control and an almost frictionless inner surface that would permit the balloon catheter to slip easily through. They also devised tiny wire tips for their balloon catheters that were shaped to make entry into arterial orifices easier.

Gruentzig was permitted although not encouraged to continue his research, to do cases at University Hospital in Zurich, and to train young Americans and Europeans who flocked to his increasingly popular live courses. Nevertheless, by 1980 he had become thoroughly frustrated with his situation. He was now past forty years old and he no longer had the patience to deal with the bureaucratic, hierarchical Swiss system of medicine. He did not receive his first full academic appointment, as a lecturer, until 1977, and only in 1979, at forty, did he receive a relatively senior post as physician in chief at University Hospital Polyclinic. During this two-year period Gruentzig traveled frequently to the United States, where he was admired and respected by the small but growing band of cardiologists who believed that the future of their field was tied to angioplasty.

One of these trips to the United States was in August 1978, at the invitation of Spencer King, whose jaundiced view of angioplasty had changed little since the 1976 American Heart Association meeting at which he told Gruentzig that his new technique would never work. Some months before inviting Gruentzig, King had received a phone call from a colleague who had just attended Gruentzig's live course and was immensely moved by its inventiveness and its therapeutic potential.

"The fellow on the phone was literally in tears as he was telling me the story," King said, thinking at the time, "this is pretty bizarre behavior for a cardiologist." But the phone call piqued his interest and he filed the information until he was asked by fellow members of a small, southern cardiovascular society to which he belonged what he thought about having Gruentzig as the speaker at their annual meeting. King said, "Why not?" and since he was the only member of the group who had met Gruentzig, he agreed to invite him to the conference, which was to be held on a resort island off the South Carolina coast.[20]

King called Gruentzig, who said he thought he could speak at the meeting and would let King know. But time passed, and with the meeting rapidly approaching and no word from Gruentzig, King was forced to scramble around at the last minute and find another speaker. The next day, however, Gruentzig called to say that not only was he coming, but that he was bringing his wife and daughter. King, the society's treasurer, apologized abjectly to the substitute, Peter Block from the renowned Massachusetts General Hospital, swallowed hard, and paid for Block and his wife to attend the meeting. Of course, the society paid for Gruentzig and his family, too, which nearly drove it into bankruptcy.

King asked a Hungarian-born surgeon who practiced in North Carolina and was known for his cutting humor to moderate the session at which Gruentzig spoke. Gruentzig straightforwardly shared his experience doing angioplasty, which at that point had a success rate of about 60 percent. The surgeon, Francis Robicek, then mocked Gruentzig's presentation with a deadpan parody in which he treated angioplasty as if it were a drug, for which such a low success rate would be unacceptably poor.[21] Gruentzig felt that he had been sandbagged. But according to King, he liked many of the members of the society and, overall, enjoyed the weekend.

The next time King saw Gruentzig was in January 1980, when he attended Gruentzig's now semiannual course. Afterward Gruentzig and King sat next to each other on a train heading for a postcourse group outing in the Emmenthal Valley. Gruentzig began telling King how dissatisfied he was with things in Zurich and that he was going to immigrate to the United States. He said he had an offer from the Cleveland Clinic, where Mason Sones was very eager to lure him, and feelers from other U.S. medical centers.

King, by now a convert to angioplasty, asked him, "What about Emory?" Gruentzig said he didn't know anything about Emory. King invited him to visit the next time he was in the United States, which, as it happened, was going to be in a week. King, then chief of the catheterization laboratory at Emory, went back to Atlanta and made a sales pitch to R. Bruce Logue, the chief of cardiology, and to the key decision-maker, J. Willis Hurst, the chief of medicine.

Hurst was skeptical. He had heard Gruentzig speak once and thought he was a prima donna and that it was a pretty wild idea to try to bring him to Emory. But when Hurst met the charismatic Gruentzig, he was won over. He joined the recruiting effort, aware that if Emory were going to get Gruentzig they would have to play catch-up ball, engage in tough negotiations, and overcome some formidable bureaucratic obstacles. Gruentzig was leaning toward Cleveland because of Sones and the surgical experience there.

Moreover, Gruentzig's European credentials were inconsistent with U.S. licensing requirements. This meant that they would very likely have difficulties getting him an immigration visa that would allow him to work in the United States, and that he would have to take a series of state examinations, which he was adamantly opposed to doing. Myler, who wanted Gruentzig to come to San Francisco, had discussed the matter with officials in Sacramento and was discouraged about the possibility of getting him a California medical license without taking the exams. At this point Hurst and his colleagues had no idea whether they could get Gruentzig an immigration visa and a Georgia medical license without his having to pass the usual examinations for foreign-trained doctors.

It didn't take long for Gruentzig to discover that he liked the atmosphere at Emory, which was more relaxed than at the Cleveland Clinic. Emory would be a serious contender if Hurst and King could figure out how to clear the bureaucratic hurdles. Then King had a stroke of good luck: During lunch with Gruentzig at the men's grill of Atlanta's Piedmont Driving Club, the kind of dark, paneled old-boy setting in which deals were done in the days before affirmative action, he saw a familiar face at the next table. It was Griffin Bell, President Jimmy Carter's attorney general. The two men did not know each other well, but they served on a board together at nearby Mercer University.

King invited Bell over to his table and introduced him to Gruentzig and his two other luncheon companions, Logue and Charles Hatcher, Emory's chief of surgery. King heaped praise on Gruentzig's contribution to medicine and told Bell that they were trying to recruit him to Emory. Bell said, "If there's anything I can do, let me know." King unhesitatingly replied, "Well, as a matter of fact, we're having some trouble with his visa." Bell said, "I can't really do anything about that, but I did appoint the chief of the Immigration and Naturalization Service. And my law firm has people who work on these things."

King, not an unworldly man, jumped at Bell's suggestion that Emory hire Bell's Atlanta law firm, King & Spaulding, to work on the visa matter. This was done, and within a couple of months Gruentzig got his immigration visa based on his "unique talents." Other connections were found who were able to arrange a Georgia medical license for Gruentzig without his having to take any examinations. When asked how they had managed to get these highly unusual exemptions for Gruentzig, Willis Hurst smiled and said, "By making the case that he would become a national treasure."[22] Neither he nor King would elaborate further, but King categorically denied that Coca-Cola, Atlanta's largest corporation and a major Emory benefactor, played a role, as has been widely rumored.

Hurst also enticed Gruentzig with an offer of half of his large office suite until additional space became available. Together, these inducements, which the Cleveland Clinic and Myler failed to match, had persuaded Gruentzig to come to Emory. He moved to Atlanta and began his career at Emory in October 1980 as professor of medicine and radiology, and director of interventional cardiovascular medicine.

Although Emory's reputation for coronary care was not as illustrious as that of the Cleveland Clinic, it nevertheless had a first-rate cardiac surgery program and a catheterization laboratory dating back to 1942, when there were probably only two others in the world, one in New York and one in London. Although they were just beginning to do angioplasty at Emory, the cath lab was staffed by four excellent interventional cardiologists, including King and John Douglas, whose touch with a catheter is reputed to equal or surpass that of Minnesota Fats with a cue stick. Moreover, Hurst, who had been Lyndon Johnson's cardiologist, was a towering figure in American medicine who had written a well-known cardiology textbook.

The cosmopolitan, faintly dandified Gruentzig was a curiosity for Atlanta, which in its mores and social customs was still something of a provincial southern city. He was romantically handsome with thick, dark hair, dark brown eyes, long lashes, and a slim mustache. He spoke with a pronounced German accent, dressed with casual European elegance, drank just a bit too much, kissed women's hands, and flirted, sometimes shamelessly, with the wives of his colleagues, among others.

Gruentzig rode a motor scooter to work, drove his Porsche at reckless speeds, and sang and played the flute. When he purchased a weekend house on Sea Island, off the Georgia coast, he bought a plane to fly back and forth, eventually upgrading his single-engine model to a high-powered twin-engine Beechcraft Baron.

After he bought the bigger plane, which was much more demanding to fly, Simon Stertzer, also a pilot, cautioned him about it. But Gruentzig, with his trademark panache, said, "We're not like the rest of these doctors who are falling out of the sky. We're used to stress."[23] While at Emory he also divorced his wife, Michaela, and married one of his students, Margaret Anne Thornton, who was almost twenty years younger than he was.

When Gruentzig moved to Atlanta, the focus of angioplasty moved with him from Europe to the United States. With the help of Myler, Stertzer, Simpson and others, a registry of cases had already been started at the National Institutes of Health. And young, highly skilled operators led by Geoffrey Hartzler in Kansas City were moving ahead of the professionally cautious Gruentzig to do double-and triple-vessel cases. In California, John Simpson was looking for a way to exploit his ideas about how to build a better catheter.

At Emory, Gruentzig continued his semiannual courses, and now three hundred to five hundred physicians typically attended.[24] Within three years of its first use, coronary balloon angioplasty went from a futuristic procedure to near state-of-the-art medicine, albeit still practiced by a relative few. The real explosion in cases would occur in the mid-1980s, topping one hundred thousand for the first time in 1986.

During the 1980s, two important changes in the field were taking place simultaneously. A relatively small number of research-oriented cardiologists, mostly on medical school faculties, and a handful of clinical scientists and engineers, mostly at small medical-device companies in northern California, were working to advance the technology of angioplasty. They were trying to improve the steerability of catheters and reduce their size, to make smaller balloons that could be inflated under higher pressure without bursting, and to make both catheters and balloons easier to see under fluoroscopy. They were also experimenting with new devices to remove or disintegrate plaque, not just squash it against the wall of an artery the way a balloon does.

At the same time, a large number of cardiologists were becoming interventionalists because it was becoming clear that this was where the action and the money were. By 1991, angioplasty overtook bypass surgery to become the most common invasive treatment for coronary artery disease in the United States. And by 1992–93, the median income of an invasive cardiologist in a cardiology group practice was $385,037, compared to $314,482 for a noninvasive cardiologist in a similar group, and $200,000 for a general surgeon. The mean salary for academic cardiologists was $154,000.[25]

Andreas Gruentzig had truly set in motion a revolution. In 1979, a total of 2,000 Americans had coronary angioplasty done by a handful of operators. In 1995 a total of 408,000 angioplasties were done by 6,000 operators in the United States. In some ways this was not what Gruentzig had hoped for. He considered coronary angioplasty a highly specialized technique that required exceptional skill and judgment, and he did not believe that everyone could do it.

In the period just after he invented the procedure, Gruentzig was in a position to control the supply of balloon catheters, which in the beginning were manufactured one at a time in Zurich by a small company called Schneider. He was very careful who got them. Even his favorites, such as Myler and Stertzer, could get only a couple at a time, and they had to reuse them. The reason was not greed, but rather Gruentzig's concern that the procedure be done only by those he believed could meet his exacting standards.

Under the U.S. system of paying for medical care, however, there was too much money at stake to keep a lid on a procedure as potentially lucrative as angioplasty. No one man could serve as keeper of the flame. Angioplasty's rapid growth was driven by a strong economic incentive independent of whether the pace of growth was conducive to a net therapeutic benefit or not. Almost certainly, the doctors doing angioplasty were convinced that they were doing good. But in Canada, where as a result of governmental controls, which eliminate economic incentives for doing angioplasty, among other things, it is performed about one-eighth as often as it is in the United States. The same is true for bypass surgery.

No definitive comparison has been made of the treatment outcomes for Canadian and American patients, but a study of thousands of elderly patients in the United States and in Ontario, Canada, found that despite the huge difference in the number of angioplasties and bypass surgeries, mortality rates for elderly patients with coronary artery disease who had suffered heart attacks were about the same in the two countries.[26] And a multicountry study showed that despite the much more frequent use in the United States of both angioplasty and bypass surgery to treat unstable angina, U.S. patients did no better in terms of death or heart attack rates.[27]

In other words, these studies were unable to discern a significant survival benefit for the vastly greater number of angioplasties—and bypass operations—done in the United States as compared to Canada and several other countries. The studies do not address long-term survival, mortality for younger patients, complications of angioplasty, or quality of life.

In the early eighties Gruentzig remained confident about the future of angioplasty as his own work at Emory advanced on several fronts. During his years there, along with King and Douglas, he built a world-class interventional-cardiology program. He also continued research he had presciently begun years earlier in Switzerland. Gruentzig had experimented, for example, with lasers to disintegrate arterial blockages and, according to King, as early as 1972 with a primitive drilling technique.

King described the device Gruentzig fabricated as a wire with an elliptical form at one end and an electric drill at the other. "When spinning," King wrote, "the wire developed the form of an ellipse, similar to an eggbeater, and displaced the atherosclerotic material against the artery wall." He dropped the drill project, however, to press forward with the development of a more effective balloon catheter.[28] Others, including John Simpson, would eventually pick it up. Gruentzig was also interested in stents, intravascular ultrasound for imaging inside coronary arteries, and learning why as many as 40 percent of arteries on which angioplasty had been performed either closed abruptly or clogged again soon afterward, the phenomenon called restenosis.

By 1984 Gruentzig had concluded that it would make sense to perform angiography on a large, randomized sample of asymptomatic patients—as an outpatient procedure—to demonstrate the distribution of coronary artery disease in the population. At Christmastime he decided to make the point that this would be easy to do by having an angiogram himself.

At 5:00 P.M. he climbed up on a lab table. One of the interventional cardiology fellows did the procedure as ordered. Gruentzig then climbed down, went home, picked up his wife, and at 7:00 P.M. turned up at Willis Hurst's door for the departmental Christmas party. Gruentzig was delighted with his theatrical example, but to this day no one has conducted an angiographic study of asymptomatic humans.

It is worth noting in passing that Gruentzig's arteries, despite his habit of consuming prodigious amounts of sausages and other fat- and cholesterol-laden delectables, were clean as a whistle. This should not be taken as an argument for eating large amounts of fat, but rather as an indication that a great deal is still not understood about the mechanisms of atherosclerosis.

It is also worth noting that Gruentzig was not just a world-class innovator and researcher; he was also a caring clinician who liked to look after patients and was good at it. One of his last patients, Stanley Hinden, was a colleague of mine when I was a reporter and editor at the *Washington Post*. He and his wife, Sara, shared with me their recollections of Gruentzig at the bedside.[29]

In the summer of 1985 Hinden, who was then fifty-eight years old, left home one morning with Sara to attend the birthday party of their grandson, Teddy. Immediately after getting behind the wheel of their car, Hinden felt sick. They went back upstairs, and he lay down to rest. After a short while he felt better, and they went to the party. Sara said nothing, but she was worried that Stan might have had a silent heart attack. Sara Hinden reads medical fiction and was familiar with some symptoms of coronary artery disease. One thing that worried her was Stan's ashen pallor; another was the suddenness with which the episode had occurred.

Over the next few days, without mentioning his heart, she nagged Stan to get a checkup. He called their family doctor, who was out of town, and made an appointment for two weeks later. Acting on her suspicion, Sara called the doctor's office without Stan's knowledge and asked that they do an electrocardiogram. The EKG showed a troublesome variation from the last one Stan had had. His doctor was concerned and referred him to a cardiologist, who gave him a stress test to measure how well his heart was pumping.

Based on his poor performance in the stress test, the cardiologist sent him for an angiogram at George Washington University Hospital. The angiogram showed several blockages, including one that was total. Everyone agreed that Hinden had had a heart attack and that he should have angioplasty. The invasive cardiologists at George Washington said they could do it. At the time, however, angioplasty was done rarely in Washington. It was new enough that neither Sara nor Stan had ever heard of it. Hinden was willing to have it done, but he and Sara were concerned that the George Washington cardiologists did not have enough experience doing it.

At about this time, Hinden's cousin, who worked for a drug company, sent him some information she had collected on angioplasty. Stan and Sara had already begun interviewing Washington cardiologists who were doing the procedure to find out how many cases they had done. They got answers such as "three," "five," and "ten," all of which, on the basis of common sense and gut feeling, they considered inadequate.

Then, among the clippings Stan's cousin had sent, they found an article about Gruentzig. Just two hours from Washington by air, they realized, was the inventor of the procedure and one of the most experienced operators in the world. They made up their minds quickly to try to get Gruentzig to take Stan's case. They picked up his angiographic film from George Washington and shipped it to Atlanta. Gruentzig reviewed it and agreed to see Hinden. Gruentzig told him it was not an emergency and asked them to be at Emory on August 11, with the procedure scheduled, if all went well, for the following morning.

Stan and Sara flew to Atlanta on the appointed day. Shortly after arriving, they were advised of the risks associated with angioplasty and told that a surgical team would be available if anything went wrong. They were also given the disquieting news that there was no guarantee that Gruentzig would be able to do his case. In the afternoon Gruentzig came to talk to the Hindens.

"It was love at first sight as far as I was concerned," Sara said years later. "First of all, he was very handsome. Secondly, the man walks in and he doesn't mince words, but he doesn't placate you and he doesn't talk down to you. His whole manner and atttitude was, 'I'm the expert. If I can't do it, nobody else is going to be able to do it. But we're going to do something.' He was very handsome, very debonair and very self-assured. I mean you just had to believe that you had made the right choice."

That evening, however, Gruentzig returned and said, "I have some unpleasant news." He explained to Stan and Sara that one of the blockages was hard to get at because it was located at a difficult bend in the right coronary artery. He said this kind of a curve was known in the trade as a shepherd's crook, and when you had it, the chances of perforating the artery increased dramatically. He said he would have to make a specially shaped catheter tip to get at the blockage, but he was confident that he could do it.

Early the next morning Gruentzig appeared at Hinden's room. He told Stan and Sara that it had taken much of the night, but he had made what he needed and they would proceed. Hinden was wheeled from his room to the brightly lit catheterization laboratory. Surrounded by assistants and fellows, with Hinden watching on a TV monitor but unable to see much because his view was blocked by lab equipment, Gruentzig took eighty-five minutes to clear the blockages. When he was done he came out of the lab, put his arm around Sara's shoulder, and told her Stan had done fine but would probably have to stay an extra day with a sandbag over the incision in his groin to stop the bleeding.

In two days Hinden flew home to Washington. He did not suffer from heart trouble again until eleven years later, when he had successful bypass surgery complicated by a stroke from which he fully recovered.

On the morning of October 28, 1985, just two and a half months after the Hindens returned to Washington, a rumor swept through Emory Hospital and beyond. Andreas Gruentzig's Beechcraft Baron had gone down in a storm in rural Monroe County, Georgia. Willis Hurst had urged Gruentzig not to fly. Simon Stertzer had urged him to stick to a simpler, one-engine aircraft. Margaret Anne's mother had warned them about the bad weather.

But Gruentzig, as he so frequently did in his personal life, pushed the envelope. Despite the wind and rain, he decided to take off from the little airport on St. Simon's Island because there was a patient in the hospital in Atlanta he wanted to check on. The rumor was true. Gruentzig, forty-six, and his physician wife, Margaret Anne, twenty-seven, were killed in the crash.

His death sent a shock wave through the cardiology community. And if the Hindens are at all representative, its impact was felt by thousands of patients and their families. Twelve years later, Sara Hinden, who said she didn't much like doctors in general, showed genuine emotion when she talked about Gruentzig and the care Stan had received at Emory.

The year of Gruentzig's plane crash, Mason Sones, Charles Dotter, and Melvin Judkins also died. It was truly the end of an era. The legacy these men left collectively is called invasive cardiology. It includes selective coronary angiography, angioplasty, and other catheter-based therapies, including stenting.

The value of angiography had been established by 1967. It made bypass surgery possible. Over four years and in a thousand patients, Sones showed that it worked. Stents were still a year from being tried in humans. Angioplasty was being widely used, and its technology was consistently being improved. But it had not been systematically tested in randomized clinical trials.

During the last eighteen months of his life, Gruentzig pushed hard for a trial comparing angioplasty to bypass surgery for patients with disease in more than one artery. The National Heart, Lung, and Blood Institute was sympathetic to the idea, but his own institution was less so. This was especially true of the cardiovascular surgeons, who thought that Gruentzig had been brought to Emory to do angioplasty on patients with single-vessel disease and, in their opinion, that was enough.

As is common with initial grant proposals, this one was not immediately funded. After Gruentzig's death, however, Spencer King submitted a revised version that received NIH support. The Emory Angioplasty vs. Surgery Trial (EAST) got under way in 1987 (see chapter 11). It was the first of seven major studies in the United States and abroad designed to test the relative efficacy of a treatment that already had been done more than three hundred thousand times in the United States.

By the time EAST was gearing up, improved catheters and new devices to extend the scope of angioplasty were already in the works. Remember John Simpson, the young cardiology fellow at Stanford whom Myler brought to Zurich? He had at that time already begun experimenting with a catheter design that would make it relatively easy for angioplasters to go places in the coronary arteries that were impossible to reach with the early Gruentzig catheters.

Simpson would also make other important contributions, not all of which were clinical or technical. One of these may have changed forever the relationship between physician-researchers and the medical-device industry, further complicating the already interesting ethical issues surrounding interventional cardiology.

10

The Interventionalist as Entrepreneur

Wil Sampson works at home in a large, darkly paneled study with an oriental carpet on the floor. Leaded-glass windows look out onto an ample front garden. Two oversize computer screens glow dimly in the room, which is flooded with sunlight on a warm April morning. His spacious house in affluent Saratoga is a Californian's dream of English Tudor.

Sampson was not born rich, but he was ambitious and persevering. He worked his way through engineering night school in Connecticut by holding a day job at United Technologies. It took ten years. Then he worked for a small medical-device company in Needham, Massachusetts, two and a half hours from his home in South Boston. He broke the evening commute just where the traffic got heavy by stopping off to take an M.B.A. in small-business entrepreneurship at Babson College.

In the late 1970s he took a job with a company that manufactured catheters, and a couple of years later he was lured to California to join what was to become the first major medical-device company in Silicon Valley as its first engineer. Now he has a stake in a company working on a new concept for minimally invasive heart surgery. He is also a passionate advocate for the California way of doing business.

"There's a mind-set in this valley," he said, "that the sky's the limit. Look at the history of California. California is made up of those people who were dissatisfied with the way things were where they came from. That personality trait carries into this state as people who are willing to take risks, to give up their families, to leave the infrastructure behind, to do something different.

"There is a makeup of personality of people out here that perpetuates this thinking—we're going to do something different, we're going to step outside the known boundaries of behavior, of family, in a lot of the things that were so comfortable and predictable . . . a continuing mentality of challenging the status quo."[1]

Sampson denigrated the East as traditional, conformist, unenterprising, and stagnant in its approaches to problem-solving and business. "It's always been done this way," he said mockingly, taking aim at what he views as the smugness of eastern certainty and the conventionality of eastern thinking. His close-set, pale blue eyes crinkled slightly at the corners as he shifted to the California mind-set to ask questions such as: "You tried it how? Tell me again: Exactly what did you do?"

"Now let's change the ground rules," Sampson continued. "If it's been done this way for all these years, let's throw it out the window and do it a different way. If you do it the same way," he concluded, "then predictably you're going to get the same result."

Almost as a footnote, Sampson zeroed in on an attitude toward proprietorship that he sees as emblematic of the difference between the seaboards: "On the East Coast a job applicant says, 'Okay, can you tell me a little bit about the salary and the position that I'll get?' On the West Coast it's, 'How much stock do I get? And what's the vesting?' " He admires what he views as the sophistication of the western approach and believes that this outlook both nourishes and thrives on a freewheeling, fast-acting

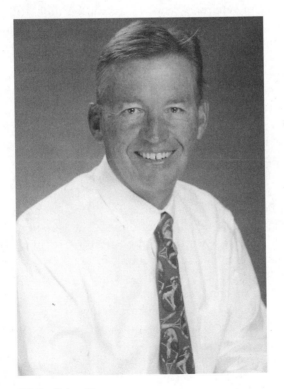

10.1. John Simpson.

entrepreneurial system that encourages risk-taking, rewards success handsomely, and, most importantly, tolerates failure.

In Silicon Valley, years of puttering in a garage on projects that never pan out are often the prelude to starting up a company that is sold in a few years for tens or even hundreds of millions of dollars. Opportunity is never more than an introduction away in the valley. It came for Chuck Taylor when Judie Vivian put him in touch with Federico Benetti. Wil Sampson's opportunity, like that of so many other medical-device entrepreneurs, was provided by John Simpson and Ray Williams.

In the mid-1970s, however, when Sampson was working for the catheter company back East, the chances of Sampson, Simpson and Williams teaming up in a business venture would have seemed extremely remote. At the time, Simpson was completing his medical training at Duke University in Durham, North Carolina.

John Simpson grew up in Lubbock, Texas, started college at Texas Tech, where he did poorly, and transferred to Ohio State, where he both fell in love with science and decided he wanted to be a large-animal veterinarian. He did reasonably well at Ohio State but did not get into any of the nation's handful of veterinary schools. Instead he took a Ph.D. in immunology at the University of Texas's graduate school of biomedical sciences in Houston and over time concluded that he had the wherewithal to practice medicine on human beings.

He was sure throughout medical school, internship, and residency at Duke that he would practice medicine. When Simpson finished his training, he followed a traditional career path for young, promising physicians. He accepted a specialty fellowship at a good academic medical center. In his case it was in cardiology at Stanford.

A year into Stanford's traditional, pharmacology-oriented training program, Simpson noticed an announcement for a lecture on a radical new method of treating peripheral artery disease. "This is a weird thing," he thought, but he said to a young colleague, "If we're going to waste our lunch we might as well waste it over this."[2] The situation was somewhat reminiscent of the time when the young Andreas Gruentzig's chief, Walter Siegenthaler, took him to a small meeting in Frankfurt, where he was exposed to Eberhardt Zeitler's work on peripheral angioplasty.

At the Stanford meeting, as it happens, Gruentzig was the main attraction, presenting *his* work on peripheral angioplasty. But he and Richard Myler, who accompanied him, also presented some very early coronary angioplasty data.

"I had never heard of treating vascular disease with catheters at that point," Simpson said. "It was laughable. I said, 'This guy uses a catheter to fix a diseased artery? Yeah, right.'" When Gruentzig finished talking about opening blockages in leg arteries, he and Myler reported to the group of about thirty polite but highly skeptical Stanford cardiologists on the inflation of balloons in coronary arteries. These were done in patients whose chests had been opened for bypass surgery. They said they improved blood flow through the arteries, but they had no slides to prove that the blockages actually had been reduced.

"I thought the concept could be either awesome or just bizarre," Simpson said. "It could really be incredibly dangerous, or it could be incredibly effective. I told my wife, 'This guy's either going to revolutionize the treatment of coronary disease or he's going to jail.' I was sort of favoring jail at the time."

Simpson also noted that Gruentzig was charismatic, gracious, and politically savvy: "He said all the right things to the right professors." Over the next few years these qualities, as much as Gruentzig's inventiveness and clinical rigor, would transform coronary angioplasty from a frightening curiosity into a standard form of treatment.

At about the same time as the presentation at Stanford, Gruentzig and Myler brought their slide show to the University of California, San Francisco. William Parmley, then chief of cardiology at UCSF, remembers the meeting well. He was impressed with the smooth, self-assured Gruentzig, especially with his intensity. He was also impressed with the slides Gruentzig and Myler showed of the cases they had done. But like their Stanford colleagues, and most cardiologists at the time, Parmley and his colleagues at UCSF were skeptical of the procedure: "That can't possibly work as well as they think it can," Parmley said. "The worry was once you blew up that balloon, what did you really do to the plaque, where does it go, do you get emboli, could you rupture a coronary artery, would you get [clot] formation and all of the bad things you can think of?"[3]

Young John Simpson remained ambivalent about the new procedure. He didn't do anything, however, or even think much about it, until several months later when he was working on a diagnostic catheterization and a piece of plaque broke loose, causing the patient to suffer a major heart attack. He told a colleague that if they'd had Gruentzig's catheter they might have been able to push the plaque up against the arterial wall avoiding the heart attack. As a result of this experience he asked the chief of cardiology, Don Harrison, to introduce him to Myler, which Harrison did.

Soon Simpson began observing and assisting with Myler's cases at St. Mary's Hospital in San Francisco. He asked Myler how he could meet Gruentzig, and Myler generously invited him to breakfast with Gruentzig, who was speaking at the American Heart Association meeting in Miami in late November.

Simpson went to Miami and attended Gruentzig's talk, at which, among other things, the still relatively unknown young German presented the first human coronary angioplasty not done as an adjunct to surgery. Gruentzig spoke in a small room that was not full. "This time," Simpson said, "I thought it was for real." It was going to be, he said to himself, "Gruentzig's last chance to present to an empty seat."

At breakfast the next morning Simpson listened respectfully as the two more experienced men talked. He was excited and now certain that he wanted to be included among the pioneers of what he believed was going to be a truly groundbreaking therapy. Gruentzig told Myler that he was trying to get the Schneider Company to make enough balloon catheters so that a few interested investigators could try out the procedure. Simpson wanted to be among them and said so. Gruentzig seemed receptive.

In January 1978 Simpson traveled to Europe with Myler to see Gruentzig and Martin Kaltenbach do coronary angioplasty. Harrison let him go but made him pay his own way because he viewed the trip as, at best, a skiing boondoggle. They went first to Frankfurt, where Gruentzig and Kaltenbach did the procedure, accomplishing what at the time was considered a major success. They reduced a 90 percent narrowing in a coronary artery to 70 percent. "To us, it was revolutionary," Simpson said. "We declared coronary disease extinct at that moment." But the cases in Zurich were harder, and to the best of Simpson's recollection, none of them worked.

Simpson does fondly remember drinking wine in the late afternoons and into the night and listening to the war stories of the older cardiologists. And on the next-to-last or last night, with everyone mildly under the influence of the wine and fellowship, he remembers Myler promoting the founding of the International Dilatation Society. He acknowledges that he was named Keeper of the Cork they all signed that evening and regrets that he can no longer find it.

When Simpson returned to Stanford, he ordered the devices from Schneider. His goal was to do some experiments and define the issues associated with angioplasty that might need to be tested in clinical trials. Not long afterward a set arrived, including sheathes and guiding catheters through which the balloon-catheters are inserted. But the most important component of the system was missing: There was no balloon.

Simpson by this time had enlisted another cardiology fellow, Ned Robert, to work with him. When the catheter set arrived without the balloon, Simpson, naive but undaunted, proposed to Robert that they make one while waiting for the Schneider balloon to arrive from Zurich. Of course, they had no idea how to go about it and for all practical purposes had no success, although they did make a crude balloon with which they carried out some rather clumsy dog experiments.

They waited several months, but when no balloon arrived, they finally concluded that not only hadn't it come, but that Gruentzig probably had had second thoughts about sharing his discovery with them and that it never would come. They next went to established companies such as United States Catheter and Instrument and tried to get them to manufacture balloon catheters for them, but no one was interested in supplying their minuscule needs. They decided that if they were going to do angioplasty, they would have to figure out how to make the catheters and balloons themselves.

Their cardiology colleagues at Stanford thought they were out of their minds, but they went ahead anyway. They bought tubing from a number of suppliers and in almost total ignorance experimented with various balloon materials, including latex, which, no matter how much air is blown into it, exerts virtually no force, and Teflon, which melts at temperatures lower than those needed to shrink it. But they learned quickly about the properties of materials and techniques for modifying them according to their needs.

Eventually they found a company called Raychem, which made a slippery polymer called RNF-100, which was used as electrical insulation in the U.S. Air Force's state-of-the-art fighter jet the F-4 Phantom. The Raychem sales engineer said that Simpson and Robert could heat the material, and stretch it or shrink it to their requirements. The tubing was irradiated to lock in a chemical bond, which gave it memory, meaning that when the heat or pressure sources were removed it would return to its original shape and dimensions.

A balloon could be created integral to the catheter tube itself by heating short segments of the tubing, and the balloon's ends could be sealed without using adhesive. This was important because Simpson and Robert had not solved the difficult technical problem of bonding a balloon to the end of the catheter. Subsequently, the Raychem sales engineer who taught Simpson and Robert these techniques sued them, claiming that his contribution entitled him to be a coholder of the patent they had been awarded. After years in court, the engineer lost.

Simpson and Robert set up a little shop in Simpson's kitchen. "It drove my wife friggin' crazy," Simpson said. "It smelled awful. We had three little kids running around the house. She said, 'You are crazy. What are you going to do with this? Can't you go out and get a job?' We had no money. My mortgage payment in California was more than my salary [as a cardiology fellow]. That put me in a jam and made my father not too happy because I was borrowing from him. He also said I ought to get a [real] job [as a practicing physician]. Actually I accepted a job with a practice in Jackson, Mississippi, and reneged on it."

Despite the financial pressure, Simpson and Robert stumbled toward their goal by trial and error. Then one day they came up with an idea that seemed natural to them but would revolutionize angioplasty. They decided to run their balloon catheter over a movable wire, much as was done with a diagnostic catheter they were used to using. This would make the balloon catheter easier to manipulate and eventually, they hoped, truly steerable. The Gruentzig catheters, which had only a short, fixed wire attached to the tip, were not steerable and therefore very difficult to manipulate into the orifices of the coronary arteries.

They had to be pushed through stiff guiding catheters with preshaped curves on their ends. That might have worked just fine if all coronary anatomy were the same, but it isn't. There is considerable variability among individuals. The movable-wire hypothesis was a clever solution to the steering problem. Turning it into a workable device, however, would require a lot of engineering.

The wire would have to have several qualities to work. It would have to be stiff enough to function as a rail, but fine enough to slip through a catheter that itself was fine enough to fit into a 3mm coronary artery. It had to be visible on X-ray film. It had to rotate easily so that its tip could be steered into hard-to-reach openings in the coronary system.

At the same time, the tip had to be hard enough not to break but soft enough not to damage the arterial wall. And a balloon catheter had to track over the wire easily. To accomplish this trackability required coiling another wire over the core like a guitar string. None of this had been done before. Their first wire was bought off the shelf from Cook Industries and didn't come close to meeting all the specifications. But it was something they could work with.

By spring 1978 they had built some primitive catheters using a coaxial design, meaning that the tube containing the wire was placed inside the tube with the balloon built into it. They used this design because it was technically difficult to duplicate Gruentzig's so-called double-lumen tube, which had side-by-side channels.

In early 1979, Simpson took one of his catheters to Zurich, but Gruentzig was unimpressed. He said the catheter was too bulky and the balloon was too short. He didn't seem to care one way or the other about the wire, except that its presence in the inner tube prevented the injection of contrast dye through the catheter and eliminated the ability to measure blood pressure between the blockage that was being opened and the aorta.

Gruentzig considered these inabilities major drawbacks because he believed that without a pressure measurement it was impossible to know how stable the lesion was, and without the contrast dye it was hard to tell how much blood flow there was through the artery. As a result, Gruentzig labeled the Simpson-Robert catheter "the blind system." In the end, though, it turned out that the pressure measurements that Gruentzig thought were so important actually were imprecise and therefore not terribly useful, and contrast dye *could* be injected through the guiding catheter to calculate blood flow.

When Simpson got home from Zurich, he and Robert went back to the drawing board in an effort to refine the wire, the catheter, and the balloon. They tried their catheters on dogs, cadavers, and even a baboon. Skepticism remained high among their colleagues, including the chief of cardiology, Don Harrison. The only moral support they got was from Stanford's great heart-transplant surgeon Norman Shumway, who urged them to continue their work.

By mid-1979 their fellowships ended and they accepted junior faculty positions at Stanford so they could continue working on the catheter. At this stage the idea of starting a company seemed both alien and totally unrealistic to them. They knew that the costs involved in getting a new product through the FDA and to market were very high, and they didn't have much idea what venture capital was.

In October they tried out the Simpson-Robert catheter for the first time at the Veterans Administration Hospital where Robert was on staff. They were terrified. The patient lived but was not much improved. "Out of the first ten cases," Simpson said, "I'd say a couple worked a little bit." But "about the ninth case," Simpson said, a patient had to be rushed into emergency bypass surgery, and "that just about brought the program to its knees."

During this period Simpson and Robert were trying to find a company that would manufacture their catheter under license. Simpson made the first foray on his own. He went to USCI. The executives he met with asked him to tell them what he and Robert had done to date and what they were planning to do and said that they would then tell him what they had done and what their plans were. Simpson talked for an hour in great detail about polymers, wires, everything. When he was done the USCI executives told him they hadn't done anything yet. Being an intelligent man, he felt like a fool for divulging so much information to a company that might have no qualms about using it on its own.

Among the many things he didn't know was that a young engineer named Wil Sampson was heading a special catheter-review project for USCI. Sampson's group was evaluating whether the Massachusetts company should sign an agreement with Schneider to become the U.S. manufacturer and distributor of Andreas Gruentzig's balloon catheter. Clearly this new technology represented both medical and business risks, but Sampson reasoned that "to make progress in medicine, you have to stretch the boundaries of what people are comfortable with."[4]

USCI would soon turn the handmade Schneider catheter into a mass-produced device. Along the way they would also improve it by making it smaller and changing its fittings and radio-opaque markings. Two weeks after meeing with Simpson, USCI announced a deal with Schneider that gave them the rights to manufacture the Gruentzig catheter in the United States.

At this point, things were looking a bit bleak for Simpson, Robert, and their invention. But just before they did the procedure for the first time on a human patient, Simpson and his wife had attended a benefit horse show at the Menlo Circus Club. At the benefit, their patent lawyer, Harold Hobach, introduced them to Ray Williams, who was helping out parking cars that evening. Williams had worked for IBM and as a financial officer with Kaiser Health Plan, but by the time he met Simpson, he was a highly sought-after Silicon Valley entrepreneur and investor, mainly in the computer industry.

Hobach had already alerted Williams that Simpson and Robert were working on an improvement for a controversial but promising new way of treating coronary artery disease. Simpson knew nothing about Williams, however. All he saw was a dusty parking lot attendant, to whom he was not about to entrust his precious invention. Simpson told Williams in cursory fashion what he was doing, and the two men parted.

Williams went home, thought about it, analyzed the economic potential of the idea, and decided that it was marginally worth pursuing. But he was up to his ears in computer business and not eager to take anything else on. His wife, however, thought the idea sounded like it might help people. In response to her prodding, he decided to look at it. For the moment, though, the ball was in Simpson's court. He was supposed to call Williams.

But Simpson still did not grasp the importance of Williams' interest. He did not know that bright young men with clever ideas were lining up to work with Williams. Nor did he believe that starting a business was a good idea. So he didn't call. Instead, he went to a company called Datascope in New Jersey. Datascope offered an up-front payment and a small royalty, which sounded reasonably good to Simpson and Robert. But a lengthy document followed that in the view of the patent holders was too complicated and gave the company too many outs if things didn't go well.

A similar scenario ensued with Meditech, a small company run by John Abele, the man who told Richard Myler about Gruentzig and who would go on to found the medical-device giant Boston Scientific Corp. Simpson and Robert turned down this offer, too. After that, they went to a company called Bentley Labs. Carl Simpson, who ran the catheter laboratory at Stanford and who assisted John Simpson and Robert, described how that negotiation fell apart:

"John Simpson is very low-key," he said. "You sometimes wonder, are you dealing with a full deck here or is this guy just very cagey?" The negotiator for Bentley finally got irritated at the slow pace of the talks and said, " 'John, come on. You're acting like you just fell off a turnip truck. Let's really talk a deal here.' This really pissed John off," said Carl Simpson, who is unrelated to John. "There was no more talk with Bentley Labs."

At this point the two young cardiologists concluded that the only way their improved balloon catheter was going to become a practical reality was if they made it themselves. And at about that time Williams called Simpson to ask why he hadn't heard from him and if he was still interested in working together. The answer was "yes," and the three men met at the Stanford catheterization laboratory.

They all remember just how alien the idea of business was to the two doctors. "God, is that really a possibility?" Robert thought.[5] Simpson said, "It's hard to explain how naive I was at the time." And according to Williams: "They kind of sat there and looked at me. I don't think they knew a stock certificate from a corporate bylaw."[6] But they came to an agreement that day under which Williams would provide the cash and own 50 percent of the stock, and Simpson and Robert would supply the patent and split the other 50 percent.

Simpson remembers Williams as a wellspring of optimism. There was no obstacle that could not be overcome, including money. In the beginning, Williams just took out his checkbook and wrote, eventually advancing the fledgling business about $250,000. And later he raised—from venture capitalists—the millions needed to keep the new company going during product development and the lengthy path to regulatory approval.

At last Simpson and Robert could move out of Simpson's kitchen, to the delight of his wife; stop begging Raychem for free tubing; and hire some help to assemble catheters. They moved into a twenty-by-twenty office in Harold Hobach's Palo Alto building and hired Simpson's next-door neighbor, who knew nothing at all about catheters, to start assembling them. Apart from her lack of experience, she had to cope with so much static electricity in the air that all of the early catheters had blue shag from the room's carpet all over them.

Several months later they moved to a fifteen-hundred-square-foot combined manufacturing and office space in Santa Clara. While all this was going on, Simpson and Robert continued doing angioplasties at a rate of about one a month, using the state-of-the-art catheter at that particular moment. Simpson remembers many failures, but he also remembers one case as a spectacular success. They reduced a blockage in a patient's left anterior descending artery from about 99 percent to about 30 percent.

While the two cardiologists kept up their responsibilities as medical faculty members and continued to work on the catheter design, a business was beginning to take shape. In November 1979 they hired Carl Simpson, the former Stanford catheterization laboratory manager, who by then was working for Hewlett-Packard. Simpson had an undergraduate degree in microbiology, an M.B.A, and had studied some chemistry and electrical engineering. He also had worked as an X-ray technician and planned eventually to be a biomedical engineer.

Carl Simpson's title was vice president for marketing. The incipient enterprise was called Advanced Cardiovascular Systems. Both labels were somewhat grandiose. In fact, Carl Simpson did a little of everything, from drafting a regulatory strategy and repairing equipment to taking out garbage and sweeping floors. He had, however, both the managerial and the technical experience to begin putting together a company. He hired a handful of people, and they began to work on all aspects of the product while he also thought about things such as the regulatory process, sales, and marketing.

Sometime later, Ray Williams received a phone call from Wil Sampson. Sampson called Williams because he had heard that Williams was investing in medical-device companies. While working for USCI during the day, Sampson was moonlighting in his basement, trying to put together a company of his own to make catheter tubing and other devices. When Williams was on the East Coast on other business, he stopped by to visit Sampson. He wasn't interested in Sampson's business, however; he was interested in Sampson. Wil Sampson was a bona fide catheter engineer, exactly what Advanced Cardiovascular Systems needed.

But as soon as Williams began to talk about ACS, Sampson stopped him. He regarded any conversation about his joining a company that would be competitive with USCI as a conflict of interest. Williams told him to relax; that things were done differently in California; that people were free to pursue their skills. He invited Sampson out to have a look, but Sampson demurred.

Williams went back to California, and Sampson went back to his basement. But after several months, with things apparently going nowhere, Sampson reconsidered and flew to Santa Clara to visit ACS. He was offered a job, but after testing the Silicon Valley housing market, he decided he couldn't afford to take it. A few months later, however, he met Williams again, at a heart meeting in Miami. Williams urged him to come out for a second look. Sampson said okay. He decided he would ask for what he thought he needed to live well in California and take the job if he got it. He didn't expect to, but he did.

The first day he arrived for work, in March 1981, he said to Carl Simpson, " 'Well, Carl, what do we do from here?' 'I don't know,' Simpson replied. 'That's why you're here.' " Next Sampson asked, " 'Where's your manufacturing area?' 'Don't really have one,' " Simpson said, leading Sampson over to an eight-foot-long wooden bench where two women were blowing up balloons with the help of a bottle of nitrogen gas and a hot-air gun. A balloon popped and one of the women said, " 'Oh, damn, we've lost another one.' " Sampson said he thought he could automate the balloon-blowing operation and asked Simpson for a screwdriver. Simpson said, " 'We don't have any tools here,' " at which point Sampson shook his head and thought, "Oh, my God, what have I done with my career?"[7]

Sampson went straight from ACS's tiny plant to Sears, Roebuck that first day. "I walked down the aisle," he said, "and I'm putting in socket sets and screwdrivers and every possible tool that would relate to this industry. The salesman, I think, had a record day."[8]

Sampson's arrival more or less marked the beginning of the transition of ACS from a mom-and-pop business with half a dozen employes to a serious high-tech company with a full staff. When he came on board, ACS had, in the Silicon Valley lawyer Casey McGlynn's phrase, "married the clinician to the engineer."

Sampson was the person they needed to help them gear up to perfect and mass-produce tubing, balloons, and wire, the key components of the product. ACS had no in-house capability to make any of these things when he arrived, and in the beginning lacked the money as well as the expertise to do so. But by the time Sampson joined the company, Ray Williams was no longer the sole source of funding; by then venture capitalists who were sold on the idea and believers in Williams had invested several million dollars, and ACS could buy materials, invest in more sophisticated equipment, and hire the professionals and skilled labor it needed.

A key concern for ACS at this stage of its development was how to guarantee a secure supply of plastic tubing to make catheters. Ordinary assembly-line tubing would not be good enough. For ACS's purposes the tubing had to be strengthened by exposure to radiation, in precisely the right dose, so it would be tough enough without becoming brittle and would have memory. ACS had been buying tubing in small quantities from Raychem. But Raychem had decided that it would no longer supply ACS.

This meant that ACS would have to buy off-the-shelf tubing and irradiate it, a delicate process requiring a great deal of precision to get maximum strength without brittleness. No one at ACS had any idea how to do it. They got lucky, though. Wil Sampson met and was able to hire an engineer named Deepak Gandhi, who knew how to irradiate tubing. When ACS began producing its own tubing, Gandhi took it to Boston, bought time on an electron beam, and gave it the needed strength and memory.

Another difficult task was getting the guidewires just right. They were working with fine lengths of stainless steel wire, using one piece as a core and coiling another around it. The finished product looked like a very thin guitar string. But they couldn't make these fine wires steerable enough, and they couldn't get the tips soft enough to allay their concerns about perforating or dissecting arteries. No one at ACS had figured out how to make the wires sufficiently steerable and the tips sufficiently soft.

Over time, however, the engineers and clinicians, working together, developed several techniques. If they tapered the wire, it became more steerable, and if they snipped off the tip of the core and let the springlike outer wire go floppy at the end, it would, in Wil Sampson's analogy, be as soft as an overcooked noodle.

Then they learned by trial and error how to use heat to take the bias—a natural tendency to flop 180 degrees one way or another—out of the wire. This enabled them to control the rotation of the catheter tip so it could be steered through switchbacks and doglegs into the coronary arteries' openings. It was far from perfect. The tip needed to be easier to guide, and the steerability had to be much better. But these were steps in the right direction.

By heat-treating the wires to just the right degree, they could get a one-to-one response. In other words, however much they turned the control end, the movement at the business end would be identical, which made it much easier to maneuver the balloon catheter into the target artery. They also learned to make the core's tip flat so it would buckle like a ribbon on contact with the arterial wall. To gauge the softness, Wil Sampson devised a simple test that involved pressing the tip of the wire into the tip of his tongue. If it hurt, the wire wasn't soft enough. The ACS engineers also figured out how to make the catheter tip radio-opaque so it could easily be seen under fluoroscopy as it moved through the arterial system.

These were the creative days at ACS. Once the product began making its way slowly through the FDA review process, however, attention shifted to the no less challenging task of marketing a catheter that Andreas Gruentzig had labeled "blind" and that was in competition with a device Gruentzig had invented himself; that had been improved upon substantially; that was being manufactured and sold by USCI, a major force in the medical-device industry; and that was supported by Richard Myler, angioplasty's leading apostle on the West Coast, and Simon Stertzer, his counterpart on the East Coast. Moreover, by 1982 Gruentzig had come around to the advantages of a movable-steerable wire, and USCI was already making an over-the-wire catheter that was better than the one ACS had so far developed.

The difference this innovation made for interventional cardiologists and their patients, according to Spencer King, was profound. In the two years "after steerable guidewires became available," he said, "the clinical success rate increased from 79 percent to 91 percent and the emergency bypass surgery rate decreased from 7.2 percent to 2.8 percent."[9]

However, the market ACS and USCI were competing for was minuscule. Estimates vary as to how many angioplasties were done in the United States in the late 1970s, but by 1981 the NIH registry listed only three thousand cases. And there were only about thirty laboratories nationwide in which the procedure was being done. But in the mideighties, angioplasty exploded. In 1984, forty-six thousand procedures were done, and by 1985 the number had soared to eighty-two thousand.[10] Just as with bypass surgery, angioplasty took off without having to go through clinical trials, and it was an instant cash cow for cardiologists and hospitals. What's more, it had a very appealing quality for patients: It wasn't open-chest surgery.

When the Simpson-Robert catheter was approved by the FDA on March 3, 1982, it was, like most new medical devices, still far from perfect. "The biggest problem for a long time," John Simpson said, "was the balloon profile. We could get there with the guidewires, but maybe not be able to cross the lesion." The wires, too, were far from perfect, however. There were still bias problems, for example, as a result of which John Simpson did a number of demonstration cases using USCI wires. Predictably this drove the ACS management to distraction. But the upshot was that within weeks they responded with a high-torque, floppy guidewire that by the late 1980s had become the dominant wire in the marketplace.

Even though the market was still small in the early 1980s, and the product was still being perfected, the large Indianapolis-based drug and device company, Eli Lilly decided that angioplasty had a big future and made a bid for ACS, an offer that John Simpson says he wasn't aware of until shortly before an acquisition agreement was reached. When the deal was concluded in March 1984, it was on what is known in the financial world as an earn-out basis. This means that stockholders of the company being sold receive an up-front payment and then over a set period the company must meet negotiated earnings targets to maximize the sale price.

In the case of ACS the period was five years, all targets were met, and because of increases in the value of Lilly stock, the total price paid for ACS could be valued as high as $500 million. Not bad for a three-year-old company that had barely sold its first catheter when the takeover was begun. Even though by the time the deal was done venture capitalists owned a fair chunk of the company, Simpson and Robert were now rich men, and Williams was even richer. Robert had dropped out of active participation in the company before the sale to go into full-time practice. Simpson, on the other hand, has remained an important innovator in interventional cardiology and has gone on to found several other companies.

11

Trials and Errors

In a mildly disconcerting touch of whimsy, the catheterization laboratory at Emory University Hospital in Atlanta, Georgia, has purple, lavender, yellow, green, and orange butterflies painted on its ceiling. Spencer King, dressed in scrubs and a shower cap, was at work in the lab. He was gloved, masked, and tending to a prone patient covered up to his neck with blue sheeting. The patient's head was hidden behind a curtain of wide plastic strips. A movable X-ray camera suspended from a metal arch hovered above him. A panel of four television monitors stood alongside the operating table.

The control room, like those in television broadcasting studios, was filled with dials, knobs, and monitors. A glass wall separated it from the lab, where King and two assistants were performing angioplasty on four severely diseased coronary arteries in an eighty-year-old male patient. It was a complicated case that even in 1996 many cardiologists would have sent to surgery. The TV screens in the control room duplicated those in the lab. The upper pair showed slides of the blocked arteries. One of the lower screens was blank. The other showed the catheter with its curved tip and tiny, built-in balloon advancing against a background of densely packed little vessels. They looked more like algae than arteries until a squirt of dye briefly gave them definition.

King bobbed over the patient, eyes on the TV screens, delicately manipulating the catheter with his fingertips, inching the balloon through a tortuous channel to the blockage. The operator's image through the control room window was slightly eerie, something like a praying mantis playing a video game. From time to time King asked in a soft, southern accent for a new slide showing a different view. A sound system wafted his voice into the control room, where an efficient young woman changed the slides as quickly as if King's brain waves had gone straight to her hand.

King stepped back from the table and removed a new catheter from a long plastic coil. He reshaped the tip slightly to ease its entry into a tiny lateral artery, slipped it through a sheath in the patient's groin, into a guiding catheter, and carefully maneuvered it through the femoral artery toward its target.

An assistant directed the patient, who was under local anesthetic: "Sir, can you put your right hand behind your head and your left hand down by your side? There you go." King twisted the catheter. The screen flooded with dye. "If you feel any chest pain, that'd be normal now. They're working with the balloon." What looked like a Pollock drip painting came into view on the screen. "Big breath in! Big breath in! Now breathe normally. How are you feeling?" The patient indicated with a slight hand motion that he was okay.

Meanwhile, the image on the screen had changed to a forest—a tangle of dark branches against a background of sunlight. A horizonlike curve rimmed by a bright, narrow band filled the top of the screen. "Any pain at all in your chest with that?" King asked. I couldn't hear the patient's response. The procedure was over.

Seconds later King was in the control room, cap, mask, and gloves off. A colleague breezed through and said there was a 100 percent chance that the procedure would have to be repeated. King agreed that it was virtually certain that this patient would be back within six months with some recurrence of at least one blockage. But he said it might not need to be treated.

On the way back to his office he stopped to tell someone that he would rather do another case that day than hold it over until the next day. He also stopped in the waiting room to chat with the family of one of his patients. He seemed about as relaxed as a man who had just finished a day of fly fishing and was looking forward to cooking and eating his speckled trout.

Back in his office in Emory's Andreas Gruentzig Cardiovascular Center, King described the case. The patient had two severe blockages in the right coronary artery, severe blockages in two diagonal-branch arteries, and a milder blockage in the left anterior descending artery. "These are the kinds of things that ten years ago would have been quite a *tour de force*," King said. "We would have made a big deal of a case like this and probably would have turned it down. But now with the very flexible wires, and very flexible catheters and small-profile balloon-catheters, we can get into all those little side branches and open them reasonably well, as we did today."[1]

Spencer King can. So can many of the best interventional cardiologists who perform hundreds of interventions a year. But what about the average operators in community hospitals around the country who do ten or twenty angioplasties a year? Many of them wouldn't try. And there is widespread agreement that they shouldn't. But others might. There are no regulations to prevent it, although the American College of Cardiology and the American Heart Association are pressing for standards.

King performed this challenging four-vessel angioplasty almost a decade after subjects were randomized for the first clinical trial comparing angioplasty to bypass surgery. The trial's principal investigator was Spencer King, and its first results had been reported less than two years earlier. King's patient this day would have been rejected as a subject because at the time of randomization his case would have been considered far too difficult for angioplasty. He would have had open-chest bypass surgery.

Of all the things angioplasty has going for it, by far the most important is that it is not surgery. Who, after all, wants surgery? What patient, all other things being equal, would say saw my chest open, or even cut a little hole in it? But what if all other things are not exactly equal, which in fact is usually the case?

What if, for example, surgery gives you a nine-in-ten chance of being angina-free for fifteen years without a repeat procedure, and with angioplasty the chances are four in ten that you'll need a repeat procedure in six months? Or what if you are offered a choice between angioplasty, which involves a very small incision done under local anesthetic with little convalescent time and only a small risk of death, heart attack, or stroke, and taking pills for the rest of your life? These are the tougher, more realistic choices faced by most people with coronary artery disease.

But inconvenience, discomfort, period of convalescence, and small differences in procedural risk are not the only, or even the most important, issues. Most of all, you would probably like to know with which of these treatments, including surgery, you can expect to live longer, or live better, or be at less risk for a heart attack or a stroke. You want to know whether two prominent Harvard cardiologists were right when they wrote in 1997 that angioplasty "may not substantially reduce the risk of myocardial infarction [heart attack] or prolong life."[2]

There is no absolutely certain way to answer these questions for any given individual. But randomized clinical trials, which compare treatments to other treatments or placebos, are designed to help physicians and patients calculate the odds for mortality, morbidity, and more and more these days, for having a good quality of life.

Proponents of so-called evidence-based medicine, which relies on the careful application of clinical-trial and other study results to specific cases, say that these data, rigorously applied, will produce the best outcomes in large populations. They argue that their approach saves lives by replacing old-fashioned medical art with modern medical science. "Art kills," David L. Sackett, one of the movement's founders, bluntly told a *New York Times* reporter. "It was the art that gave us purging, puking, leeches, the gastric freeze, all that sort of stuff."[3]

Nonetheless, the collected results of the best randomized clinical trials often are either ambiguous or, when a new treatment is compared to a standard treatment, show only a small advantage for one over the other. In comparative trials large numbers of subjects are needed to get a statistically significant result, which means they are very expensive to conduct. This sometimes leads to trials with subject populations that are too small, yielding results that are not useful and wasting millions of dollars.

An alternative to clinical trials for figuring out how to treat a specific patient is called outcomes analysis. It involves searching large databases kept by academic medical centers, professional societies, and the federal government, and comparing how all patients with relevantly similar conditions fared with different treatments. Outcomes studies have the advantages of being much cheaper than clinical trials and of not excluding, for example, the very old and the very sick, as clinical trials often do. But because outcomes studies are not randomized, the patients whose records are reviewed may differ from one another in some relevant way that has not been detected by the investigators and that therefore might mislead them about the cause of the outcome—death, heart attack, etc.

Physicians can learn a great deal from randomized trial results and outcomes data, but neither provides a foolproof formula for choosing the right treatment. In deciding how to treat an individual, they also must rely on an additional range of knowledge, talent, and skill, including up-to-date awareness of progress in the field; their own clinical experience; ability to interpret and apply complex study results; adroitness in eliciting information from patients; sensitivity to subtle clinical signs; ability to administer, read, and interpret high-tech diagnostic tests such as echocardiograms, and more.

Without these other attributes, the best clinical-trial and outcomes data will be about as useful in choosing treatments as reading the best books on basketball will be in turning a schoolyard hoopster into Michael Jordan. Put another way, the most important variable in medicine about which a potential patient has any choice is the physician. And the choice of a hospital is a close second.

It would be nice to be able to assure those patients who are lucky enough to be under the care of a first-rate clinician that once they have been diagnosed and their cardiologist knows everything that can be known about their case, and all of the clinical trial and outcomes data are in hand, that the best single choice of treatment, at least in terms of longevity and quality of life, will emerge logically and inevitably. But this is not always so, for a variety of reasons. For one thing, while most diagnostic tests, if they are competently administered and interpreted, are quite good at identifying the existence of coronary artery disease and its physiological effects, they can be unreliable or even useless as guides to selecting the best form of treatment. Imaging technologies are improving rapidly but still have quite a way to go before they will be able to provide the kind of high-resolution, three-dimensional pictures needed to take the remaining guesswork out of treatment selection.

Although clinical trials "are accorded an almost religious sanctification,"[4] they are not always more helpful. While most of the major trials described in this book have demonstrable value, they also have notable weaknesses. Some of their findings are statistically insignificant or inconclusive, others conflict with one another or are hard to interpret, and still others are incomplete or out-of-date when they become available. They may also be irrelevant to the case at hand.

The conclusions of randomized studies comparing forms of treatment often sound something like this one, reported in the journal *Circulation* in July 1997: "Procedural success of rotational atherectomy is superior to laser angioplasty and balloon angioplasty; however, it does not result in better late outcomes." In other words, chances are you will end up about the same no matter which of these three treatments you get. And even the short-term difference is only about 10 percent.[5] What's more, even if you get the optimal treatment in a clinical trial, there seems to be less than a fifty-fifty chance that it will improve your chances of living longer than you would have without the treatment.[6]

It may begin to sound as if it is impossible, except by luck, to get the right treatment; or, alternatively, that it doesn't much matter which treatment you get. But such conclusions would be overdrawn. In fact, some treatments are better than others for some people; clinical trials and outcomes studies sometimes help match these treatments to the right patients, and even if they don't increase longevity, they may improve quality of life, reduce costs, or both.

Unless a case is unusually straightforward, though, it takes a well-trained, thoughtful, diligent cardiologist to evaluate it well. How many cardiologists have these qualities? John Kirklin has written that "the perpetually increasing demands on surgeons, pediatric cardiologists and adult cardiologists, and their responses to these demands, have resulted in their being, as a group, less contemplative, less able to understand intimately the special circumstances of each of their patients, and perhaps less fit to help patients with heart disease make the many complex decisions required."[7]

The cardiologists who diagnose with subtlety and accuracy, and who best understand the idiosyncrasies of each individual patient and his or her disease, may not be the most innovative researchers; they may not be the most skilled operators in the catheterization laboratory; but they may be the most valuable clinicians because they do better than others in guiding their patients toward treatment choices that are most appropriate for them. Their special gifts, which are becoming rarer all the time, are clinical judgment and clinical skills—that is to say, using the most basic methods to figure out what is wrong with a patient and the best way to fix it. Even their most research-oriented colleagues at least pay lip service to these qualities as the defining characteristics of a first-rate physician, a skilled, sensitive practitioner of the art of medicine.

Clinical judgment is not an exact science, which is where the art comes in. Each person, as Kirklin suggests, is a distinct entity, anatomically, physiologically, and psychologically, and the clinician must take account of the differences. Each person's disease is also distinct, and that, too, must be taken into account. Furthermore, since randomized clinical-trial results as reported in the medical journals provide only generalizations, there is no way of being absolutely sure, except in some relatively small number of clear-cut cases, that for patient X angioplasty is a better choice than drugs or surgery.

All we can know with certainty, and with hindsight, is that the treatment worked or it didn't; that the patient survived, or not; that he had or didn't have a stroke or a heart attack, and needed or didn't need follow-up bypass surgery or repeat angioplasty. Maybe drugs would have worked just as well as or better than angioplasty. Or maybe bypass surgery as a first choice would have given seventeen angina-free years instead of seven.

Yet, now that angioplasty has been around for more than twenty years and has become the most common form of interventional treatment for coronary artery disease, shouldn't cardiologists know more precisely on which patients it will work at least as well as surgery or drugs? The commonsensical answer to this question is an easy yes. But because common sense and science work differently, it may not always be easy or yes. To understand why this is so requires a basic grasp of four things: the conservatism of medicine; how biomedical scientists test the safety and effectiveness of new treatments; the kinds of answers these tests yield; and the rapid developments that take place in medicine while the clinical studies plod along.

Consider first medical conservatism. Doctors are trained to react with skepticism when they are exposed to a new idea or to a new drug, device, or procedure. James Herrick called it "the paralyzing influence of the dead hand of tradition,"[8] and it explains in part the reception of Herrick's papers on heart attacks, John Gibbon's heart-lung machine, Mason Sones's selective coronary angiography, and René Favaloro's bypass surgery. In these examples, the leading skeptics were the pillars of the medical establishment, the Charles Friedbergs, Willis Hursts, and Eugene Braunwalds. This is to be expected, and even Herrick would have agreed that it is not only to be expected, but probably as it should be.

In science—and especially biomedical science—it is not enough to demonstrate that something works once, or twice, or even a dozen times. It must be shown that it can be repeated successfully—and safely—thousands of times. History is littered with examples of promising cures, such as flecainide acetate for certain arrhythmias, fast-acting calcium channel blockers for angina, and the classics cited above by Sackett that sometimes turned out to be worse than the disease.

But there is a difference between perfectly appropriate skepticism and small-minded scoffing, which is what Herrick seems to have had in mind. Often what slows the progress of a promising new treatment is the latter rather than the former. Doctors get locked into a mind-set about what can and cannot be done: you cannot suture the heart; you cannot inject dye into the coronary arteries; you cannot put catheters into the coronary arteries. This negativism may close their minds to a new procedure for years.

Scoffing conservatism not only slows the acceptance of a new procedure such as angioplasty, it also puts a roadblock in front of clinical trials to test it. Because clinical trials are very expensive to conduct, frequently costing tens of millions of dollars, and not always conclusive, or even widely used in decision-making,[9] a certain critical mass has to be reached and a high barrier of skepticism scaled before it is possible to get a large study funded.

It was ten years before the first such trial comparing angioplasty to bypass surgery got under way. It was the Emory Angioplasty vs. Surgery Trial (EAST), first proposed to the National Institutes of Health by Andreas Gruentzig, and its usefulness will be assessed here. Today, a new device-based procedure like angioplasty would have to undergo at least one small trial to test its safety and efficacy before it could be used in a large, randomized clinical trial, but as late as 1978, when angioplasty was first done in the United States, this was not the case. All that was required at the time was to get approval from a hospital institutional review board—the in-house committee whose job is to protect the rights of research subjects—and to notify the FDA.

In the case of angioplasty, seventeen years had passed before the first trial results were finally reported in the peer-reviewed literature.[10] In that year, 1994, angioplasty was done 428,000 times in the United States, and it had been the most prevalent form of invasive treatment for coronary artery disease for four years. What's more, several new types of catheter-based treatment had been added to the interventional armamentarium, techniques and technology for treating complicated disease with balloon angioplasty had advanced considerably, and minimally invasive surgery was spreading rapidly and becoming competitive with angioplasty.

Of what possible use was a trial, or trials, based on old devices, old methods, and old treatment paradigms? Was the money thrown away? A closer look at BARI (Bypass Angioplasty Revascularization Investigation), a large, multicenter trial, and EAST, a smaller, single-center trial, will help answer these questions. Let's look at EAST first.

EAST

EAST was funded by the National Heart, Lung, and Blood Institute a decade after the birth of coronary angioplasty to see how angioplasty compared to bypass surgery with respect to blood flow to the heart muscle, heart attacks, and death. When its results were reported in 1994 they showed no statistically significant difference between the two procedures for any of the three end points.

In 1987 it became the first of the major angioplasty-vs.-surgery trials worldwide to get under way. An important measure of its success, in Spencer King's words, would be the extent to which it helped "patients and physicians . . . struggle with the decision of which procedure to select."[11]

The trial included as subjects only those patients whose arteries were so diseased that treatment with drugs was no longer considered an option, who had at least two blocked arteries, and who were seen as equally good candidates for angioplasty or surgery. This meant that patients with severe disease for whom surgery had been shown to increase longevity were excluded. Patients who had already had either bypass surgery or angioplasty also were excluded, as were patients with certain other characteristics, such as a recent heart attack or serious congestive heart failure.

Less than 2.4 percent of the 16,499 patients who were initially screened were enrolled in the trial. Of this original group, only 5,118 had more than two blocked arteries and no prior bypass surgery or angioplasty. Of these patients, 4,085 were excluded because they had one or more of the characteristics listed above or because of other factors.[12] Of the remaining 1,033 patients, 191 were rejected because one or the other of the two procedures—bypass surgery or angioplasty—could not be carried out safely. This left 842 eligible patients. Of these, 353 were ruled out because their referring physicians had a clear preference for one procedure or the other, leaving 489 patients available for randomization. Of these, 97 refused to participate, bringing the number of actual enrollees to 392, or 7.7 percent of the 5,118 who met the initial criteria. The remaining 450 eligible but unrandomized patients were enrolled in a registry, a detail of some importance that we will return to.

The 392 randomized subjects were representative of only a very small percentage of patients with coronary artery disease. What's more, technological advances that occurred during the seven years between randomization and the availability of EAST's first results to practicing cardiologists dramatically changed the playing field. In a 1995 cost and quality-of-life study the trialists noted that "all areas examined in EAST" were "moving targets."[13]

Better balloons and balloon-catheters, stents, atherectomy devices, Rotablators, and more had become available by the time Spencer King did angioplasty on his eighty-year-old man in 1996. Angioplasty operators could attack hard-to-reach lesions, excise long lesions, ablate calcified lesions, and insert scaffolding to keep arteries from shutting down, none of which was possible when EAST began.

New antianginal and cholesterol-reducing drug combinations were also available, and new clot-inhibiting drugs that had the potential for sharply reducing heart attacks during or just after angioplasty were about to come on the market. Intravascular ultrasound and other sophisticated imaging technologies could now be used to help evaluate the architecture and composition of lesions. Indeed, cardiac-care technology was advancing so quickly that even as the 1995 quality-of-life study was announcing that surgery was "changing the least" of all the treatments for coronary artery disease, Heartport and CardioThoracic Systems were racing toward human trials of minimally invasive bypass surgery, the biggest advance in heart surgery in thirty years.

In the years during which EAST was under way, new knowledge, like new technology, was revising the way cardiologists thought about treating coronary artery disease. It became known during this period, for example, that the lesions most likely to cause heart attacks and death were not the most obstructive, most easily identifiable ones that cardiologists and surgeons traditionally have treated. They were relatively small, unstable lesions that seemed to be profuse, were having little or no effect on blood flow to the heart muscle, and were difficult or impossible to identify angiographically.

These plaques, however, were fragile and therefore likely to rupture and promote the formation of a blood clot, which could completely close the artery causing a heart attack and possibly death. Arteries partly blocked by more stable, more obstructive plaques, on the other hand, seemed to develop a collateral blood supply through tiny blood vessels that helped prevent heart attacks by rerouting blood around the blockages.

Recognition that these vulnerable plaques cause most heart attacks is not a categorical argument against bypassing or doing angioplasty on all or even most severely blocked major vessels, however. It has been known for twenty years that while neither angioplasty nor bypass surgery prevents heart attacks, both reduce angina and increase exercise tolerance by increasing blood flow through significantly obstructed coronary arteries.

But this new understanding of what causes heart attacks does cast doubt on the value of these invasive treatments for some unknown percentage of patients, and on the usefulness of EAST's main finding. Since by 1994 it was already known that neither angioplasty nor bypass surgery prevents heart attacks—and therefore death from heart attacks—how much have we learned from EAST's combined primary end point, two of whose three components were death and heart attacks?

Despite what hindsight tells us about the pace and magnitude of technological change and the accretion of new knowledge, at the time, EAST seemed to make sense. Although angioplasty had been in use for a decade, no one knew with the certainty provided by a well-designed, well-conducted clinical trial whether it was a wise option for large numbers of patients. Good science seemed to dictate that a controlled study be mounted.

So the investigators moved ahead with their select group of patients, randomizing 194 to surgery and 198 to angioplasty. Their primary goal was to find out whether outcomes would differ based on three events: (1) death from any cause, (2) heart attack, and (3) a significant inadequacy in blood flow to a large segment of heart muscle. This combined end point was used because the number of subjects was too small to get a statistically significant result for the single end point of death from all causes alone. Secondary goals were to find out which procedure reduced angina more; which had a better (or less negative) effect on congestive heart failure; which did more to increase exercise ability; and which required fewer additional procedures, whether surgery or angioplasty.

All 392 patients were treated and examined every six months for three years, with angiograms being done one year and three years after treatment. The results were published in October 1994 in the *New England Journal of Medicine,* and the main finding was that there was no statistically significant difference between the two forms of treatment with respect to the primary composite end point of death, heart attack, and compromised blood flow to the heart muscle. One of these three things occurred in 27.3 percent of the patients treated surgically and in 28.8 percent of the patients treated with angioplasty.

There was a major, albeit unsurprising, difference, however, in an important secondary end point. After three years the number of patients who needed repeat procedures was substantially higher among the patients initially treated with angioplasty. Only 1 percent of the surgical group needed repeat surgery, and 13 percent needed angioplasty. In the angioplasty group, 22 percent needed surgery, and 41 percent needed repeat angioplasty. Surgery also did significantly better in getting blood to the heart muscle and in reducing angina pain.

From all of these results the investigators drew the overarching conclusion that "the selection of one procedure over the other should be guided by patients' preferences regarding the quality of life and the possible need for subsequent procedures."[14] This conclusion is hardly dramatic, but the findings on which it is based might help some patients in the gray zone overlapping balloon angioplasty and standard bypass surgery to identify the trade-offs between the two procedures.

However, even this is uncertain. Indeed, the EAST investigators themselves expressed doubt in 1994 that the trial had answered the main questions it had been design to answer.[15]

Another important issue discussed at length in the EAST paper, although it is not listed among the end points of the study, is the degree of revascularization, the extent to which all arteries with compromised blood flow were opened enough to restore the best possible blood flow to all segments of the heart muscle. By all measures, surgery provided significantly better revascularization.[16]

From the early days of angioplasty there has been a debate between surgeons and angioplasty operators about the virtues of "complete revascularization," with surgeons favoring this treatment strategy and angioplasters preferring to treat only what they call the culprit lesions, which is to say the ones they believe are most likely to cause angina or a heart attack.

The angioplasty operators argue that because their intervention requires only a minor incision and is done under local anesthetic, it makes sense to do only what is necessary and wait to see if additional revascularization is required. The surgeons reason that once the patient's chest is open it makes sense to take care of as much as possible to avoid having to open it again. There is also a financial dimension to the argument. An initial strategy of surgery is roughly twice as expensive as angioplasty. But repeat angioplasties can come close to eliminating the difference. One consequence of this is that interventional cardiologists can earn almost as much money as cardiac surgeons, a rarity in medicine where surgeons typically earn much more than their medical colleagues.

EAST was the first of seven trials designed to test similar hypotheses about the comparative advantages and drawbacks of angioplasty and bypass surgery in multivessel disease. The largest of these trials was the Bypass Angioplasty Revascularization Investigation (BARI).

BARI

The BARI trial, like EAST, was funded by the National Heart, Lung, and Blood Institute, and it was similar to the Emory study in its goals and randomization criteria. But it was substantially larger, enrolling 1,829 subjects at eighteen centers in the United States and Canada, and therefore substantially more expensive, costing $47.5 million. It also established a registry of 2,013 patients who were eligible for enrollment but refused randomization, and 422 who were ineligible.

Like EAST, BARI was designed to test the hypothesis that initial treatment with angioplasty rather than bypass surgery did not compromise patient outcomes. But because of its larger size and five-year term, BARI was able to produce a statistically significant result, although just barely, using the single end point of mortality from all causes. The BARI trial was also big enough to allow investigators to analyze results in subgroups such as patients with diabetes.[17]

In the protocol for their study, the BARI investigators asserted that "Evidence from this clinical trial will provide a scientific basis for choosing [angioplasty] or [bypass surgery] as the initial revascularization treatment of severe multivessel coronary disease."[18] While more forcefully phrased than Spencer King's modest expression of hope that EAST would help cardiologists "struggle with the decision of which procedure to select," the assertion by the BARI investigators amounts to the same thing.

The BARI conclusions, also published in the *New England Journal of Medicine* (July 25, 1996), were strikingly similar to EAST's conclusions published two years earlier. "As compared with [bypass surgery], an initial strategy of [angioplasty] did not significantly compromise five-year survival in patients with multivessel disease, although subsequent revascularization was required more often with this strategy."[19]

Like EAST, BARI showed that angioplasty was no riskier than surgery, but that with angioplasty there was a much greater chance that a patient would need another procedure (54% for angioplasty vs. 8% for surgery). Sixty percent of the BARI subjects and 77 percent of the EAST subjects who were randomized to angioplasty avoided surgery.

Toward the end of their first publication, the BARI investigators noted a survey suggesting that only about "12 percent of all patients who required coronary revascularization would be eligible for the BARI trial." As a result of BARI's exclusions, patients with the most serious disease—the kind that stand to benefit the most from surgery—were not randomized.

The National Heart, Lung, and Blood Institute has spent about $56.5 million on BARI and EAST. They have reached virtually identical conclusions, and their results are substantially similar to those of five trials conducted abroad. EAST and BARI were by most standards well-designed, well-conducted clinical trials for which a significant need undoubtedly was seen by many investigators at the time they began. Yet their findings are not very helpful clinically.

Instead, they raise such questions as: What has been learned from these studies and with how much certainty? How applicable are the data to saving lives and improving quality of life? Could the same or more important things have been learned for less money?

Both trials showed that an initial strategy of angioplasty rather than bypass surgery did not increase mortality or heart-attack rates. But these studies also found that compared to bypass surgery, angioplasty did not improve the overall outcome of patients with multivessel coronary artery disease, reduce their risk of suffering a heart attack, or improve their quality of life.

What the trials accomplished was to confirm with a high level of confidence what two decades of experience, collected in registries, had shown: that a decision about whether to treat patients with the same disease profile as the study subjects by surgery or angioplasty—that is, relatively straightforward cases of multivessel disease that were considered treatable by angioplasty twenty years ago—would have to be made on grounds other than mortality or heart-attack rates. These grounds might include a patient's dread of surgery, or his or her desire to avoid the repeat procedures so common after angioplasty. This confirmation was reassuring, but since it affected a relatively small number of patients, it was a minor payoff for the investment.

A combined analysis of eight trials comparing angioplasty and bypass surgery was published in 1995 in the British medical journal *Lancet*, with results closely approximating those of BARI and EAST.[20] In the same issue of the *Lancet*, a commentary strongly suggested that this study would be of little or no help to cardiologists in advising their patients on what treatment to choose. It cites many reasons why this might be so, all of which apply to EAST and BARI. Among them are the fact that only a small minority of patients suitable for either bypass surgery or angioplasty were randomized in the trials, which means that the trial results can only be applied to this small minority; the possibility that results might vary in subgroups such as women and the elderly, but that the studies' subgroups were too small for these differences to be detected; and, similarly, that there might be significant but undetectable differences between patients with two blocked arteries and those with three.[21]

The commentary also called attention to a report based on data from Duke University showing equivalent three-year survival rates for patients with two- and three-vessel disease treated with either angioplasty or bypass surgery.[22] Although the Duke report was based on a retrospective review, it covered 6,210 patients and might have been as good a measure of survival as the eight-trial analysis, which covered 3,371 subjects.

Daniel Mark, the lead author of the Duke study, has written elsewhere, however, that to properly evaluate the appropriateness of a treatment choice such as the one between angioplasty and bypass surgery takes five to ten years. It is only over this period of study, he argues, that both survival and quality of life can be fairly tested. At the same time, he points out that it is impractical to compare quality of care over such a long period because by the time the outcome can be identified, the treatment responsible for it has usually changed substantially,[23] which was the case with EAST and BARI.

At the time, angioplasty had been compared to drug therapy in three controlled studies. The first was a small single-vessel disease study known as ACME, in which only 212 patients were randomized.[24] The results of this trial, to the extent that they are generalizable at all, apply only to the very small group of patients who have a single, less-than-total blockage, who suffer from angina only while exercising, whose angina is not getting worse, whose anginal episodes are not long-lasting, and who have not had angioplasty or bypass surgery. Angioplasty was found to increase exercise tolerance and reduce angina somewhat as compared to drug therapy for these patients, but at a price of more complications and higher cost. Two subsequent trials—the Second Randomized Intervention Treatment of Angina trial (RITA II) and the Veterans Affairs Non-Q-Wave Infarction Strategies in Hospital study (VANQWISH), yielded similar results.[25]

Edwin L. Alderman, a Stanford researcher and BARI investigator, thinks that if the BARI and EAST patients had been treated with drugs they might have suffered even fewer premature deaths and heart attacks than those treated with angioplasty or surgery. And he and Javier Botas write further:

> It is possible that if modern antianginal medications [such as beta blockers and calcium channel blockers], aspirin, lipid-lowering drugs, and intensive risk-factor management had been available, the clinical outcomes with medical therapy would have been even more favorable. The implication . . . is

that, unless there are compelling anatomic or symptomatic reasons to proceed with revascularization, there is no evidence that deferral of revascularization combined with intensive medical treatment places patients at risk of premature death or infarction.[26]

It is unlikely that a large enough trial to adequately compare angioplasty to medical therapy in patients with multivessel disease will be carried out. The main reason is cost. Because heart attack and stroke rates are very low (in the range of 1 to 3 percent) for patients who are candidates for both drug treatment and angioplasty no matter which treatment they receive, it would require a very large number of subjects to find out if there is a statistically significant difference between the two treatments. A trial enrolling enough patients to meet this goal would be very expensive. The same is undoubtedly true of a trial attempting to determine whether the optimum treatment for these patients would involve using a combination of angioplasty and drug therapy, or stents.

Alderman also points out that the value of using drugs and risk-factor modification to counter atherosclerosis was "less well-publicized, less well studied and less well reimbursed than revascularization strategies."[27] In other words, these strategies are not as sexy, not as well understood, not as appealing to patients, and not as lucrative for practitioners.

12

Interventional Cardiology Expands

In 1978, at about the time John Simpson began working on his angioplasty catheter at Stanford, a young Argentine radiologist arrived in the small town of Martinez, California, about fifty miles away, to begin a residency. He was attracted to the United States because he wanted to do research, and the prospects were dim at home. His name was Julio Palmaz, and his research led to the development of the coronary stent, a device that went on the market in 1994, and in 1998—just three and a half years later—was used in half a million procedures.[1]

Not too long after arriving in the United States, Palmaz went to a meeting of the Society of Cardiovascular Interventional Radiology in New Orleans. While there he attended a lecture on percutaneous transluminal coronary angioplasty delivered by the only person in the world who had done it—Andreas Gruentzig. The audience gave Gruentzig a standing ovation. Palmaz was among the impressed. What impressed him most of all was that while Gruentzig poetically likened a good result to "a clear footprint in fresh snow," he was also willing to candidly present examples of failures of his procedure.

He remembers Gruentzig showing slides of arteries that had been split open by the balloon and clots that had formed in treated arteries. Gruentzig also reported that some arteries recoiled like rubber when the balloon was removed, again restricting blood flow to the heart muscle. Palmaz's reaction, as he recalled it in late 1997, was to ask himself: "Why not do something? It was almost an obvious thing to me, you know, like a mine tunnel that is crumbling; put something there to keep it open."[2]

The idea seemed simple enough. Indeed, it had occurred to Alexis Carrel, who experimented unsuccessfully with glass tubes in animal arteries early in the twentieth century. And in the 1960s Charles Dotter inserted stainless steel and nickel-titanium tubes in the peripheral arteries of animals, demonstrating the feasibility of what is now called stenting.[3] But in fact the concept of coronary stenting was radical and at first would be almost universally rejected by cardiologists. It was just a few months earlier, after all, that Gruentzig had become the first person to put a balloon catheter into a human coronary artery. And despite the success of this procedure, angioplasty was still seen by many cardiologists as a disaster waiting to happen. Most mainstream cardiologists viewed putting a rigid piece of metal inside a coronary artery and leaving it there as somewhere between unreasonably risky and certifiably loony.

But Palmaz didn't know that. He just went back to Martinez and began playing with bits of wire and rubber tubing. His idea was to use a balloon like Gruentzig's to expand a tiny metal scaffold that would be rigid enough to keep an artery open after angioplasty. In those days, however, a medical resident had even less free time than now. Moreover, like many physicians who have ideas about how to solve clinical problems, Palmaz had no more idea than John Simpson of the engineering problems involved, such as how to weld the tiny bits of stainless steel.

As a result, over the next few years he made little progress. During this time, however, he wrote a monograph addressing the mechanical feasibility of making a safe device tiny enough to be delivered to a coronary artery and rigid enough to remain fixed in place. He did this not with the intention of publishing it, but just to get his thoughts in order.

By early 1983, Palmaz had built a somewhat oversized model out of copper, which was relatively easy to work with because he could solder it instead of welding it, and he began trying to find a manufacturer. He had no success, partly because the model was relatively crude, but mainly because the concept had almost no supporters. Palmaz remained convinced, however, that he had something.

Then one day he wandered into his garage and noticed a worker nailing a metal lattice to studs in the wall. In a flash of insight sparked by seeing this mesh framework for applying cement, he realized that he could avoid difficult welds by making his stent out of a single piece of stainless steel wire. The basic design would be tubular, about 15mm long, with narrow slots. When expanded, the slots would become diamond-shaped.

Palmaz still had no idea how to actually fabricate a device tiny enough to fit into a coronary artery. But a couple of months later he was introduced to a retired Stanford rocket scientist named Wernher Schultz, who had arrived in the United States with Wernher von Braun. Palmaz showed him his monograph and drawings, and Schultz immediately had three or four suggestions about how to handle various elements of the manufacturing process, including arc welding, electron-beam welding, laser cutting, and photo etching. A few weeks later, however, he suffered a ruptured abdominal aortic aneurysm and died.

After the death of his recently found technical adviser, Palmaz saw no reason to remain in the small town of Martinez. He had an offer from a radiologist mentor of his named Stewart Reuter to come to the University of Texas Health Sciences Center in San Antonio, which he accepted. He continued working on the stent, but without grant money. Before long he was substantially in debt to the University of Texas.

Palmaz offered the university ownership of the patent on his stent, but no one there believed it would amount to anything, so they turned it down. He also showed his handmade device to more companies, all of which also turned it down. Meanwhile, Palmaz was testing it in dogs and getting good results.

In 1985, seven years after the idea began to germinate, Palmaz went to the Southwest Research Foundation in San Antonio in search of funds but was told that if he wanted to work in their labs he would have to bring his own money. While they didn't give him any cash, they did introduce him to another young cardiologist they thought would share his research interests. His name was Richard Schatz. "Richard was fiddling around with monkeys, balloons, and things," Palmaz said.[4] Schatz, like Palmaz, was interested in restenosis, the poorly understood process that caused arteries to close up again after they had been opened by angioplasty. He thought stents might be a solution to this Achilles' heel of angioplasty.

After a couple of failed experiments with monkeys, the two researchers switched to dogs, and the results were good: The stents kept the arteries from closing. But still there was no money, until one day Schatz told Palmaz that he had found someone who might be interested in supporting the project. This was a businessman named Philip Romano, who had founded a fast-food chain with the unlikely name of Fuddrucker's. "Philip came completely out of the blue," Palmaz said. "He had no medical knowledge, but he fell in love with the idea. He gave us a $250,000 grant, which at the time was magnificent."[5]

With Romano's money, Palmaz and Schatz were able to take the time and pay for the engineering support needed to refine the device. Schatz figured out how to make the stent more flexible by shortening it and dividing it into two or three segments. In later designs the segments were connected to one another by a single strut. These innovation made the stent easier to introduce into the coronary arteries. In November 1985 the two partners applied for a patent (granted in 1988) while continuing their animal studies.

During the mid-1980s, experiments with stents were also being conducted in France, Switzerland, the Soviet Union, and Champaign, Illinois. The first implantation in a human was done by Jacques Puel in Toulouse, France, in March 1986. In June of that year, during a live demonstration course at University Hospital in Lausanne, Ulrich Sigwart implanted a self-expanding mesh stent in the totally blocked left coronary artery of a fifty-year-old woman. Six weeks later he implanted an identical stent in her right coronary artery. Ten years later she was asymptomatic.[6] Nevertheless, for various reasons, the stents developed abroad and in Illinois were not immediately granted FDA approval and therefore could not compete in the U.S. market.[7]

By 1987 Palmaz and Schatz were ready to submit a request to the FDA for an investigational device exemption (IDE). The IDE, which constitutes FDA permission to begin testing a new device in human subjects, is granted after the federal agency conducts a preliminary review of the device itself and supporting data, including the results of animal tests. In that same year Schatz implanted a Palmaz-Schatz stent in the coronary artery of a patient in Brazil. The IDE, which was granted, permitted Palmaz and Schatz to place stents in peripheral arteries only, not coronaries.

At the same time, Romano, who had been exploring the commercial prospects of the stent, brought the device to Johnson & Johnson, which was eager to get into the cardiovascular device business. The company hired a consulting firm to evaluate the project, and they recommended against it. But Johnson & Johnson decided to take a chance on the stent even though it had not yet been approved for peripheral let alone coronary use by the FDA.

Human trials in peripheral arteries were carried out successfully, and in 1991 the FDA approved the Palmaz-Schatz stent for noncoronary use. Meanwhile, two trials comparing combined use of the Palmaz-Schatz device and angioplasty to angioplasty alone had gotten under way.[8] In 1994 they both showed that stented arteries were more likely to remain open enough to provide adequate blood flow to the heart muscle than those treated only with balloon angioplasty. Following these trials, the FDA granted approval for unrestricted use of the Palmaz-Schatz stent in coronary arteries.[9]

By this time, sixteen years after Palmaz first made his analogy between a blocked artery and a collapsed mine shaft, a consensus had formed that stents represented both a major advance in coronary care and a major business opportunity. Oddly, it was an opportunity that Silicon Valley missed. By 1999, however, companies such as Guidant (a Lilly spin-off that included the ACS division founded by John Simpson), Medtronic, and Boston Scientific, were battering Johnson & Johnson with improvements on the Palmaz-Schatz theme.

This proliferation of new devices suggested the need for a period of reflection. In 1998 Spencer B. King III, by then the incoming president of the American College of Cardiology, wrote in a special article for the college's journal that "Improved methods for evaluating these stents in an efficient, cost-effective manner are needed."

King also believes there is a need to address "off-label use," which refers to the application of a device or a drug to a situation for which it has not been specifically approved, a common—and legal—practice in American medicine.[10] Eric Topol of the Cleveland Clinic wrote in the *New England Journal of Medicine* at the end of 1998 that "in hospitals throughout the United States" stents are used for various kinds of severe coronary disease "even though there are no data to support these applications."[11]

As with bypass surgery and angioplasty, however, commerce was driving the pace. There was no reflective pause. By the end of the 1990s the field had expanded and had become fiercely competitive, but Johnson & Johnson's gamble had already paid off handsomely. The company had reaped fat profits—many think way too fat—and was positioned as the dominant player. By 1997 the Palmaz-Schatz stent, which reputedly costs less than $2 to make, was selling for about $1,600. More than two million of them had been implanted, and J&J had roughly a 75 percent share of a rapidly growing market, valued at $1.5 billion a year. And in 1998 there was a quantum leap in stent placement. In that year alone about eight hundred thousand stents were implanted in the United States.

Johnson & Johnson took a calculated business risk at a time when others thought it was unwise. Palmaz says J&J deserves a lot of credit because he and Schatz could never have taken it all the way on their own. But Johnson & Johnson's development costs would have had to have been outrageously high to justify the kind of profit margin—estimated at 85 to 90 percent[12]—that the company has been making on this product. To date no one has explained the size of the margin in anything other than monopolistic terms. Repeated calls to Johnson & Johnson yielded frustration rather than clarification on this point.

In theory, the competition for the expanding stent market should bring the price of the device itself down substantially. But the placing of a stent, or, as frequently happens, more than one stent, remains a complicated business. Besides the stents, the complete procedure usually requires the use of a balloon catheter and several other devices, all of which are expensive. Stenting also requires a slightly longer hospital stay than angioplasty or even minimally invasive bypass surgery. And only time will tell if its future is as bright as so many think.

John Simpson, for one, still worries about leaving a piece of metal in a coronary artery. He also notes that Jacques Puel, the first cardiologist to place a stent in a human being, has cut back sharply because of concerns about plaque formation within the stent itself.

Simpson believes better solutions to reblocking of arteries are likely to be developed, but not for a decade or so. However long it takes, though, the solution will almost certainly come from private industry working closely with an inventive physician. The U.S. system of device development may be fraught with conflicts of interest and potential for profiteering, but it does seem to find answers to concrete problems, such as how to get more blood to the heart.

One has to wonder, though, whether the coming together of intellectual power and money in a bottom-line-oriented enterprise translates into safer, more effective medicine, or whether it encourages overly aggressive medicine that carries more risks than benefits. Interventional cardiology may be the ideal case for studying this question because it is more than just a medical subspecialty. It is a closely linked assemblage of technology-based therapies and lucrative business opportunities.

I didn't fully grasp this until I attended the ninth annual Transcatheter Cardiovascular Therapeutics (TCT) conference in Washington, D.C., where John Simpson was being honored for his lifelong contribution to interventional cardiology, and Julio Palmaz was in attendance. This great big, world-class interventional-cardiology scientific meeting, run by a private cardiology group that practices at Washington Hospital Center, is joined at the hip with a world-class interventional-cardiology trade show. And the line between medicine and trade is blurry.

Apart from the overt commercialism of the 105 companies on the exhibition floor, physicians promote products in the plenary sessions, sometimes covertly and sometimes brazenly, and breakout sessions are explicitly devoted to pushing new products. At the end of 1997, Valentin Fuster, the incoming president of the American Heart Association, said TCT "is owned by industry. It's very troublesome."[13] And the vice chairman of the Cardiology Department at the Cleveland Clinic, Steven Nissen, said cardiology's close link to industry "isn't just a minor problem in medicine. It affects hundreds of thousands of patients and the whole way interventional cardiology is practiced" in terms of how and why treatment decisions are made.[14]

Martin Leon, the Washington interventional cardiologist who ran the meeting with the flair of a Borscht Belt tummler, praised products during the plenary sessions as they flashed by on the four floor-to-ceiling screens arrayed at the front of the arena-sized auditorium.

If Leon was outdone in theatricality, it was only by the Italian cardiologist Antonio Colombo and his patient Mario Da Vinci. Beamed by satellite directly from Milan, Colombo appeared larger than life on one of the four screens and announced to the audience that his patient, stretched out on the table in front of him and awaiting angioplasty, was about to sing. A guitarist strolled into the catheterization laboratory, and Da Vinci launched into a full-throated version of "O Sole Mio" as Colombo began catheterizing him. After a generous round of applause mixed with laughter,

Da Vinci, while undergoing the procedure, did "Come Back to Sorrento" as an encore.

To be sure, most of the satellite time was devoted to new trends in cardiology, not Neapolitan schmaltz, but the entire meeting was redolent of entertainment and salesmanship. To what extent is this four-day, multimillion-dollar extravaganza, which physicians pay $1,200 a head to attend, emblematic of the subspecialty of interventional cardiology? It's hard to say precisely, but it is probably more typical of the high-tech medical and surgical specialties than it is of medicine generally.

The conference is a major draw, with more than five thousand interventionalists attending, making it a gold mine for device companies, which spend millions of dollars on their exhibits. John Simpson's Perclose system for sealing groin incisions was featured at one of the dozens of small sessions held outside the plenary. Such sessions are run by the companies, which pick their own speakers, although the meeting's program does not mention this.

Of course, most physicians who practice interventional cardiology do not treat it as a get-rich-quick scheme. They believe in what they do, and if they do it more often than they should, usually it is not for mercenary reasons. Inappropriate angioplasties might be done, for example, because of what some cardiologists call the "oculostenotic reflex." This can be paraphrased roughly as "I see a blockage, therefore I fix it," even if there is not a physiological reason for doing it.

It is also possible, however, that greed is the right lens for viewing the dynamics of interventional cardiology understood as a business; that traditional liberal assumptions about money as a motivator in medicine are wrong. Maybe the benefits of financial incentives for talented physician-researchers outweigh the costs, at least with respect to device development.

To examine whether greed is good in interventional cardiology, consider the four ways by which interventional cardiologists can make fortunes in their field. The first is simply by practicing medicine long enough at several hundred thousand dollars a year, an option as long as the health-care financing system doesn't change. The second is by inventing new devices and licensing them to established companies, as Tom Fogarty and others have done. The third way is to start a company and run it, or to sell it in a few years—as John Simpson did with ACS—to one of the medical-device giants such as Johnson & Johnson or Boston Scientific. And the fourth is to acquire a large equity stake in a company that makes a promising new device like the Rotablator, as Maurice Buchbinder did with Heart Technology, Inc.

In each case, money, in varying degrees, is a motivator. Patients, however, have little interest in physicians' motives, unless they compromise good therapeutic outcomes. What they need to know is: Does a money-motivated system produce better health care for Americans than the practical alternatives? Does it do so without unduly compromising the safety of research subjects and patients? Does it do so cost-effectively? And does it do so in a timely fashion?

The financial relationship between research-oriented cardiologists and the medical-device industry is at the epicenter of the system. Obviously there can be no such industry without the participation of cardiologists at every stage. Cardiologists identify the research questions that need to be answered; they usually provide key insights that lead to technological solutions; they conduct the clinical trials; and they administer the new device-based treatment once it is approved for use. The relevant question therefore is not what their role in device development should be, or whether it is appropriate, but rather whether cardiologists should have a direct stake in the financial success of a device they have helped develop or test.

An ethicist's knee-jerk response to this question is likely to be no, on the ground that anything that might deflect a clinician's attention from a patient's best interests, or a physician-researcher from giving appropriate weight to a subject's best interests, is bad on the face of it. But a clinician might take a slightly different view. He or she might ask whether medical innovation would dry up if there were no financial incentives for physicians to invent devices. If the financial incentives for invention were minimal, would people like John Simpson still invent medical devices?

It is true that in the past physicians such as John Gibbon invented devices without the promise of huge financial rewards. But these are different times. It took Gibbon a quarter century and a gift from IBM to make a heart-lung machine that worked on humans. Few researchers would stick to something that long in today's medico-economic environment, and few companies would fund it without taking a piece of the action.

Thanks to entrepreneurialism, however, the pace and the volume of new-device development have increased substantially since the 1980s. The mantra of innovation, according to the science writer Stephen S. Hall, is "discovery creates value."[15] But value for whom? For the public or just for the discoverers?

I believe there are two closely linked reasons for the rapid pace of innovation. One is that interventional cardiology is perceived as a growth industry capable of generating large profits for some time to come. The worldwide market is already large and expected to expand, and the development cost for devices—compared to drugs—is relatively low.

The other reason is that interventional cardiology is technology-driven, and the nature of technology companies is to compete by replacing one generation of products as quickly as possible with the next. Just as Microsoft keeps churning out new operating systems, and Intel faster microprocessors, so cardiovascular device companies make and market new devices to ream out and ratchet open clogged arteries as fast as they can. First came balloons; then atherectomy devices with spinning blades; then little, whirring, diamond-studded burrs; then lasers; then stents; then biologically coated stents, drug-delivery stents, and so on.

Of course, just as it is not clear how much Windows 98 added to a PC owner's ease of use or efficiency, so it is not yet clear how much some of the new interventional devices have benefited the million or so patients a year worldwide who are treated with nonsurgical cardiac interventions. Innovation does not always yield improvement. Lasers, for example, have so far proved largely ineffective for opening blocked coronary arteries, although they are currently getting a second look. And the only proved benefit of stents is that they reduce the need for a repeat angioplasty.

Some new devices fill small but important treatment niches and are therefore minor but welcome additions to the therapeutic arsenal. To date, however, there have been few completed and no definitive clinical trials comparing new devices to balloon angioplasty. Twenty years after its invention, the balloon is still the standard for interventional cardiology, just as open-chest surgery remains the standard for coronary artery bypass operations.

Even the balloon, however, is being overused. Indeed, some experts charge that it is being grossly overused. Stephen Oesterle, director of interventional cardiology at Massachusetts General Hospital, believes that "50 percent of the angioplasty that goes on is unnecessary."[16] Most of the cardiologists interviewed for this book agreed in principle with Oesterle. Some thought his 50 percent figure might be high but declined to give their own estimates. A Texas cardiologist in private practice who didn't want to be identified said he thought Oesterle's number was somewhat high but that 25 to 35 percent would be a reasonable guess. Using a low-end estimate, the calculation yields 250,000 patients worldwide being treated with angioplasty they don't need. One hundred thousand of these excess cases would be in the United States, where eight times as many angioplasties are done than in Great Britain or Canada, countries where most doctors get the same pay from the national health system no matter how many procedures they do.[17]

Financial incentives to use one form of treatment over another pose conflicts of interest. It does not require a leap of the imagination to surmise that there might be a connection between the high rates of compensation for doing angioplasty and the number of times it is done. Medicare pays interventional cardiologists $863.63 for a single-vessel angioplasty and

$1,152.68 for placing one stent. Most managed-care plans pay 20 percent above the Medicare rate. Because the interventionalist's fee drops sharply if he or she opens additional arteries during the same procedure, there is also a financial incentive for doing the procedures in stages. These procedures take from twenty minutes to an hour and a half, depending on the degree of difficulty.

Another conflict of interest arises in research when an investigator with a financial stake in the outcome of a clinical trial is allowed to participate in the design of the trial, oversee the enrollment of subjects, the collection of data, or influence crucial decisions such as whether the trial should be called off before running its full course. Each of these involvements presents an opportunity for the investigator to bias the trial's outcome in a way that favors his or her interests. In the worst case, some trial subjects or future patients may die if, for example, this bias causes investigators to overlook potentially life-threatening flaws in the device or the drug.

This kind of bias can be minimized, however, even without forcing the physician in question to get rid of his or her equity. For example, a stock-holding physician-inventor, whose expertise is seen as both unique and important to the successful conduct of a trial, might serve as a consultant with no responsibility for sensitive decisions such as those related to design and subject recruitment. Distancing the inventor from the decision-making process would not eliminate all risk of investigator bias, but it would provide a safeguard.

There is no such simple solution, however, for principal investigators or others with decision-making authority. Unless these researchers are completely free of financial conflicts of interest there will always be legitimate concern, even if small, that the results might be compromised. The common practice of requiring them to disclose stock ownership rather than sell the stock is inadequate. Disclosing equity ownership may diminish the ability of investigators to bias trials—by putting their colleagues on guard—but it cannot eliminate bias entirely; nor does it in any way diminish the investigator's interest in seeing the trial prove the device safe and effective.

Similarly, such investigators should not be able to hold stock options that can be exercised when the trial is completed, nor should their close family members be able to hold such stock or stock options. There is too much at stake in a trial involving hundreds if not thousands of subjects, tens of millions of dollars, and perhaps millions of patients in the future to allow even a suggestion that conflicts of interest have compromised the outcome.

Even when investigators have neither equity holding nor consulting relationships with drug or device manufacturers, other kinds of financial considerations may bias their judgment and decisions. Baruch Brody points out, for example, that the prospect of profiting from a grant, or of losing a grant, might influence an investigator "to pressure patients to participate in clinical trials" or to continue or stop trials inappropriately.[18]

For most physicians who write about ethical issues in American medicine, conflict-of-interest problems begin and end with clinical trials. But what about a physician-inventor's conflict of interest in his clinical practice if he has gone on the road as a paid speaker promoting a new drug or device or if he owns stock in the company? Is it in the best interest of a potential candidate for an intervention, for example, to be diagnosed and treated by a cardiologist who has a financial interest in David Auth's Rotablator, or John Simpson's directional atherectomy device, both of which have limited applications?

When asked, cardiologists and cardiac surgeons seemed to agree that major shareholdings in device or drug companies can represent a serious conflict of interest for a practicing physician, but they frequently disagreed about what constitutes a major holding. One interventional cardiologist said his ten-thousand share holding in a device company was too small to influence his decisions. He did not say whether there was some amount he thought might influence his care of patients.

An amount that might strongly influence one physician's judgment or behavior might have zero impact on another's. The most effective way to eliminate this conflict of interest altogether would be to ban cardiologists and other clinicians from having any financial interest in any devices used in their practice.

There is another approach, however, that seems more practical. It entails both disclosure and changes in medical decision-making. And it deals simultaneously with several critical problems of contemporary cardiology practice. To begin with, it would substantially ameliorate the equity-ownership conflict of interest. But more importantly, it would largely get rid of a much larger and more widespread conflict of interest: self-referral. Self-referral as I am using the term can occur when a clinical cardiologist doubles as an interventional cardiologist or practices in a group with interventional cardiologists.

Both types of conflict arise when treatment choices are made. This happens because these choices determine, among other things, who gets paid and how much, and which device, or devices, if any, will be used. The choices are: Should there be any treatment at all? If treatment is needed, should it be surgery, one of a range of interventions performed by cardiologists, or drugs? Or should it be some combination of the above?

In today's medical marketplace, the critical diagnosis is often made by a cardiologist who does interventions himself, or even if he doesn't do interventions, he belongs to a group in which interventions are done. If, based on the diagnosis, the recommended treatment is an intervention other than surgery—stenting, for example—and if the patient is referred to an interventional cardiologist in the diagnosing cardiologist's group to have the procedure, it counts as self-referral.

The conflict of interest in this situation is based on the following considerations. Treatment choices are often less than clear-cut. Many patients are potential candidates for surgery, interventions, or drug treatment, and honest cardiologists might differ on which treatment would be best. The choice of treatment therefore might be influenced by financial considerations. If the recommended treatment is surgery, the group will receive nothing. And if the patient is treated with an intervention rather than drugs, the group will earn more.

Then, if intervention is chosen, a decision must be made, based on the composition, architecture, and location of the blockage, among other things, as to what the specific intervention should be. If the diagnosing cardiologist, or any of his partners, has a financial interest in a device company, there is another conflict of interest.

Chances are overwhelming that patients will be unaware of any conflicts of interest. What's more, even those who happen to have this knowledge are unlikely to be willing or able to do much about it. One reason for this is that even today, or perhaps especially today, in the impersonal world of managed care, patients want more than ever to trust the doctors in whose hands they find themselves.

While many are better informed about medicine than typical patients twenty years ago, most still want to believe their doctors can make them whole again. These patients often do not want to raise hostile-sounding questions that threaten to shatter a fragile bond with a specialist they might never have seen before, and to whom they have been referred by a primary-care physician they might not know much better. Moreover, even if they know about specific conflicts of interest, it is only in rare cases that they know enough to intelligently question a cardiologist's recommendation and adequately evaluate the response.

There are two complementary ways to protect patients' interests and to defuse conflict-of-interest concerns in these circumstances. One is to institute a policy of full disclosure, and the other is to change the way treatment choices are made.

First, patients should not be forced to ask whether physicians have financial conflicts of interest relevant to their treatment choice; they should be told as a matter of course. If, for example, they are possible candidates for balloon angioplasty, rotational atherectomy, or directional atherectomy, and if the cardiologist owns stock in a company that makes any of the devices used in these procedures, patients should be advised of that. They are then at least put on notice that the cardiologist has a conflict of interest that might favor angioplasty, or atherectomy generally, or one kind of atherectomy in particular.

The notification should be in writing, and it should explain in clear English the significance of the conflict. Moreover, it should be presented to the patient in a way that encourages questions about alternative forms of treatment and does not discourage the patient from seeking another opinion. In most cases such disclosure will not outweigh a physician's authoritative recommendation of one device over another, nor will it turn all patients into sophisticated, coolheaded health-care consumers. But it should improve some patients' chances of getting appropriate treatment.

And second, consultative decision-making should be institutionalized. Before the days of interventional cardiology, when the choice was just between surgery and drugs, a close call was often made by a cardiologist in consultation with a surgeon. Older cardiologists and surgeons still speak favorably of this system, and some use it. There is even a mild groundswell of opinion that something like it might help resolve today's conflict-of-interest controversy. The 1998–99 presidents of the American Heart Association, Valentin Fuster,[19] and the American College of Cardiology, Spencer B. King III,[20] support this kind of approach.

More and more practices today are made up of both clinical cardiologists, who do noninvasive diagnostic tests and prescribe drugs, and invasive cardiologists, who do invasive diagnostic tests, therapeutic interventions, and prescribe drugs as adjuncts to their interventional treatment. Interdisciplinary consultation requires a separation of the income streams of the clinical and the invasive cardiologists.

Probably the best way to acomplish this would be by having clinical and invasive cardiologists practice in separate groups, a voluntary change that would have to be encouraged by professional societies. Clinical cardiologists would still diagnose patients and either treat them with drugs or refer them to an invasive-cardiology group for angiograms or other invasive diagnostic tests. When test results favor catheter-based interventions and adjunctive drug therapy, the interventional cardiologists would carry out these treatments.

But before any patient was treated interventionally or surgically, except in emergencies, one clinical and one interventional cardiolgist and a surgeon would review the diagnostic-test results and try to reach a consensus on a treatment choice. These consultants would not have to leave their offices to consult with one another. All of the patients' test results, including echocardiograms and angiographic film, would be available to them on their computer screens to review at a convenient time. The consensus recommendation would then be presented to the patient by the diagnosing clinical cardiologist. He or she would also specify the other options examined and explain why they were rejected.

If a consensus did not emerge, the clinical cardiologist who brought the case to the board would then present to the patient the options considered, pointing out their advantages and drawbacks, and make his or her own treatment recommendation. Neither the decision-makers nor colleagues in their practice would be eligible to perform the recommended procedure. Cardiologists and cardiac surgeons would serve as decision-makers on a rotating basis.

The system need not be cumbersome or impractical, although it would depend on the willingness of busy physicians to volunteer some time. The biggest problem it would face would be acceptance by interventional cardiologists because it would require them to share their decision-making authority with others and probably would result in a significant reduction in the number of interventional procedures done.

Medicare, insurance companies, and HMOs, on the other hand, would like such a change precisely because it would reduce the number of expensive procedures. And they, of course, are in a position to put pressure on invasive cardiologists, most of whom depend on them for the majority of their patients.

A related proposal, by Fuster and Ira Nash of Mount Sinai Medical Center in New York, while primarily aimed at reducing the number of cardiologists and increasing the numbers of primary-care physicians, would also address the conflict-of-interest problems. Fuster and Nash's idea is to offer a five-year post-medical-school training program that would board-certify young physicians in internal medicine with special competence in cardiovascular disease.

Physicians who have completed the program would be qualified to do noninvasive cardiac diagnostic tests, with the exception of the most advanced imaging techniques, and to evaluate and manage "prevalent cardiovascular illness."[21] These specially trained internists could care for most heart patients, thereby cutting back on the need for fully trained clinical cardiologists.

Under the scheme proposed here these internists could serve on the decision-making panels in place of clinical cardiologists, thereby increasing the pool of physicians available for this key task designed to eliminate self-referral. It might also reduce the oversupply of interventional cardiologists, most of whom also do clinical cardiology,[22] which would lower the number of interventional procedures.

With fewer procedures being done, managed-care organizations would have an easier time identifying the best operators and the worst. Lack of access to HMO patients, combined with stricter practice guidelines and certification examinations now being developed by the American Heart Association and the American College of Cardiology, would then squeeze the least-qualified interventionalists out of the marketplace.

However, if a hundred thousand or more unnecessary angioplasties and other interventional procedures such as stenting really are being done annually in the United States, this suggests that something more than just the financial interests of some cardiologists, or even the oversupply of interventional cardiologists, is responsible for the excess. Treatment decisions, after all, are based on many variables, some or all of which may outweigh financial considerations. These include patients' preferences, variance in physicians' clinical judgment, the quality of evidence drawn from clinical trials and case registries, and the proficiency with which the evidence is applied to specific cases. These factors almost certainly influence quality of care much more than financial conflicts of interest.

13

How Healing Can Harm

The past thirty years have been a time of remarkable progress in treating the symptoms of coronary artery disease. Bypass surgery, various catheter-based interventions, and a plethora of new drugs have become available to stock the shelves of a previously all-but-bare armamentarium. But with only a few exceptions, these new treatments are what Lewis Thomas has called "halfway" technologies;[1] while improving quality of life, they do not extend it.

At a more basic level, a new consensus has emerged in recent years about what triggers most heart attacks. For decades it had been assumed that there was a direct relationship between the degree of arterial narrowing caused by the slow buildup of fatty and fibrous material and the risk of a heart attack. Now almost all cardiologists are convinced that the composition of the arterial plaque and its vulnerability to rupture and clot formation, not the degree of narrowing it causes, correlate most closely with risk.

And at last researchers are beginning to unravel the complex interaction of physical and biochemical forces at the root of atherosclerosis—the disease that precipitates the event—although multiple perplexities remain. These developments have made the nineties an exciting and generally optimistic decade for heart researchers.

But investigators remain bedeviled by two unsolved mysteries. The first is a detection problem: how to identify the vulnerable plaques—custardy on the inside and fibrous on the outside—that are usually unsymptomatic until they rupture, setting off the devastating chain of events that causes most heart attacks. The second is how to stop the deadly, inexorable atherosclerotic process itself. When these two questions are answered it will be possible to identify trouble on the way in unsymptomatic patients and take preventive measures.

The disease process is complex. New elements keep being identified. But its end stage in most cases is a blood clot, an aggregation of cellular and extracellular materials normally produced by the body at the site of an injury to keep the injured person from bleeding to death. If blood did not clot in response to injury, wounded soldiers, victims of car accidents, and people who slit their fingers in the kitchen would die from loss of blood. Because hemophiliacs lack clotting factors in their blood, they may die from superficial cuts. However, if a clot forms in response to an injury inside a major coronary artery and blocks it for too long, instead of saving the injured person, the clot will kill him or her.

Because it has been well established for about twenty years that clots cause most heart attacks, drugs have been mobilized to dissolve them. This treatment, called thrombolysis, or thrombolytic therapy, works—when it works at all—roughly speaking in the first six hours after the attack. In recent years emergency angioplasty, sometimes combined with stenting, also has been used to quickly open arteries blocked by clots. Perhaps as many as twenty-five thousand lives are saved annually as a result of these two treatments.[2]

Primary angioplasty, as it is called, appears to reduce brain hemorrhages better than thrombolytic therapy.[3] But like all other treatments to date, neither thrombolytic drugs nor primary angioplasty saves everyone. They do not attack atherosclerosis, they undermine collateral circulation that may be providing blood flow to the heart muscle, they do not prevent deadly clots from forming, and they may even cause them by showering debris downstream (thrombolysis) or rupturing a vulnerable plaque (angioplasty). And, of course, they do not guarantee that a patient will get to a hospital fast enough for the treatment to do any good, or that the patient will get to a hospital where the treatment can be done. In 1997, for example, only 21 percent of American hospitals had facilities to do angioplasty, and not all of those could do emergency angioplasty.[4]

Now, however, the research focus has shifted. The rest of our story of treating coronary artery disease, except for the emergency role of clot-dissolving drugs and angioplasty, is not about relatively primitive plumbing-type solutions analogous to rerouting corroded pipes or removing hair balls with snakes or Drāno. It is about ending corrosion and blockages by manipulating the living cells in the walls of arteries and those that circulate in the blood, which is to say controlling the disease process. Late in the twentieth century, cardiologists have refocused their research on James Herrick's prescient insight into clots as the cause of heart attacks—an insight most of them largely ignored for about a quarter century. This means they can finally move beyond palliation and get on with the business of prevention and cure.

While Herrick believed that blood clots caused heart attacks, he could only demonstrate their presence in coronary arteries at autopsy. This was not good enough to prove that they were a cause of death, or even, for that matter, of heart attacks. Indeed, various postmortem studies after Herrick showed no clots in some heart-attack deaths. It was not until 1980 that the University of Washington's Marcus DeWood, by performing angiography on 517 patients in the early stages of heart attacks, showed that in most cases clots had totally blocked the vessels. The essential correctness of Herrick's hypothesis was proved.[5] DeWood's findings also provided the intellectual underpinning for generalizing a brilliant clinical innovation by a physician in Göttingen, Germany, named Peter Rentrop.[6]

Rentrop was doing an angiogram on a patient who had had a heart attack some time before and was again suffering from chest pain. While on the table under local anesthetic with a catheter inserted through his femoral artery, its tip lodged in one of his coronaries, the patient suddenly showed signs of having another heart attack. A quick squirt of dye displayed a clot blocking the right coronary artery. Rentrop and his colleagues instantly decided to try to get blood to the heart muscle by pushing the stiff guidewire of their angiography catheter through the clot. It worked. The patient's pain quickly subsided.

Over the next year, Rentrop continued to experiment. First he continued to poke guidewires through clots obstructing coronary arteries. In later patients, after creating an opening with the wire, he infused a protein known to dissolve clots. And finally he tried the protein, known as streptokinase, alone. In the summer of 1979 he restored normal blood flow to a patient with a totally blocked left anterior descending coronary artery with an infusion of streptokinase.

Streptokinase had been known for its clot-busting ability since 1933. Two American cardiologists, Sol Sherry and A. P. Fletcher, had experimented with it intravenously on a human patient as early as 1959. Like so many effective drugs, it is derived from an unlikely source—streptococcus bacteria. It works by converting a factor in the blood into an enzyme that dissolves the clot-forming material. It was first used to stop a heart attack in progress by a Russian team in 1976. But like most medical developments published in Russian-language journals, including the work of W. P. Obrastzow and N. D. Straschesko, who described heart attacks two years before Herrick, and Vasili Kolessov, who did an internal mammary artery bypass operation on a beating heart in 1964, it went largely unnoticed outside the Soviet Union.

Taken together, the work of Sherry and Fletcher, DeWood's study, and Rentrop's clinical experiments created the new field of thrombolytic therapy in the West. In the 1990s, emergency use of clot-busting drugs such as streptokinase and newer agents such as tissue plasminogen activator (tPA), first genetically engineered in 1982, has become state-of-the-art medicine, although many cardiologists contend that both treatments are

often used inappropriately.[7] And a number of potentially better thrombolytic drugs are currently in clinical trials.[8]

The conflict-of-interest-laden story of the fierce competition for market
dominance between the manufacturers of streptokinase and tPA, and the
coteries of high-powered cardiologists working with them, has been told
well by Baruch Brody in his book *Ethical Issues in Drug Testing, Approval
and Pricing: The Clot-Dissolving Drugs* (New York: Oxford University
Press, 1995) and need not be repeated here.

This rest of this chapter will look instead at promising new research that
is currently under way. As I write, clinical investigators are exploring exciting possibilities such as bypassing blocked arteries biologically, a process
known as angiogenesis. Using two different proteins known as growth
factors, researchers in the United States and Germany have made tiny new
vessels grow around blockages in coronary arteries to replace part of the
lost blood flow, mimicking a process that sometimes occurs naturally. This
is, in effect, bypass surgery without the surgery.

Others researchers are tracking the causes of atherosclerosis, the underlying disease that causes heart attacks, sudden cardiac death, some strokes,
and some heart failure, an eventually fatal stretching and weakening of the
heart muscle that prevents it from pumping blood efficiently. Their interim
goal is to figure out how to stabilize vulnerable atherosclerotic plaque so
that bits will not break off, leading to blood clots, heart attacks, and death.
Their ultimate goal is to get rid of plaque altogether.

This is the first full-fledged attack on coronary artery disease itself. Because the disease process is so complex, the quest could go on for decades.
Different groups are attacking the problem from different directions. Some
researchers are looking for answers encoded in the genes. Others are probing cellular and molecular activity deep inside the layers of the arterial wall.
Still others are tracking hostile intruders in the bloodstream. And others
are working on the physics of visual imaging.

Through these investigations, they are learning how the body's over-
reaction, or misplaced reaction, to injury in the coronary arteries can cause
deadly cascades of activity. The work is going well enough so that some
researchers are beginning to believe that in their lifetimes dreams about
eliminating a disease that kills more people in Western societies than any
other will come true.

Valentin Fuster, an intense, Barcelona-born cardiologist who came to
the United States almost a quarter century ago, is in the forefront of this
research. Fuster has blunt features, a wide forehead, iron-gray hair, and
despite his long years in the United States, a strong Spanish accent. He is
the embodiment of gravitas. It is evident that he neither suffers fools nor
squanders his time on anything extraneous to his professional mission.

Medicine runs in Fuster's family. His grandfather, who served as rector of the University of Barcelona, was a physician. His father practiced psychiatry in Barcelona. And his brother is a well-known neuroscientist at UCLA. His own ambition as a youth was to be a professional tennis player. But like John Gibbon, who wanted to be a poet, he thought better of it. And like his brother, he practices far from his ancestral roots in Catalonia, today an affluent region of northeastern Spain but once a powerful seafaring, commercial nation. Although he has elected to live and work in the United States, Fuster is unambiguous about his identity. When asked his nationality, he unhesitatingly says Catalan, not Spanish.

As a student in Barcelona he rejected psychiatry because it wasn't concrete enough for him. Instead, when his medical-school mentor had a heart attack at age forty-five, Fuster decided to specialize in cardiology and make room in his career for research. He wanted to learn more about the causes of coronary artery disease and heart attacks.

Fuster is director of the cardiovascular institute at Mount Sinai Hospital in New York, professor of medicine, and dean for academic affairs at the Mount Sinai School of Medicine. In 1998 he became president of the American Heart Association. His route to the pinnacle of American cardiology took him from the University of Barcelona's medical school, from which he graduated *magna cum laude,* through Edinburgh, Scotland, where he was a resident and earned a Ph.D. in biology (awarded by the University of Barcelona).

Like Andreas Gruentzig, Fuster accepted a job with an institution that was able to get him into the United States. He had an offer to work with Eugene Braunwald at the University of California, San Diego, but when his entry was delayed, he went instead to the Mayo Clinic, which produced a visa. His original plan was to spend a year at Mayo, but he stayed eleven years. Then he went to Mount Sinai as chief of cardiology, and except for a stretch from 1991 to 1994 as Mallinkrodt professor of medicine at Harvard Medical School and chief of cardiology at Massachusetts General Hospital, he has remained at Mount Sinai.

Fuster wants to know how to prevent heart attacks and how to eliminate the disease that causes them. "What we see," Fuster said, "is that whenever a patient comes in with chest pain he ends up in a cardiac catheterization laboratory, he ends up with a procedure, and at the very end, you ask, why?"[9]

An obvious answer to this question, of course, is that it is better to relieve symptoms than to do nothing at all. But Fuster's question is intended to probe deeper than that. First, he wants to know, are procedures being done when drugs, or perhaps nothing at all, might work as well? And at an even deeper level, he wonders whether there isn't something wrong with a system in which young cardiologists are trained to do technical interventions but lack the skills and data necessary to understand how much—or how little—good their interventions do.

Fuster is unwilling to speculate about how many excess angioplasties and surgeries are done annually, but like just about every other thoughtful cardiologist, he is convinced that too many are done.

Fuster has followed in the footsteps of two nineteenth-century Germans who first zeroed in on the causes of the disease, and the pathologist Russell Ross, who linked their hypotheses 130 years later to his own work on injury response mechanisms such as clot formation, smooth muscle cell proliferation, and inflammation.[10] Fuster was among the first to follow up on Ross's discovery that an element in the blood called a platelet played an important role in clotting.

In examining this role, he built on the fact that platelets released proteins during the clotting process to develop a test to detect the presence of these proteins—a noninvasive way to identify clot formation in progress. Soon thereafter he did a study in pigs demonstrating that when their platelet function was impaired, the pigs became resistant to atherosclerosis. This was one of the first times anyone had demonstrated the important role played by platelets in the development of atherosclerosis.

Although the precise nature of this role remained unknown, Fuster and his colleague James Chesebro were able to show that drugs such as aspirin that interfered with platelet function could prevent vein segments used to bypass blocked arteries from clogging. Fuster was also among those to follow up on Ross's recognition that angioplasty and other treatments involving threading catheters through coronary arteries sometimes caused injuries that led to clotting. To deal with this problem they recommended anticlotting therapy after these interventions.[11]

The administration of antiplatelet drugs and anticoagulants after catheterization to prevent reblockage of the vessels is now standard. New antiplatelet agents such as abciximab, which is marketed as Reopro, have proved especially effective in reducing clotting, but they are expensive, and their added value has not been demonstrated to the satisfaction of everyone.[12]

Fuster and his colleagues, along with others, such as James Willerson at Texas Heart Institute in Houston, were beginning to build on Ross's insight that atherosclerosis was a disease process that began with a very small injury to the wall of an artery and progressed as the body mobilized its internal mechanisms to repair the damage. In other words, the body's natural response to injury, which at another site would constitute normal healing, in a coronary artery can constitute deadly disease. The theory goes like this:

When blood is driven through the coronary circulation under the pumping pressure of the heart, it rushes through the arteries, exerting what are called shear forces on the vessel walls. At points where the arteries bend or branch, the pattern of flow changes. This small change in the force and direction of flow can cause a minute injury, or create conditions leading to the adhesion of bad cholesterol (low-density lipoprotein) to the arterial wall. Other factors, such as chemical irritants in tobacco smoke that enter the bloodstream, can cause similar injuries. These injuries set in motion a chain reaction that includes the deposition of fats and platelets at the injury site, an accumulation of fibrous material, and the release of growth factors that cause the proliferation of smooth muscle cells in the arterial wall. These materials then combine to form lesions on the wall that are fatty on the inside and fibrous on the outside.

As these lesions increase in size they narrow the arterial channel. Some of the lesions are composed mainly of hard, fibrous material. These are likely to be stable and for many years benign. Eventually they may narrow an artery enough to reduce blood flow to the heart muscle and cause angina, especially if the partially blocked vessel is large. Other lesions, however, are composed mainly of soft, fatty material, with only a thin, fibrous cap. These can break easily, exposing material to the flowing blood that stimulates the formation of clots that can suddenly and completely block the artery, causing a heart attack.

Fuster and his colleagues are among numerous researchers around the world currently looking for a way to identify vulnerable plaques and then to stabilize them, thereby preventing the cracking and fissuring of the cap that appear to be responsible for most heart attacks. But ultimately they want to understand the process by which the plaques are formed so they can prevent them from developing in the first place.

Fuster's team is international and includes two Spaniards (both Catalan) other than himself; a German; a Lebanese-born, French-reared American; an Israeli-born American; and several native-born Americans. The group includes cardiologists, physiologists, and a physicist who works on ways to create images of plaques that will identify their composition and structure, making it possible to determine whether they are vulnerable.

They work in a high-rise medical center tower on the edge of East Harlem in Manhattan. Some of their activities take place in the basement, where the big, barrel-like magnetic resonance imaging machines are installed, and some of the work is done on the top floor, where the experimental animals are housed. It is here, for example, that Mercedes Roque, a tiny, dark-haired research fellow who is from Fuster's alma mater in Barcelona and who barely looks eighteen, does angioplasty on pigs in a special catheterization laboratory reserved for these animal experiments.

Roque is studying why some arteries reclog in the first couple of months after having been opened with catheter-based interventions such as angioplasty or stents. This narrowing process—restenosis in medical jargon—seems mainly to involve the proliferation of smooth muscle cells and connective tissue, not fats. As a result, the plaque formed is hard and stable, not soft and vulnerable. Radiation can be used to destroy the mechanism that produces the excess tissue, but Fuster is uncomfortable with the risks associated with radiation, so his team is exploring another treatment option—blocking the cell cycle, a principle similar to one that has opened up new approaches to cancer therapy.

In the basement imaging laboratories, the team's ultimate goal is to figure out how to identify the most dangerous plaques in living human subjects. To do this, a way must be found to look inside the vessel wall and the plaques themselves. It will not be enough to see where these plaques are, or how big they are, or how they are shaped. It will also be necessary to know their structure and composition—how much is soft or even liquid fat; how much is hard, fibrous shell; how much is calcium. What is the architecture of the plaque? Where are its weak spots? This is the work taking place below the street, on pigs, rabbits, and genetically altered mice. Fuster is excited about it. "We can already see the artery," he said, "the lumen [channel] and the wall. In five or ten years we'll have technologies that will tell us by direct visualization where the plaque is."[13]

Since Mason Sones accidentally discovered in 1958 that it was possible to make X-ray movies of individually selected coronary arteries without killing the patient, coronary angiography has been the best source of information about blockages. In recent years, however, it has become clear that angiography is not good enough. It does not spot all blockages in the coronary arteries, and more importantly, many of the ones it misses, either because they are relatively small or not in the biggest arterial channels, are more likely to cause heart attacks than most of the ones it identifies. These are, of course, the vulnerable plaques.

Moreover, angiography only shows in shadowy form the diameter of the inside of the partly or completely blocked artery, and even this view may be misleading if the entire arterial segment shown on angiography has been narrowed, leaving a round, smooth, normal-looking channel.[14] Also, angiography tells nothing about the condition of the arterial wall or the structure or composition of the plaque protruding from it.

As a result, cardiologists have been seeking an imaging technique that will give them more information. Over the past decade they have experimented with several methods, some of which are invasive, involving incisions and added risk. Therefore, like angiography, they are unlikely to be used unless a patient already has severe symptoms such as angina, or already has had a heart attack. In other words, these tests will not lead to preventive treatment that might stop a first heart attack, about a quarter million of which are fatal every year in the United States alone.

All of these methods are limited in their ability to identify and elucidate the structure and composition of plaque and arterial walls. They are based on technologies as old as sonar, which was developed to detect German U-boats in World War II, and as contemporary as fiber optics, developed for modern, high-speed communications. Among the noninvasive methods being explored are the use of radioactive substances to label specific molecules such as low-density lipoproteins and platelets so they can be detected by nuclear imaging technologies such as CT or PET scans; Doppler wires that measure the velocity of blood flow to help determine if anything is impeding the flow; and so-called heart scans, which use electron-beam computed tomography to measure the calcium content of plaques.

One fiber-optic technique developed in the past decade is called angioscopy. It uses a direct-vision device called an angioscope—a lens-tipped optical-fiber bundle on a catheter—which is attached to a color camera and a high-powered light source. The catheter is inserted into the femoral artery in the same way an angioplasty balloon is introduced and then threaded up to the coronary target. Once in place, the system provides color pictures of the surface of the lesion and the surrounding arterial wall.

The current angioscopy catheter is relatively thick and therefore difficult to use. But angioscopy can identify yellow plaques, which appear to rupture easily, and also surface fissures and clots. Although the angioscope was designed as a diagnostic tool, John Simpson and Paul Yock are trying to incorporate a fiber-optical bundle such as the ones used in angioscopy into a thinner atherectomy catheter, thereby producing what they call a therapeutic device with "an eye on board."[15]

A second invasive technique, intravascular ultrasound, uses a tiny transducer mounted on a catheter to bounce sound waves off the inner walls of coronary arteries. When translated by a computer, this sonar message provides a clear, cross-sectional view of the arterial wall, any plaque that has formed on it, and the remaining channel through which blood can flow. Because the elements of plaque have different densities, the sound waves echo back at different wavelengths. These differences make possible some degree of distinction among fat, fiber, and calcium in the atherosclerotic lesion. But ultrasound does not do a really good job of delineating the structure of plaques, nor does it adequately differentiate between fat and fiber in plaque and clot material.

Fuster and his colleagues are concentrating on magnetic resonance imaging (MRI), both because it is noninvasive and because they are convinced that eventually the technology can be refined to the point where it will be able to discriminate well enough between fatty and fibrous tissue to identify vulnerable plaques. The underlying principle on which MRI is based was discovered in 1946 by physicists working independently at Stanford and Harvard.

Magnetic resonance imaging is a three-dimensional imaging technique that differentiates tissue structure according to the magnetic properties of protons.[16] It relies on a powerful magnet—usually a superconductor—to create a magnetic field. The fields generated by these superconductors are ten thousand to eighty thousand times stronger than the earth's magnetic field. The patient is placed in the field, which exerts a force on the protons in the hydrogen atoms in his body. These spinning, electrically charged protons—weak little magnets themselves—are attracted by the powerful external magnet, which lines them up parallel to its own field. When they are aligned, about half of the protons have their north and south poles oriented in the same direction as the external field, and about half are oriented in the opposite direction. As a result, the protons pointing down and the protons pointing up neutralize each other's magnetism.

There are, however, a thimbleful of unneutralized leftovers. The reason there are leftovers is that it takes slightly less energy to point in the same direction as the strong external field than it does to point in the opposite direction; therefore, a few more protons take this path of least resistance. Because there are no protons to neutralize the magnetic field created by these extra protons, all of which are pointing upward, the patient himself is now slightly magnetized in the direction of the external magnetic field. But because his magnetism points in the same direction as the field's, it is indistinguishable from the field's magnetic force; therefore it can't be split off and measured, which is what has to happen to make it useful.

To be useful for imaging purposes, a way had to be found to change the direction of the patient's magnetism. This is done by introducing an electromagnetic pulse with the same frequency as the patient's protons. This pulse exchanges energy, or resonates, with the extra protons in the same way that tuning forks resonate with sounds on their frequency. The resonance has several effects. Most importantly, it changes the direction of some of these protons so they are no longer parallel to the external magnetic field. This means that their magnetism, which generates an electrical current known as a signal, now can be measured.

The next step is to determine where on the cross section of the body being imaged the signal is coming from. Because the strength of the external magnetic field determines the frequency, or rate of rotation of the protons, this can be done by varying the strength of the field over each point on the cross section. Each gradation in magnetic force yields a signal with a slightly different frequency. This variation in frequency can be measured, making it possible to identify precisely where on the cross section the signal originates.

Different tissues, depending on factors such as their molecular structure, anatomical surroundings, and water content, return to their normal magnetic states at different rates when the external electromagnetic pulse is switched off. Diseased tissue, for example, usually has a higher water content than normal tissue. This difference produces a measurable variation in its rate of return to a normal state, making it identifiable.

A computer correlates the time-related, tissue-identifying information— that is, the rate at which a specific tissue returns to its normal state—with the spatial information based on frequency differences that situate the tissue precisely in the body. The result is a three-dimensional visual image that provides information about the location, architecture, and structure of the tissue in question.

Fuster became interested in applying this form of imaging to the coronary arteries because of MRI studies his brother was doing on the brain. Despite its weaknesses, magnetic resonance angiography has shown fairly good results in locating plaques, although it tends to overestimate their lengths.[17] However, Fuster and his colleagues are betting that in the next decade it will leapfrog the invasive technologies and make possible clear, consistent identification and characterization of vulnerable plaques.

If this happens it will be a development comparable in magnitude to Sones's discovery of selective coronary angiography. It will mean that patients at high risk for plaque rupture and heart attacks can be identified and given cholesterol-lowering drugs, which appear to stabilize their plaques by initiating a process in which hard connective tissue replaces soft, thrombogenic fat. Fuster's own research suggests that preventive action of this kind could eliminate some heart attacks and deaths, although it is not clear how many.

There are several problems that remain to be overcome, including MRI's relatively poor overall resolution, and motion of the artery during the exam. As a result, MRI cannot yet characterize the composition of plaque in the tiny coronary arteries of a living subject. It is also difficult to image the entire circumflex artery, a major vessel, much of which traverses the back of the heart, and parts of other large arteries. In addition, MRI is relatively expensive, and therapeutic interventions such as angioplasty currently cannot be done while the patient is encased in the machine.[18]

These are the problems that the researchers at Mount Sinai, and their colleagues elsewhere, are trying to solve. Others are betting that a different technology—optical coherence tomography (OCT), which uses reflected infrared light to produce very-high-resolution pictures of tissue, including plaque and arterial walls—will do the job sooner and better. These investigators are convinced that OCT will be able to overcome all of the draw-backs associated with MRI. Researchers at Harvard Medical School have reported that OCT can image the structure and composition of plaque in living subjects with greater resolution than any other available technique.[19] But OCT also has a major drawback: like angiography, angioscopy, and ultrasound, it is catheter-based and therefore invasive. Its use is accompanied by more than negligible risk.

In the Mount Sinai basement, two members of Fuster's research group—Meir Shinnar, an Israeli-born, American-educated mathematician and physician, and Zahi Adel Fayad, a Lebanese-born, French-reared, American-trained biomedical engineer—are trying to refine MRI technology to the point where it can do two things: (1) replace most invasive angiograms, and (2) consistently identify if not all then at least some of the most vulnerable plaques. But there's still a long way to go, and some leading researchers are convinced that MRI will never be good enough.[20] The resolution of standard angiography is still several times better than that of MRI, which means that while MRI has the clear advantage of being noninvasive, it cannot yet replace angiography as a means of identifying blocked coronary arteries.

One of the main obstacles that must be overcome to accomplish these objectives is, quite simply, motion. The coronary arteries are constantly moving. The beating of the heart agitates them; so does the pulsing flow of blood, and so, too, does the steady rising and falling of the diaphragm caused by breathing. The movements caused by these three sources blur the image unless it is compensated for in some way.

Researchers have already figured out how to get around the blurring caused by the blood-pulse and heartbeat movements. An electrocardiogram machine is synchronized with the MRI machine to trigger the release of energy that initiates the "snapshots" of the artery. The shutter, if you will, is only allowed to click at the single instant during the heart's pumping cycle when there is virtually no motion.

Compensating for the motion caused by breathing, however, has been harder to do. Until now the main technique has been to stop it altogether by getting patients to hold their breath. But to get as complete a set of pictures of the coronary arteries as is currently possible can take up to an hour. The patient is required to stop breathing from twelve to twenty seconds every minute. For some patients with coronary artery disease this burden is just too great.

One reason it takes so long to get a full set of images is that each image is a two-dimensional slice along a single plane. Since the coronary arteries wind their way through many planes, it requires many images to get a complete, three-dimensional picture of a single artery. The pictures can be taken faster, but at an unacceptable price—loss of resolution.

An experimental system called navigator echo tracks the breathing motion of the diaphragm. This technique synchronizes the diaphragm's movement to the magnetic resonance image itself, much as the electrocardiogram synchronizes the heartbeat to the clicking of the shutter, thereby compensating for the motion of the artery caused by breathing. This improves image resolution and provides greater consistency than a series of breath-holds, any one of which might differ from others.

Another problem that needs to be solved is how to differentiate adequately between the target in magnetic resonance angiography—blood flowing through the coronary arteries—and background tissue and structures such as veins or the chambers of the heart that obscure the view. Unless the blood can be imaged clearly, sites where flow is blocked cannot be identified. To accomplish this goal, experiments are being conducted with a contrast substance called gadolinium, which improves the signal-to-noise ratio, providing greater resolution in a shorter imaging time. Also, techniques have been developed to suppress the brightness of fat and other surrounding tissues, thereby enhancing the contrast between the blood and these tissues.

Other problems also remain to be solved. The processing and display of images are still inadequate. MRI cannot be used if a patient has a pacemaker. Metal stents act as a shield that distorts the image of the vessel (stentmakers now are experimenting with plastic materials). And about 10 percent of patients are too claustrophobic to go into the constricting, tubular machine.

While they continue working on imaging methods, Fuster and his colleagues also have been studying the malign role played by a chameleonlike scavenger with two identities and three names. In its simplest form, it is called a monocyte. Under normal conditions this microscopic bit of cytoplasm rounds up viruses and other potentially dangerous intruders in the blood. But it responds to wounds in coronary arteries perversely by instigating the atherosclerotic process.

Some monocytes infiltrate the wound and engorge themselves with cholesterol, which turns them into troublemaking macrophages (literally, big eaters, from Greek). In their new guise it appears they collaborate with other constituents in the wall to begin the process that results in the formation of vulnerable, or easily ruptured, plaque. Other monocytes remain in the bloodstream. These cells seem to work with the sticky platelets and other circulating cells to promote rapid clotting.

The atherosclerotic process is complicated and begins early in life. It involves a dozen or more interacting elements. Usually it takes decades for a plaque to develop to maturity, although sometimes new plaques seem to develop in just months. To understand what Fuster and others are trying to do requires at least a basic idea of how this process works, beginning with what an artery is and what goes on inside it.

Although analogies with plumbing are commonly used to describe the heart and circulatory system, there are crucial differences. The most important distinction between an artery or vein in a human body and a pipe behind a bathroom sink is that the former is living tissue and the latter is inert metal or plastic. When a pipe corrodes or cracks under stress, it cannot repair itself because, unlike human tissue, it has no cells that are automatically activated to patch it. This is both good news for humans—our physiological repair mechanisms usually help keep us alive and well—and bad news—when these mechanisms get out of control in the coronary arteries, they can cause a heart attack.

Coronary arteries have three layers that are called, from the inside out, the intima, the media, and the adventitia. The intima is largely made up of cells that regulate the passage of substances from blood into the arterial wall and ward off clotting. The media consists mostly of smooth muscle cells that enable the vessel to expand and contract. The adventitia is a protective layer of tough, fibrous connective tissue. The channel in the artery through which oxygen-rich blood flows to the heart muscle is called the lumen.

For several years Fuster's group had concentrated on responses to injury taking place within the two inner layers of the artery wall, the intima and the media. But early in 1998 their interest suddenly shifted to previously unsuspected activity in the circulating blood. What led up to this change in focus is essentially the story of what is currently known about the atherosclerotic process, and a fairly typical example of the blend of design and serendipity that leads to scientific discoveries.

Atherosclerosis begins early, although no one is certain exactly how early. Studies done on American soldiers killed in the Korean War showed that most had plaque in their coronary arteries. There is rough agreement among cardiologists and pathologists that the disease process starts with a minute wound to a coronary artery, which sets in motion a complex effort by the body to repair the damage. The precise way in which the wound is inflicted, the nature of these healing responses, how they get out of control, and exactly what role they play in the development of the plaque and blood clots that cause heart attacks are still more matters of conjecture than consensus. What follows is a description of the atherosclerotic process that most researchers would consider plausible even though they might disagree on some details.

When an injury to an artery occurs, cells die and are replaced by new ones. This process of cell death and replacement makes the intima more permeable during a period from about two weeks until twelve weeks after the injury. During this time, circulating fats such as cholesterol can enter the cell wall in either of two ways: directly through receptors on the outer cells of the intima; or indirectly, when the fats are smuggled in by monocyte-macrophages already inside the intima. These scavenger cells envelop the fats—mainly low-density lipoprotein—as they try to breach the wall and carry them across the gap resulting from the injury.

Fats and smooth muscle cells then begin to accumulate at the injury site. The cholesterol-laden macrophages contribute to the buildup by releasing chemicals called growth factors that stimulate the production of more smooth muscle cells that migrate to the injury site. Then the macrophages die, leaving behind fatty deposits that form the core of the plaque.

At the same time, clotting factors, including platelets, accumulate at the site, possibly because they are attracted by toxic products released by the monocytes that are already there. Like monocytes, the platelets secrete growth factors, which promote additional buildup of unwanted smooth muscle cells.

While all this is going on, the fats that have accumulated inside the arterial wall stimulate the release of chemicals that attract even more monocytes. Once inside the wall, these ravenous cells, like their predecessors, envelop all the fat they can find. Before long, the newly arrived and longtime-resident fat-filled monocytes—all having turned into macrophages, excreted their toxins, and died—are aggregated with the smooth muscle cells, collagen, and other fibrous materials to form atherosclerotic plaque.

All atherosclerotic plaque, as we have seen, is not created equal, and this is the beginning of the next part of the story. In recent years many researchers have contended that stable, fibrous atherosclerotic plaques, even when they narrow major arteries by more than 70 percent, constitute what in effect is a benign disease—that is, the disease progresses very slowly. Moreover, it does not pose an acute threat even when it closes an artery completely because it does so only after collaterals have developed to carry blood around the blockage. The minimal flow provided by these tiny conduits generally prevents a heart attack from occurring.

Plaques with only a thin fibrous cap to contain a soft, unstable, fatty core are another matter, however. They are liable to break at any time, initiating a process that often leads to a fatal blood clot. Fuster and others are interested in the composition and structure of such plaques because these are the elements that are likely to determine whether they rupture, and if they do, whether they will stimulate a large, totally obstructive clot that can kill. Researchers are also interested in finding out whether the substantial number of plaques that are relatively small and hard to identify are more likely than large, easily identifiable plaques to be fat-filled and therefore unstable and dangerous.

The most vulnerable plaques tend to be crescent-shaped, with a soft core composed largely of cholesterol, some of it in a liquid form known as cholesterol esters. The fibrous cap surrounding the soft, fatty core is relatively thin to begin with and may have been weakened further by the presence of macrophages, which release various toxic products such as free radicals, which might make the cap even more prone to rupture. The shape of the plaque, the location of the fatty core within the plaque, and other factors that influence the physical stresses to which the cap is subjected also contribute to the plaque's overall vulnerability.

When a plaque ruptures, the fatty material in the core is exposed to the flowing blood. This material—oxidized fats, macrophages and cellular debris—is highly thrombogenic, which is to say, it reacts with elements in the blood to form clots. This clotting process, unlike plaque formation, is extremely rapid. A clot can form within seconds, and if it blocks the artery completely, it can cause a heart attack within minutes. More often than not, however, the clot does not close off the artery, there are no symptoms, the event goes unnoticed, and healing takes place. But a lesion remains that can rupture again. And the existence of one vulnerable plaque suggests that there very likely are others, planted in the vessel wall like enemy agents under deep cover waiting to be activated.

For years researchers studying vulnerable plaques had concentrated on activity within the arterial wall such as the atheroma-producing role of lipoprotein (a), a genetic variant of low-density lipoprotein that accumulates in fibrous plaques. In the past couple of years they also began studying the role played in plaque and clot formation by monocytes that had infiltrated the wall. But toward the end of 1997, something unexpected happened that caused Fuster to turn his attention to the bloodstream, with a view to understanding the effect of circulating cholesterol on clotting.

Fuster was puzzled by the fact that ruptured plaques were found in only two-thirds of the people who had heart attacks. What, he wondered, had caused the clots that caused the heart attacks in the other third? Many of the patients who had heart attacks without ruptured plaques had very high cholesterol, but he did not understand why this should be so, or even if it was relevant.

Then Fuster read a journal article[21] suggesting that a simple erosion of plaque, exposing only relatively nonthrombogenic fibrous material, rather than a rupture, which exposes highly thrombogenic fatty material, could cause a clot. For this to happen, he reasoned, the blood must clot very easily. This realization triggered another question: Why should the blood of people with high cholesterol clot more easily than anybody else's blood?

To find out, he conducted a small, blinded study in which the blood of human subjects with high cholesterol was exposed to a standard sample of plaque taken from a pig. This was done in a tiny perfusion chamber invented for the purpose by Juan Badimon, one of Fuster's colleagues at Mount Sinai. The chamber is a small, innocuous-looking, two-piece, clear plastic block a couple of inches long and perhaps an inch wide and an inch high. It has a holder for the pig plaque and a channel for the blood to flow in, come into contact with the plaque, and flow out.

To do the experiment, a cannula is inserted into the vein of a subject, a small amount of the subject's blood is run over the plaque in the chamber, and the researchers observe the clotting as it occurs. What they are learning is that the higher the subject's low-density lipoprotein, the more clotting takes place. They then treat the same subjects with two different cholesterol-lowering drugs and pass their blood through the chamber again. In every case, irrespective of which drug they have taken, their blood no longer clots at all when it comes into contact with the pig plaque.

"What I'm telling you," Fuster said, "is that things are not as simple as saying everything's in the vessel wall. One of the most powerful antithrombotics is a statin [cholesterol-lowering drug], and one of the most powerful thrombotic agents is cholesterol. And it has nothing to do with the vessel wall. So this led us to change our way of thinking. We [now] believe that clotting factors in circulating monocytes are affected by the cholesterol. You have circulating blood that is explosive in a way."[22]

Fuster's point is that clotting, the most common end stage of the atherosclerotic process, can occur if a person has high cholesterol even if that person has no plaque that is vulnerable to rupture. But this is not the sole insight that is likely to flow from the Mount. Sinai group's research. Fuster has begun to wonder, for example, why certain proteins that are markers for inflammation are elevated in persons with coronary artery disease. If the inflammatory process associated with atherosclerosis occurs, as has been thought, deep within the arterial wall, why do signs of inflammation show up in the blood?

Even more interesting, perhaps, is that these experiments support the once widely ridiculed hypothesis that infections can cause heart attacks. In a small study, traces of the chlamydia pneumonia virus were detected in 30 percent of atherosclerotic plaques.[23] Since monocytes transport these viruses through the bloodstream, and since monocytes in the blood are very likely implicated in plaque rupture and clotting, it appears that infectious agents such as chlamydia pneumonia viruses could play a part in the atherosclerotic process. For example, once inside the monocyte, the virus might activate it much as cholesterol does, starting the chain of events that leads to a clot and a heart attack.

Over the years, with the identification of new risk factors such as homocysteine, fibrinogen, and lipoprotein (a), Fuster has revised downward from 25 to about 10 the percentage of people without identifiable risk factors such as family history, high cholesterol, smoking, obesity, and a sedentary lifestyle, he believes get coronary artery disease. The implication is clear: If more people changed their behavior, fewer people would die. But as of the mid-1990s, only 15 to 25 percent of Americans who know best that they are at risk—those who have undergone bypass surgery or angioplasty—are on intensive cholesterol-lowering and risk-management programs.[24]

Two controllable lifestyle-related risk factors that he is particularly concerned about because they appear to play a significant although far from perfectly understood role in the atherosclerotic process are smoking and excess homocysteine. Smoking, which everyone agrees increases heart-attack risk, appears to contribute to unwanted clotting in the coronary arteries, and it causes blood vessels to constrict.

Homocysteine, a breakdown product of an amino acid called methionine, which is a component of animal protein, has been suspected of being implicated in cardiovascular disease since 1933. But no one has proved it in a controlled, randomized clinical trial, or demonstrated the mechanism at a laboratory bench. Many population studies, however, such as the Framingham Heart Study and the Harvard Physicians' Study, have shown a strong association between high levels of homocysteine and coronary artery disease.

Many cardiologists are now convinced that homocysteine levels that are too high represent a cardiovascular risk comparable to high cholesterol or moderate to heavy smoking. But most Americans with high cholesterol don't know it, or know it and do nothing about it; fifty million Americans smoke, and even though exercise and relatively small amounts of three B vitamins can easily keep homocysteine under control, most Americans have never heard of homocysteine, and they don't eat the readily available foods such as beans, leafy green vegetables, and orange juice that provide the B vitamins.

14

What Shall We Make of All This?

[M]edical care has become a commodity transacted as a
business and organized as an industry;[1]

Medical consumerism—like all sorts of consumerism, but
more menacingly—is designed to be unsatisfying.[2]

There is intelligence enough, and some brilliance, too, in
this era of medicine. What about wisdom?[3]

In the past half century the world has witnessed a revolution in treating
heart disease. Clinicians collaborating with engineers and entrepreneurs
have devised brilliant solutions to previously insoluble problems. Recently
a heart was completely detached and removed from a young man's body,
a tumor was excised, and the organ was returned to its natural setting in
the thoracic cavity. The patient is doing fine. And researchers have announced that they can stimulate the body to create new blood vessels, an
advance that could lead to bypassing blocked coronary arteries without
surgery.

Fueled by vast infusions of cash and a new spirit of entrepreneurialism, cardiac research in the United States (and in Western Europe and
Japan) has metamorphosed into a multibillion-dollar academic-industrial-
governmental enterprise. Because a similar expansion has occurred in other
fields of research, the country's medical economy and American medical
practice are being remodeled.

Some of the most impressive technical advances have been made in treating coronary artery disease, with bypass surgery, angioplasty, and stenting
among them. But paradoxically, it is not clear how well this new medico-
industrial complex serves patients in general and patients with coronary
disease in particular. A 1997 RAND Corporation study reports that "there
are large gaps between the care that people should receive and the care

they do receive."[4] Do we pay a price in quality of medical care for the emphasis we place on commerce? Are we replacing clinical judgment with costly technology?

Sherwin B. Nuland, a professor of surgery at Yale University and author of several fine books on medicine, including *Doctors: The Biography of Medicine* and *The Wisdom of the Body,* neatly capsulized the essential change in the American system of doing medicine. He observed that until very recently what clinicians did at the bedside drove medical research, but now what scientists do in the laboratory drives clinical practice.[5]

Before the end of World War II, most physicians in the United States were general practitioners who were on the whole well respected, who were rewarded for long hours of hard work by modest fees from their patients, and whose relatively simple methods of practice did not raise expectations that they could work miracles. They were generally paternalistic, which their patients not only expected but also desired, and they were trusted.

Such medical practice flowed naturally from a sense of professional duty that was commonplace. It still exists here and there, perhaps especially in rural areas. Clifford Smith, a seventy-two-year-old family doctor in McGregor, Iowa, who in 1998 still made regular house calls, said, "I grew up thinking medicine was about service, and that's just the only way I know."[6] But if the Clifford Smiths are not extinct, they are rare enough so that no one can be blamed for thinking they are.

Medical research in the immediate postwar period was not a lucrative calling, either. It was done on a small scale often by full-time medical scientists without clinical practices, because in those days practice left little or no time for secondary activities. Money was scarce. At the federal level just before World War II, biomedical research was a marginal activity. A National Institute of Health (NIH) was created in 1930 to promote investigations of chronic illnesses such as cancer and heart disease. But it was funded at a mere $43,000, which even for the time was a microscopic sum.[7]

In the early 1940s, out of wartime necessity, an important change occurred. The United States began awarding contracts to academic medical centers and laboratories around the country. This system worked well and, as a result, the postwar NIH was expanded and charged with sponsoring research—mostly at universities—on a grander scale than any previously known effort. By 1950 the now pluralized National Institutes of Health received a federal appropriation of $43 million, a thousand times more than the original appropriation of twenty years earlier. Funding topped $1 billion in 1970 and $11 billion in 1995, by which time the NIH had grown to twenty-six institutes.[8]

As the U.S. economy boomed in the postwar years, the drug and medical-device industries took off as well, and soon they, too, were funding biomedical research outside their own walls, mainly at university medical centers. These centers were delighted to have still another source of revenue, which paid not only for the research but also for university overheads. Research grants brought both prestige and a steady cash flow to universities such as Harvard, Stanford, Johns Hopkins, and Duke. With so much public and private money available for research, drug and device development drew more attention, and some of the best and the brightest flocked to it.

By the early 1980s, however, a new breed of business-oriented physician-researchers that included men such as John Simpson, Wes Sterman, and Tom Fogarty was beginning to reshape the relationship of research to practice. Unlike John Gibbon, Mason Sones, and René Favaloro, all of whom conducted their research primarily in the context of patient care, these men, while not strangers at the bedside, are first and foremost inventors and entrepreneurs. As Robert Petersdorf has noted (see chapter 7), "the culture of the biomedical [research] enterprise was changing from a primary emphasis on scholarship to a focus on entrepreneurial success."

There was a new recognition among physicians that, Hippocrates notwithstanding, they were engaged in commerce and that, in the words of William F. May, "The spring of action in a commercial society is money."[9] Most physicians remained full-time clinicians, but the shift toward entrepreneurialism in cardiac medicine has had a trickle-down effect that has wrought change throughout the specialty.

Scientific discovery and invention provided intellectual excitement and previously undreamed-of economic opportunity. The big academic medical centers were soon competing for the money, and for the stars, the big-time clinical researchers who brought it in. The fruits of their labor, whether drugs, devices, or new procedures that created a need for new devices, were then marketed by the fast-growing biomedical companies. The inventors quite naturally shared in the proceeds, and often participated in the companies, as stockholders or even officers. Innovations that once ambled at a leisurely pace from a doctor's bedside observation or improvisation to a lab bench and eventually into general practice were now being conceived and developed at breakneck speed.

Practicing cardiologists and cardiac surgeons are often overwhelmed by the rate of change. They find it difficult to keep up with the literature and to absorb into their practices the new drugs and devices—and the new indications for old drugs and devices—that seem to pop up almost daily. And even though the underlying impetus for new products, from the latest in intravascular ultrasound to the most recent iteration of the coronary stent, is still patient need, the standards by which their success is measured is no longer just easier, more reliable diagnosis, symptom relief, or cure; market share and profit margins have skewed the calculation.

The changes are making cardiac medicine look more and more like a bottom-line-oriented, consumer-driven industry. For example, as soon as angioplasty and minimally invasive bypass surgery captured the imagination of the press, the public, and the Wall Street analysts, pressure was exerted on practicing physicians to deliver these treatments. For a variety of reasons, including intellectual commitment and money, they did so, possibly sooner than was safe and certainly before it was clear how much good the treatments would do. This was true a decade or two earlier of traditional bypass surgery. As late as the beginning of the 1980s, 14 percent of bypass operations were done for inappropriate reasons, according to a RAND Corporation estimate.[10]

Another contemporary example of how research and industry push patient care is the intense promotion of high-priced anticholesterol drugs for millions of people with what are currently considered moderate cholesterol levels. Alan Garber, director of the Center for Primary Care and Outcomes Research at Stanford, told the *New York Times* that "the pressure is really on to use these [drugs]" and as a result "the public will be clamoring for them, too." But Garber also noted his uneasiness about prescribing cholesterol-lowering drugs for large numbers of people who may be at low risk for coronary artery disease because nothing is known about their long-term side effects.[11]

Despite the warnings of conservative doctors such as Garber, however, once the publicity and marketing steamroller gets going, medical prudence can sometimes be crushed. Appropriately, Garber made his cautionary remarks at a meeting of cardiologists and venture capitalists, a not uncommon coming together in the life of a research-oriented physician.

The new emphasis on research also has attenuated the relationship between some of America's smartest (if not always wisest) doctors and their patients. Many still maintain clinical practices, usually in large groups and in effect on a part-time basis. Their status and sometimes their income are tied more to research than to patient care. They are consulting for industry, attending scientific meetings that sometimes are combined with trade shows, and often have industry sponsors, presenting papers and overseeing one or more laboratories.

This frequently means that their patients get short shrift or are treated by two or three different physicians. In other words, the physician's caring role as understood from the time of Hippocrates in the fifth century B.C. has given way, among some of the best minds in medicine, to a new professional lifestyle centered on research and lubricated by money.

The size and wealth of the biomedical research enterprise and the technological imperative to apply its results have contributed substantially to driving up the cost of health care in the United States by fostering the overuse of high-tech medicine.[12] Eric Topol of the Cleveland Clinic has called interventional cardiologists "medical-technology junkies."[13] Part of the attraction is undoubtedly an understandable belief that these sophisticated new tools represent scientific progress and are the instruments of better care. But it is also true that physician compensation is often linked to using them.

Angioplasty, stenting, and minimally invasive bypass surgery are good examples of popular procedures based on expensive devices whose use is spurred in part by financial incentives. Efforts to remove these incentives by capitation, for example, which means paying doctors a fixed amount per patient annually, have been introduced. But they are far from universally accepted, and it is not clear that they will replace the procedure-based payment system.

In the meantime, the high cost of health care has led to the scrapping of most fee-for-service medicine, which is said to encourage too much care at too high a price, and replacing it with managed care, which is said to encourage minimal medicine to keep costs down. Managed care did slow the rise in health-care costs, but costs are going up again, and physicians are unhappy with the way managed care has changed medical practice.

They complain that managed care has reduced their professional autonomy because they are only paid for procedures that often-unqualified employees of managed-care organizations authorize; that HMOs or insurance companies determine which patients can be hospitalized and for how long; that they are forced to operate under gag rules that prevent them from discussing relatively expensive forms of treatment; that their practices are overwhelmed with bookkeeping and other bureaucratic requirements of HMOs, insurance companies, and federal programs such as Medicare and Medicaid; that frivolous malpractice suits cause them to practice defensive medicine; and in some cases that they are working more for less pay. Moreover, they say they cannot be strong advocates for their patients for fear that the plans that control the patient pools will blackball them. For many physicians, these drawbacks make practicing medicine more onerous than satisfying.

Against this background, let's return to the question with which this chapter began: How well are patients and society being served by the commodified system of cardiac medicine that has developed in the United States since the end of World War II?

One seemingly straightforward answer can be provided by mortality statistics. Between 1963 and 1994 the annual number of deaths from coronary artery disease in the United States was cut in half. Part of the decline was due to changes in diet and lifestyle, but part was due to high-tech treatments and new drugs. No one can say with precision or certainty how much of the reduction should be attributed to each cause.

The numbers leave little doubt, however, that technology driven, industry funded, research-oriented cardiac medicine has produced benefits: a better understanding of the effects of risk factors such as smoking and cholesterol; a range of effective new drugs including statins, beta blockers, calcium channel blockers, ACE inhibitors, and antioxidants; and interventions such as bypass surgery, angioplasty, and stenting.

However, the overall number of people in the United States suffering from coronary artery disease, 14 million, and the number of heart attacks annually, 1.5 million, have not declined. Moreover, because of the aging of the U.S. population, the absolute number of cases is likely to increase in the next decade, and there are likely to be more hard-to-treat cases in the mix.

Also, in something like two-thirds of all cases, invasive treatments such as surgery and angioplasty are being used without good evidence that they provide any survival benefit over drugs. Where a benefit is provided, it is in pain relief and exercise tolerance. But it comes at a price: a combined risk of death, nonfatal heart attack, stroke, and infection adding up to 6 or 7 percent in the case of surgery, or a 20 to 40 percent likelihood of one or more repeat procedures in the case of angioplasty and angioplasty combined with stenting—and the repeat procedure after a failed angioplasty might be surgery. Furthermore, medical science still fails to prevent most heart attacks, and the underlying causes of most heart attacks are just beginning to be understood.

That's the overview. In sum there is significantly less mortality than there was thirty years ago and a somewhat lower incidence of disease, but no reduction in disease prevalence, the likelihood of increased prevalence in the next generation, a death rate that remains high, and about a million invasive procedures a year that are relatively risky, expensive, and to some extent overused. Meanwhile, the search for a cure for coronary artery disease is just beginning.

In the first decade of the new millennium research in its current entrepreneurial form will almost certainly remain the primary engine driving cardiac medicine. The focus may be shifting away from palliative, device-based treatments toward cure-oriented genetic, molecular, and cellular manipulations. But private entrepreneurs who either collaborate with physicians or are physicians themselves will continue to create the high-tech products, whether they are drugs or devices, for profit.

Wes Sterman, a founder and director of Heartport Corporation, which makes the devices and instruments needed to do on-pump, minimally invasive bypass surgery, succinctly captured the spirit of the medical entrepreneurs when he characterized disease as a business opportunity. He believes that this unsentimental outlook promotes innovation. He acknowledges that conflicts of interest and market-oriented biases are unavoidable in such an approach, but he considers these conflicts and biases trivial compared to the benefits of such a dynamic, efficient means of uniting capital with clinical science and engineering.

There are, however, some serious negative consequences that flow from treating disease as a business opportunity. For example, practicing physicians are being flooded with new technologies, not all of which have been adequately tested, faster than they can absorb them. This happens in part because technology companies, whether they make computers or catheters, survive by innovating. One logical correlate of innovation is obsolescence. Therefore, even before a complicated new artery opening system is fully integrated into practice, a new one is churned out to supplement or replace it.

This might be fine for cutting-edge cardiologists and cardiac surgeons who thrive on such challenges, but it is not the best thing for average practitioners with average skills operating in small, understaffed community hospitals, or for their patients. But patients often do not know that their local, minimally trained interventional cardiologist, who does fewer than thirty single-vessel balloon angioplasties a year, should not try to do complicated stent placements or use new devices without proper training.

All they know is that they've seen an (often hyped-up) version of the new device or procedure in the news media or maybe even on the Internet, they want it, and they tell the local cardiologist, in effect, "if you can't or won't do it, I'll find somebody else who can and will." This creates pressure to use the latest technology, whatever it is, from rotational atherectomy to stenting to on-pump or beating-heart minimally invasive bypass surgery.

Although no one has tried to quantify the human and financial cost of failed interventions done by inadequately qualified operators using technologies they have not mastered, a recent study has shown that there is a direct correlation between how often an operator does angioplasty and his or her success rate.[14]

There are also strong financial, ego, and status-linked incentives to use these technologies. As a result, excess procedures are being done to the detriment of patients and at a substantial economic cost to society.

A classic conflict of interest exists for a small number of high-profile practicing cardiologists and cardiac surgeons who have financial ties to the manufacturing side of the cardiac drug and device industries as patent holders, licensors, company owners or officials, scientific advisers, and so on. These conflicts are especially egregious when the physician has a significant financial interest in a device or drug used in his practice. But patients usually have no way of knowing that such conflicts exist.

There are also economic incentives to act contrary to patients' interests that arise when members of a group practice both diagnose disease and perform interventional procedures. Angioplasty pays the rent, after all, not drug prescriptions or referrals to surgery. These conflicts exist for high-profile physicians with links to industry and for the large majority of cardiologists who have no such connections.

But other factors can compromise patients' interests, too. For example, ego and status considerations can motivate cardiologists to buy advanced devices and do complicated procedures that are beyond their training and skill levels. Cardiologists sometimes do procedures on patients referred to them because "they do not want to embarrass and alienate the sources of the referrals."[15] And an even more subtle reason for using the latest technology is a tendency in the presence of uncertainty to err on the side of action,[16] possibly for reasons of conscience, but possibly to avoid a malpractice suit for having failed to use what was available.

Entrepreneurialism also encourages capital to flow to the drugs or devices with the biggest profit potential, not necessarily those most needed. This is not to say that venture capitalists and biomedical entrepreneurs should feel guilty about pursuing large, profitable markets. Venture capitalism and entrepreneurship are not eleemosynary enterprises. And many of the most profitable solutions the entrepreneurial system produces are good solutions. When appropriately used, this is true of both bypass surgery and angioplasty. And it probably will turn out to be true of stents, which so far have posted some impressive clinical results.

But the fact that there is no one to blame does not mean that there isn't a problem. Private industry is not motivated to find low-cost solutions to low-volume problems (several thousand rare diseases[17]), no matter how humanly significant they are. As a result, little basic or clinical research is being done on diseases that affect relatively few people, such as Hunter's syndrome, which causes cardiovascular, respiratory, and hearing disorders; hereditary hemorrhagic telangiectasia, a platelet disorder; and long QT syndrome, which causes sudden cardiac death in young athletes, among others. The financial incentives simply are not there. The chief executive of one California biotechnology company put it succinctly: "In a business setting you have to consider the commercial value of a product."[18]

Filling this venture-capital gap is an appropriate role for the federal government. The NIH could place a higher priority than it currently does on funding basic research and clinical research and development—including clinical trials—on treatments for diseases that private industry does not view as good business opportunities.[19] If the government underwrites research and development costs, industry should be willing to produce drugs and devices for small markets, and it should be able to sell them at relatively low prices and earn a profit.

Where there are profits to be made without public support, however, a good case can be made that private industry will identify the problem and, with or without the help of academic researchers, do the job better than government-financed academic medicine.

But the drug and device industries do not come close to funding all of the basic and clinical research that is needed. The government pays for important laboratory research and for large, randomized clinical trials conducted by academic investigators. In 1997 the NIH spent $4 billion on clinical trials.[20] And between 1985 and 1996 the National Heart, Lung, and Blood Institute, one of the twenty-six NIH components, funded almost $900 million in cardiovascular studies alone.[21]

Drug and device companies pay for many trials—according to some estimates, more than half—but they consider information on how much they spend for this purpose to be proprietary and do not disclose it. Industry money makes more trials possible with less bureaucracy, but the conflicts of interest in industry-sponsored trials are more substantial than in government-sponsored trials. Industry sponsors also offer financial incentives to investigators. For example, they pay capitation fees per enrolled patient-subject that are two to five times greater than those paid by the NIH.[22] And sometimes they use unqualified physicians in private practice as researchers.

When clinical researchers are beholden to drug or device companies for their funding they may be more likely to pursue an outcome favorable to the company's commercial interests, less likely to publish results unfavorable to the company's interests, and less likely to share their results with other researchers because of the company's concern that proprietary information will be disclosed.

Investigators are only part of the problem. Institutions can also become beholden to the companies. In fact, academic medical centers may be more vulnerable to conflicts of interest than individual investigators. According to a draft report by the inspector general of the Department of Health and Human Services, these centers are so dependent on the revenue flow from clinical research that they sometimes put pressure on their institutional review boards (IRBs) to go easy on the drug or device company that is paying for the research, even if this entails shirking their basic duty to safeguard subjects' safety, privacy, and right to informed consent.[23]

The implication is that if a medical center gets a reputation for being difficult to deal with, industry's research money will simply go elsewhere.

At a time when many academic hospitals are barely surviving, these beleaguered, understaffed human-subject committees form a pretty thin line of defense.

IRBs have little or no ability to do more than review protocols, and their mandate does not extend beyond protecting human subjects. Once trials are under way, unless a subject dies, they rarely become involved again. The NIH has an office that investigates complaints concerning human subjects, but it has only a handful of investigators, most of whom are neither physicians nor bioscientists. The FDA investigations unit is also badly understaffed. What's more, none of these watchdog organizations is adequately equipped to monitor investigator or systemic bias, intentional or otherwise, in the conduct of trials or in the interpretation of data.

Since the likelihood that Congress will pay for enough well-trained monitors to protect against abuse seems vanishingly small, another way needs to be found. One approach has been suggested by Gary Ellis, head of the NIH's Office for Protection Against Research Risks (OPRR). Ellis proposed that academic medical centers might create a new job category: research monitor. These full-time slots would be filled by physicians or biomedical scientists with special training in the design and conduct of clinical trials. They would follow trials from beginning to end, with a specific mandate to eliminate or at least minimize bias.[24] To protect the monitors from institutional pressures, medical centers might form consortia under which monitors would work at institutions other than their own.

Better training for clinical researchers and monitoring of trials would undoubtedly improve the quality of the results. But these relatively small fixes fail to address larger questions, such as, for example, whether it even makes sense to conduct clinical trials to test new devices—as opposed to drugs—especially when the technology is changing so fast that the trial results are likely to be outdated by the time they become available.

The experiences of the past thirty years with bypass surgery, angioplasty, and other interventional devices for treating coronary artery disease suggest that the answer, at least sometimes, might be no. A combination of very large databases; more detailed, precisely targeted data collection, and the use of advanced statistical techniques may soon make at least some randomized trials superfluous.

Where does all this leave us? Millions of Americans have enjoyed collectively tens of millions of pain-free, active years because of the drugs, devices, and procedures developed to treat coronary artery disease since the 1960s. Many lives have been extended and many heart attacks and deaths from heart attacks have been prevented, although no one knows for sure how many individuals have benefited and how many years of life have been added overall. And now, at the millennium, a concerted attack is at last being made on atherosclerosis.

The research focus is now prevention and cure, not symptom relief. Promising data are being reported from laboratories around the country. The goal of eliminating coronary artery disease is no longer fantasy or science fiction, although no one is quite ready to fix a date for its demise.

A large part of the credit for these advances must go to the dynamic, industrial-academic-governmental hybrid that is America's biomedical-research enterprise, and especially to visionary entrepreneurial physicians, businessmen, and engineers. Other important therapies, of course, such as thrombolytic drugs, continue to be developed through collaborations between traditional academic clinical researchers and biotechnology and drug companies. And still other clinical researchers are working on problems whose commercial payoff is not quite in sight yet.

But entrepreneurialism and its progeny, high-priced, high-tech treatments, are not without malignant side effects. The entrepreneurial doctor is likely to be biased toward the treatment he has helped develop or promote and whose profitability he may share in. The full-time practitioner with no financial interest in the drug or device has to keep up with a torrent of often hyped mass media and journal articles and video news releases to stay one step ahead of his patients; he is under pressure from HMOs and insurance companies to see more and more patients; and he must deal with direct consumer pressures to use the latest drug or device. All of this can overwhelm his ability to make wise treatment decisions.

Meanwhile, virtually all physicians must balance various roles and interests instead of just practicing traditional medicine with a clear duty to treat their patients' medical welfare as paramount. Many contemporary cardiologists are entrepreneurs with economic interests in drugs and devices, guardians of society's medical resources, and gatekeepers and business managers for HMOs and insurance companies. In this last role they are under economic pressure to, at worst, undertreat, and at best, keep the cost of treatment down.

What's more, many contracts between third-party payers and physicians "hold the doctors, not the health plans, liable in malpractice suits over denial of care," and doctors in some of these contracts "give up the right to sue the health plan if it refuses to pay for a service."[25] In the context of these multiple conflicts, the welfare of individual patients is compromised, at least some of the time.[26]

Yet, despite all these strains and stresses, for most people, most of the time, the American medical model probably delivers better technology and care than other systems elsewhere, with less bureaucratic hassle and less waiting time for major procedures. This is not to excuse its many flaws. It is simply to state a fact.

The level of technology and care the system at its best can provide, of course, is actually delivered only to those who have some kind of medical insurance. It does not embrace the more than forty million uninsured. This American disgrace results from the same two ingrained American beliefs that are responsible for industry's excessive influence on health care—that self-interest is the best incentive for achieving social goods, and that individuals have only minimal responsibility for the common good.

To foster fundamental change in American health care requires more than cost-cutting schemes, even elaborate ones such as managed care. It requires a move away from these beliefs—a fundamental shift in values. We must come to grips with the fact that the free market, self-interest, and American individualism, as potent a combination for economic growth as they have been in the twentieth century, do not provide all the answers. Until we do, we will muddle along with doctors who are enjoying practicing less and therefore are practicing less well, or less ethically, or not practicing at all, and periodic, ill-conceived attempts such as the Clintons' to bring about reform.

None of this is meant as a plea to restructure or even to increase regulation of the drug and device industries, which for the most part are doing what they are supposed to do—make and market good products and provide a fair return for their investors. Nor is it meant as a plea for physicians who are doing research to give up the bench for the bedside. The researchers are making an important contribution that we cannot afford to lose. And it is not meant as a plea for physicians as a class to be more compassionate, or more skilled. Most physicians are well-meaning and competent, but they operate under a truly burdensome system.

It is rather a plea for all of us, including industry, researchers, and practicing physicians, to reexamine our priorities and to reconsider what we as a society want or even think we deserve from our health-care system. If the answer is a system more focused than the current one on both healing and helping patients and promoting health generally, we must figure out how to return patients and practicing physicians, not biomedical researchers and industry, to its center. We must find a way to transform medicine from the industry it has become into a caring profession again.

Appendix A:
Designing and Mounting Clinical Trials

Controlled, randomized clinical trials are the most highly valued means of testing new drugs, devices and procedures. A sophisticated consumer in the medical marketplace needs a basic understanding of how clinical trials work; what their strengths and weaknesses are, how their results are used, for what purposes, and by whom, and what alternatives to them exist, if any.

Here's how the National Institutes of Health defines a clinical trial:[1]

> A scientific research study undertaken with human subjects to evaluate prospectively the diagnostic, prophylactic, or therapeutic effect of a drug, device, regimen, or procedure used or intended ultimately for use in the practice of medicine or the prevention of disease. A clinical trial is planned and conducted prospectively and includes a concurrent control group or other appropriate comparison group.

There are four criteria in this definition: (1) The trial must be conducted with human subjects; (2) the trial must be designed to determine whether the drug, device, regimen, or procedure does what it is intended to do safely and effectively; (3) the trial must test the drug, device, regimen, or procedure prospectively—that is, on a newly selected group of subjects, and evaluate its effects on them; and (4) the trial must compare the results of the test group against another relevantly similar group given a standard treatment or a placebo, or an appropriate historical control group. An animal study is not a clinical trial, nor is a study that simply analyzes the medical records of patients previously treated.

There are two more criteria that clinical trials usually need. The fifth criterion is randomization, a means of guaranteeing that there is no bias in the allocation of subjects to the groups being compared. Randomization maximizes the likelihood that any difference in outcome between groups is due to the treatment the subjects received, not other factors, such as age or the severity of their disease. It is the same method used by political pollsters seeking to get a representative sample of the general public. For randomization to work, the allocation of subjects must be adequately concealed from the investigators. If it is not, investigators will be able to influence the assignment of subjects to the treatment or placebo group, thereby biasing the trial's results.

Rigging treatment assignments is probably rare. Although no one knows with precision how common the practice is, there are numerous examples cited in the medical literature. Motives are varied and can involve both ignorance and malice. One investigator acknowledged cheating in this way because he "wanted experience in vaginal rather than abdominal hysterectomies."[2] He might have had little idea of the extent to which his actions could compromise the trial's results. More commonly, though, investigators favor a particular outcome, either because they believe it to be valid, or because they have a financial or other interest in it.

Sometimes it is as simple as checking a bulletin board where the allocation sequence is posted. Usually, though, a bit more ingenuity is required. There have been cases of researchers checking the relative weights of envelopes containing assignments, holding the envelopes up to intense incandescent bulbs found in radiation laboratories to read the contents, or rifling files for the randomization code. The author of a study in the *Journal of the American Medical Association,* from which these examples are taken, concludes by saying: "Researchers need to realize that humans, if given the opportunity, frequently subvert the intended aims of randomization."[3]

The sixth criterion is known as double blinding, which is a means of guaranteeing that neither the subjects nor the investigators know who is actually getting the experimental treatment and who is getting the alternative treatment or placebo. Double blinding is intended to eliminate investigator bias in data collection during the trial. It, too, of course, can be subverted by investigators willing to resort to cheating. And for obvious reasons it cannot be used when medical devices are being compared. Two pills can be made to look identical, but a stent and an angioplasty catheter cannot. The investigator need only look to see which form of treatment is being used.

Once researchers decide that a new treatment needs testing and that a large-scale clinical trial may be warranted, they must formulate a hypothesis. For example, the hypothesis of a multicenter trial comparing angioplasty and bypass surgery, the Bypass Angioplasty Revascularization Investigation (BARI), was that trying angioplasty before bypass surgery in a predefined set of patients would not compromise these patients' health status during a five-year follow-up period.[4]

After the investigators have agreed on the hypothesis and framed it clearly, they must design a study that can reasonably be expected to test it. Before actually beginning work on the study design, however, they will often try to determine whether a reasonable alternative would be to analyze patient records stored in databases, or to conduct some other type of study that could cost less than a tenth as much as a clinical trial.

Investigators must also determine if there are ethical obstacles to conducting the trial, such as compelling evidence that the new treatment is safer and more effective than standard treatments and therefore should be made available to patients who need it without delay. If there are no ethical hurdles, or if those that exist can be surmounted, the researchers then must design a trial whose results will satisfy standard statistical tests of validity.

For a clinical trial's results to be valid it must be extremely unlikely that any difference detected between the treatment being tested and the alternative treatment or placebo was generated by chance. The sample size must be large enough to ensure this result, the trial must be long enough to adequately test the treatments, and the methods by which the data are collected and analyzed must be sufficiently rigorous. There are well-established norms for meeting these criteria.

The design itself has several fundamental elements. Curtis Meinert of Johns Hopkins University lists ten in his book *Clinical Trials: Design, Conduct and Analysis* (New York: Oxford University Press, 1986). Here they are, with jargon removed and slightly explicated:

1. A concise statement of the trial's objectives. A typical objective might be to determine whether initial treatment with drugs rather than bypass surgery compromises the five-year outcome of patients with two blocked arteries.
2. Specification of the event or events, such as death, heart attack, or the need for additional procedures, that will be used to evaluate the treatments being tested.
3. Specification of the treatments to be tested, such as balloon angioplasty and bypass surgery.
4. The proposed sample size and its statistical justification.
5. Specification of how long patients will be followed up after treatment.
6. Criteria for inclusion and exclusion of subjects, such as the number of diseased arteries, age, general health status, etc.
7. A method of randomization.
8. A schedule of examinations for all subjects before and after treatment.
9. Specification of a system for collecting and analyzing data.
10. Specification of an organizational and decision-making structure.

The draft design document, including Meinert's elements, a plan for obtaining the informed consent of subjects, and other factors specific to the proposal, such as whether it will be a single or multicenter trial, then becomes the basis for a grant application.[5] If the investigators are seeking federal funds rather than industry support, this is a slow, complex, and often frustrating process, involving intensive peer review. It is, however, the process academic researchers must go through to get the large sums of public money needed to conduct large clinical trials, and it is one reason why it takes so long for the trials to get under way. It typically takes a year for a proposal to be reviewed, and more often than not the first version is rejected. It is not unusual for two or three years to go by between the first draft of the trial's design and the beginning of subject selection.

Thus the first clinical trial comparing a new treatment to an established therapy or placebo may not begin until five to ten years after the first experimental use of the new treatment—three to six years to overcome medical conservatism and two to four years to work through the review process, get the study funded, and actually begin the research.

Appendix B:
What Patients Need to Know

Today, coronary bypass operations are as familiar to most Americans as appendectomies. Angioplasty and stenting are almost as well known and even more prevalent. Important questions remain, however, about who should be treated surgically, who with a different intervention, and who with drugs. These include:

What protection if any will a specific interventional procedure such as surgery or angioplasty provide against heart attacks and disease progression that drugs alone won't? How will a particular treatment choice affect quality of life with respect to work, exercise, freedom from pain and discomfort? At what point should a procedure be done? If the treatment selected is surgery, for example, should it be avoided for as long as possible to put off the added risk of reoperation, which is increasingly common in the United States' aging population?

And potential candidates for revascularization procedures such as bypass surgery and angioplasty need to know the short-term—that is, operative and immediate postoperative—survival odds for each treatment that might be an option for them; the chances in the operative or immediate postoperative period of suffering a serious side effect such as a heart attack or a stroke; and which treatment if any is most likely to extend their life.

The answers to these questions depend on things such as the severity of the coronary disease, anatomical features, and risk factors such as old age and the presence of related conditions such as diabetes. Because there is no consensus among cardiologists and cardiac surgeons about the answers, it is especially difficult for someone like David Allison, in the immediate wake of a heart attack, to deal with them (see chapter 1).

While certainly less acute, the pressure to decide what to do is also great when elective bypass surgery is recommended to a mildly symptomatic patient who might never have given a thought to the possibility of undergoing surgery, and who may not need it. A well-informed patient, however, can improve his or her chances of surviving surgery (possibly by not having it); avoiding bad nonfatal events such as heart attacks and strokes, and getting good long-term results (see chapter 8).

To better understand your cardiologist's treatment recommendation, ask him or her to describe the general outline of your particular case—how many blockages you have; how severe they are; how difficult it should be to open them; what degree of opening angioplasty would provide (surgery completely bypasses blockages); in which arteries the blockages are located and what part of the heart they supply with blood; and whether you have developed a collateral blood supply that offsets some of the loss resulting from the blockages. You might also ask what other risk factors you have, such as fragile arteries resulting from diabetes. Then ask your cardiologist to explain why he or she thinks a particular treatment is the best option for you.

Ask your cardiologist to support his or her recommendation with clinical trial results and data from the tens of thousands of cases collected in registeries maintained by the National Institutes of Health, Duke University, the Cleveland Clinic, and the Society of Thoracic Surgeons, among others. And most importantly, ask your cardiologist to explain how his or her own experience supports his or her clinical judgment. Then, if your cardiologist hasn't already done so, ask him or her to make clear why he or she rejected the other treatment options. If there is anything you haven't understood, ask him or her for clarification. Everything you need to know can be expressed adequately and concisely in lay language, as Paul Corso demonstrated in explaining treatment options to Lewis Hollander (see chapter 8).

You must then decide whether to accept your cardiologist's recommendation or to seek another opinion. Unless you are completely comfortable with the advice you are getting—and perhaps even if you are—you should get at least one more professional opinion. It is not an affront to your cardiologist to do this. If he or she is resistant, this should be taken as an argument for getting another opinion.

While there are circumstances in which, by consensus, surgery is the best option—for example, a severe obstruction of the left main coronary artery, or severe disease in three or more arteries combined with a poorly functioning left ventricle—in most other circumstances, the judgment of good cardiologists may differ as to what constitutes the best form of treatment.

If you do get a second opinion, you should try to get it from someone who is board-certified (i.e., has passed a relevant specialty examination) and who went to a different medical school and trained at a different hospital from your cardiologist (who also should be board-certified). You should be able to get information about physician certification and training from the state medical society or from various local or regional Internet physician databases. You might also consider a fresh diagnosis. Remember that David Allison was told he did not need a procedure because the third of his heart muscle supplied by the left anterior descending artery was dead. But that turned out to be wrong, and he had a successful angioplasty.

The second critically important decision is the selection of a surgeon or interventional cardiologist, which will determine not only who performs the procedure but also where it will be performed. The choice of a hospital is important partly because some are better equipped and organized for heart surgery, angioplasty, and stenting than others, but mainly because interventions in general and heart surgery in particular are team enterprises. Ideally, you want a surgical team—surgeons, nurses, anesthesiologists and anesthetists, and perfusionists (heart-lung machine operators)—who are not only skilled and experienced, but also who have worked together a lot. The same holds true for an interventional cardiology lab team.

New York and Pennsylvania publish risk-adjusted performance data on both cardiac surgeons and hospitals where bypass surgery is performed, and a nonprofit coalition of health-care purchasers in California and Arizona began ranking hospitals in 1998. But these data and rankings are far from infallible, and similar data are not available for interventional labs. Criticisms include using only mortality as a guide to quality, inadequate risk assessment, and unreliability of data. But they are not a bad rough guide. Elsewhere, the best option is to seek out the judgment of several cardiac surgeons and cardiologists.

The more serious your disease, the better the odds are that the right choice will improve your chances of surviving surgery or another procedure. And for the long term, on the highly likely assumption that you survive the operation, the right choice might buy you many more additional years of angina-free active life. Some important things a potential surgical, angioplasty, or stent patient needs to know follow in the form of eight questions, with the optimal answers in parentheses:

1. How many bypass operations or interventional procedures do the operators and hospitals do annually? (More than a hundred for a surgeon or interventional cardiologist, and more than a thousand for a hospital.)
2. Do they take the hardest cases? (Yes.)
3. What is their overall mortality rate? (Less than 3 percent [for surgeons] and 1 percent [for interventionalists] if they do a large volume and take the hardest cases; otherwise, even lower.)
4. What is their overall event (heart attack and stroke) rate? (Less than 5 percent if they take the hardest cases; otherwise, lower.)
5. How many cases like yours do they do a year? (This information may be hard to get, and the specific number will depend in part on how common

or rare your case is. Look for a surgeon and a hospital with high volume and good mortality rates and some experience with your specific combination of disease factors.)

6. What is their mortality rate for cases like yours? (Compare an operator's or a hospital's success rate in treating cases like yours, especially if it is rare, with those of the other surgeons, interventionalists, or hospitals to whom you might go.)

7. What is their event rate in cases like yours? (Same as for 6.)

8. How do their overall mortality and event rates compare with rates of other surgeons, interventional cardiologists, and hospitals to whom you might go? (Their rates are as good as or better than the available alternatives.)

I know of no statistical program or decision-making model that will crunch the numbers and spit out the right choice. But if—with the help of your cardiologist, primary-care physician, or state medical society—you can get the answers to these questions, or most of them, you have the most pertinent information for selecting a surgeon or an interventional cardiologist. In preparation for such a decision, should you ever have to make it, it would be wise to discuss these issues with your doctors before the need arises.

If you still cannot decide, here, too, there is no reason not to ask for other opinions. You might also go to the library and check the *Dartmouth Atlas of Health Care* to see how your city or region compares to others in terms of the number of bypass operations done annually. The rate varies dramatically, with too much surgery being done in some places and too little in others. If your area is an outlier, you can factor that into your decision.

Finally, there is the question of what kind of surgery you should have if you choose surgery. The options are standard open-chest coronary artery bypass surgery using a heart-lung machine; less-invasive surgery using a heart-lung machine; and beating-heart surgery done either through a small incision or in an open chest, but without a heart-lung machine.

Some critics of less-invasive surgery contend that surgeons cannot work as precisely when their vision is limited by a small incision. Some surgeons believe the heart-lung machine is the source of most surgical morbidity, and therefore they oppose using the machine except when absolutely necessary. And most surgeons agree that the beating-heart method, especially through a small incision, cannot be safely used to bypass arteries on the back surface of the heart.

Lewis Hollander's experience with Stuart Seides and Paul Corso as described in chapter 8 can serve as a model for selecting the right kind of surgery.

Notes

Preface

1. *Fact Book, Fiscal Year 1995*, National Heart, Lung, and Blood Institute, p. 35.
2. *1997 Heart and Stroke Statistical Update*, American Heart Association, p. 28.
3. *1997 Heart and Stroke Statistical Update*, American Heart Association, p. 10, for coronary artery disease statistics and p. 3 for comparative statistics on AIDS, breast cancer, and lung cancer.

Chapter 1: A Heart Attack

1. Anne Michaels, *Fugitive Pieces* (New York: Vintage International), 1998, p. 117.
2. Interview with David Allison, (May 7, 1997), Washington, D.C.
3. Allison interview.
4. Allison interview.

Chapter 2: The Revolution of 1912

1. Mary Gordon, *The Company of Women* (New York: Random House, 1980). p. 254.
2. William Butler Yeats, *The Collected Poems of W. B. Yeats* (New York: Macmillan, 1959), p. 39.
3. Edgar Allan Poe, *Edgar Allan Poe*, Raven Edition, vol. 2 (New York: P. F. Collier & Son, 1903), pp. 352–59.
4. Alfred P. Fishman and Dickinson W. Richards, eds., *Circulation of the Blood* (New York: Oxford University Press, 1964), p. 201.
5. Aristotle, *On the Parts of Animals*, Book 3, chap 4 (New York: Garland, 1987), p. 68.
6. Blaise Pascal, *Pensées*, sec. IV, no. 277, Harvard Classics, vol. 48 (New York: P. F. Collier & Son, 1910), p. 99.
7. Sir Thomas Lewis, *The Mechanism of the Heartbeat* (London: Shaw & Sons, 1911).
8. Associated Press, "Art Sleuth Spots Ancient Image of Heart," *New York Times* (September 9, 1997), p. C6.
9. Michael Servetus, *Christianisimi Restitutio*, a tract published anonymously in 1553.

10. For a fuller account see André Cournand, "Air and Blood," in *Circulation of the Blood: Men and Ideas*, ed. Alfred P. Fishman and Dickinson W. Richards (New York: Oxford University Press, 1964), pp. 18–22.

11. William Harvey, *Exercitatio anatomica de motu cordis et sanguinis in animalibus*, Harvard Classics, vol. 38 (New York: P. F. Collier & Son, 1910), p. 131.

12. Harvey, William, *Exercitatio anatomica de motu cordis et sanguinus in animalibus*, Chauncey Leake translator (New York: Charles Thomas, 1928), Part 2, p. 25.

13. René-Theophile-Hyacinthe Laennec invented the stethoscope in 1816. See Stanley Joel Reiser, *Medicine and the Reign of Technology* (New York: Cambridge University Press, 1978), p. 25.

14. Robert Hooke, "A General Scheme or Idea of the Present State of Natural Philosophy . . ." in *Posthumous Works of Robert Hooke*, ed. Richard Waller (London: Samuel Smith and Benjamin Walford, 1705), pp. 39–40.

15. Giovanni Battista Morgagni, "The Seats and Causes of Diseases," repr. in Fredrick A. Willius and Thomas E. Keys, *Classics of Cardiology* (Malabar, Fla.: Robert E. Krieger, 1983), pp. 185–86.

16. William Heberden, "Some Account of a Disorder of the Breast," *Medical Transactions*, 2, Royal College of Physicians, London, (1772), p. 59. Heberden first used the term "angina pectoris" in a lecture to the Royal College of Physicians in July 1768.

17. W. Bruce Fye, "Acute Myocardial Infarction: A Historical Summary," in *Acute Myocardial Infarction*, 2d ed., B. J. Gersh and S. H. Rahimtoola, eds. (New York: Chapman & Hall, 1997), pp. 1–15.

18. Telephone interview with Bruce Fye (January 15, 1997).

19. Paul Dudley White, "Angina Pectoris: Historical Background," in *Angina Pectoris*, ed. Oglesby Paul (New York: Medcom Press 1972), 1, 9.

20. J. O. Leibowitz, *The History of Coronary Heart Disease* (Berkeley: University of California Press, 1970), p. 174. Sprague's estimate is relative to the population "at risk," determined by average age and freedom from other causes of death, especially tuberculosis and other infectious diseases.

21. R. J. Bing, "Atherosclerosis," in *Cardiology: The Evolution of the Science and the Art*, ed. Richard J. Bing (Chur, Switz.: Harwood Academic Publishers, 1992), p. 127. See also Louis J. Acierno, *The History of Cardiology* (New York: Parthenon Publishing Group, 1994), p. 97.

22. Leibowitz, *The History of Coronary Heart Disease*, p. 9. Also see Acierno, *The History of Cardiology*, p. 287.

23. Aristotle, *On the Parts of Animals*, p. 71.

24. Christian Albert Theodor Billroth, as quoted in Robert G. Richardson, *The Surgeon's Heart: A History of Cardiac Surgery* (London: William Heinemann Medical Books, 1969), pp. 28–29. Richardson notes that in the preface to the ninth edition of his textbook, Billroth wrote, "I have not followed the advance of medical science as closely as one should who was to present the results of recent workers to a new generation of students." His point seems to have been that at some later date Billroth might have reconsidered this remark, which, as far as is known, he did not repeat.

25. Julius H. Comroe, Jr., *retrospectroscope* (Menlo Park, Calif.: Von Gehr Press, 1977), p. 121.

26. Paget is cited in Harris B. Schumacker, Jr., *The Evolution of Cardiac Surgery* (Bloomington: Indiana University Press 1992), p. 3.

27. L. Rehn, "Penetrating Cardiac Wounds and Cardiac Suture," *Archiv Klinischer Chirugie* 55 (1897): 315–29.

28. L. L. Hill, "A Report of a Case of Successful Suturing of the Heart, and Table of 37 Other Cases of Suturing by Different Operators with Various Terminations and the Conclusions Drawn," *Medical Record* 62 (1902): 846–48.

29. Thomas Kuhn, *The Structure of Scientific Revolutions*, 2nd ed. (Chicago: University of Chicago Press, 1970), p. 24.

30. Steven Weinberg, "The Revolution That Didn't Happen," *New York Review of Books* 45, no. 15 (1998): 48–52.

31. Ronald L. Eisenberg, *Radiology: An Illustrated History* (St. Louis: Mosby-Year Book, 1992), pp. 210–11.

32. Stephen L. Johnson, *The History of Cardiac Surgery 1896–1955* (Baltimore: Johns Hopkins University Press), 1970, p. 16.

33. Ibid., pp. 18–19.

34. The material on Alexis Carrel in this chapter is based on chapter 6 of Steven G. Friedman, *A History of Vascular Surgery* (Mount Kisco, N.Y.: Futura, 1989).

Carrel's Nobel prize was awarded specifically for his work in suturing blood vessels and transfusion and transplantation of organs, all in animals.

35. Ulrich Sigwart, "Introduction," *Endoluminal Stenting*, ed. Ulrich Sigwart (London: W. B. Saunders, 1996), p. 2.

36. Julius H. Comroe, Jr., *Exploring the Heart* (New York: W. W. Norton, 1983), p. 185.

37. The young woman became a nun and lived thirty-four more years. Friedman, *A History of Vascular Surgery*, p. 76.

38. Comroe, *Exploring the Heart*, p. 189.

39. Kuhn, *The Structure of Scientific Revolutions*, p. 24.

40. James B. Herrick, "Clinical Features of Sudden Obstruction of the Coronary Arteries," *JAMA* (59, no. 23) (1912): 215–20. A similar article, written by the Russians W. P. Obrastzow and N. D. Straschesko, was published in 1910 ("Zur Kenntniss der Thrombose der Koronararterien des Herzens, *Zeitschrift für Klinischer Medizin* 71: 116) and cited by Herrick. For a fuller discussion of this article see J. O. Leibowitz *The History of Coronary Heart Disease* p. 12. Leibowitz notes that neither the Herrick nor the Obrastzow and Straschesko articles were original, nor did they claim to be. What sets them apart, Leibowitz wrote, "is their way of approach: explicit, definitive and unreserved in expression, and free from obscurity of meaning. In contrast, most of the best clinicians immediately preceding them only implied the diagnosis of coronary thrombosis, the notion being contained in the mind, without being clearly formulated."

41. James B. Herrick, "An Intimate Account of My Early Experience with Coronary Thrombosis," *American Heart Journal* 27, no. 1 (1944).

42. James B. Herrick, *Memoirs of Eighty Years* (Chicago: University of Chicago Press, 1949), p. 196.

43. James B. Herrick, "Thrombosis of the Coronary Arteries," *JAMA* Vol. 72, No. 6 (1919): 387–94. This paper was published in 1919 but was delivered in 1918.

44. Herrick, James B., An Intimate Account," p. 15.

45. Marcus DeWood, et al., "Prevalence of Total Coronary Occlusion During the Early Hours of Transmyocardial Infarction," *New England Journal of Medicine* 303 No. 16 (1980): 897–902.

46. In an address given on the inauguration of the faculty of science at the University of Lille on December 7, 1854, Pasteur said: *"Dans les champs de l'observation le hasard ne favorise que les esprits preparé."* This remark is usually translated something like, "Where observation is concerned, chance favors only the prepared mind."

Chapter 3: Creating the Platform

1. The endocrinologist was Herbert McLean Evans.

2. J. McLean, "The Thromboplastic Action of Cephalin," *American Journal of Physiology* 41 (1916): 250–57.

3. R. DeWall and R. J. Bing, "Cardiopulmonary Bypass," in *Cardiology: The Evolution of the Science and the Art,* ed. Richard. J. Bing (Chur; Switz.: Harwood Academic Publishers, 1992), p. 60.

4. Julius H. Comroe, Jr., *retrospectroscope* (Menlo Park, Calif.: Von Gehr Press, 1978), pp. 92–94.

5. Unless otherwise indicated, the account of Forssmann's self-catheterization and subsequent career is based on his autobiography, *Experiments on Myself: Memoirs of a Surgeon in Germany* (New York: St. Martin's Press, 1974).

6. *Experiments on Myself,* p. 82.

7. The nineteenth-century leaders in studying animal hearts were Claude Bernard, the great French physiologist who dubbed the method cardiac catheterization, and two other Frenchmen, Jules Marey and Étienne Chauveau.

8. Advisory Committee on Human Radiation Experiments, *Human Radiation Experiments* (New York: Oxford University Press, 1996), p. 84.

9. *Experiments on Myself,* p. 83.

10. *Experiments on Myself,* p. 84.

11. This account also benefits from an interview with Forssmann conducted by Lawrence K. Altman and published in his book *Who Goes First? The Story of Self-Experimentation in Medicine* (New York: Random House, 1987), p. 43.

12. In his autobiography Forssmann said Romeis "almost tried" to pull the catheter out of his arm, but in his later interview with Altman, Forssmann said Romeis actually tried to pull it out. *Who Goes First?* p. 44.

13. According to Forssmann's autobiography, the tip of the catheter was in his right ventricle, but he told Altman that it was in the right atrium because the catheter was too short to reach the ventricle. *Who Goes First?* p. 45.

14. Werner Forssmann, "Probing the Right Ventricle of the Heart," *Klinische Wochenschrift* 8 (1929): 2085–87.

15. *Experiments on Myself,* p. 86.

16. James V. Warren, "Fifty Years of Invasive Cardiology (Werner Forssmann (1904–1979)," *American Journal of Medicine* 69 (1980): 12.

17. *Who Goes First?* p. 50.

18. They hardly make mothers like that anymore.

19. *Experiments on Myself,* pp. 107–8.

20. *Experiments on Myself,* pp. 162–63.

21. D. B. Melrose, B. Dreyer, H. H. Bentall, and J. B. Baker, "Elective Cardiac Arrest," *Lancet* 2, no. 21 (1955).

22. Robert G. Richardson, *The Surgeon's Heart: A History of Cardiac Surgery* (London: William Heinemann Medical Books, 1969), p. 252.

23. D. B. Effler, L. K. Groves, F. M. Sones, Jr., and W. J. Kolff, "Elective Cardiac Arrest in Open-Heart Surgery: Report of Three Cases," *Cleveland Clinic Quarterly* 23, no. 105 (1956).

24. R. DeWall and R. J. Bing, "Cardiopulmonary Bypass," in *Cardiology: The Evolution of the Science and the Art,* ed. Richard J. Bing (Chur, Switz: Harwood Academic Publishers, 1992), p. 55. Also in 1929, according to Harris B. Schumacker's *The Evolution of Cardiac Surgery* (Bloomington: Indiana University Press, 1992), p. 247, the Russian S. Brukhonenko did experiments on dogs that led him to write the following about the artificial circulation of blood: "If this method were perfected could it not be used in the domain of medicine and especially in the case where it is essential to replace, even if it be temporary, the insufficient work of the *human* heart?" Brukhonenko goes on to say that *"in principle* the method of artificial circulation may be applicable to man (in certain cases and perhaps even for performing certain operations upon the temporarily arrested heart). . . .

25. Steven G. Friedman, *A History of Vascular Surgery* (Mount Kisco, N.Y.: Futura, 1989), pp. 79–81.

26. This anecdote was written by Marjorie Gibbon Battles, John Gibbon, Jr.'s, mother, in a letter to Harris B. Schumacker, M.D., and cited by Ada Romaine-Davis in *John Gibbon and His Heart-Lung Machine* (Philadelphia: University of Pennsylvania Press, 1991), p. 10.

27. John H. Gibbon, Jr., "The Development of the Heart-Lung Apparatus," *Review of Surgery* 27, no. 4 (July–August 1970), Unless otherwise noted, the story of the heart-lung machine as told in chapter 2 is based on this account by Gibbon, the principal inventor of the machine.

28. Ada Romaine-Davis, *John Gibbon and His Heart-Lung Machine* (Philadelphia: University of Pennsylvania Press, 1991), p. 21.

29. "The Development of the Heart-Lung Apparatus," p. 232.

30. Harris B. Schumaker, Jr., *The Evolution of Cardiac Surgery,* p. 17.

31. J. H. Gibbon, Jr., "Medicine's Living History," *Medical World News* 13 (1942): 47.

32. "The Development of the Heart-Lung Apparatus," p. 233.

33. "The Development of the Heart-Lung Apparatus," pp. 234–35.

34. *The Evolution of Cardiac Surgery,* p. 244.

35. *The Evolution of Cardiac Surgery,* pp. 249, 251.

36. It wasn't until 1937 that clinical-grade heparin was available for use in humans.

37. Francis D. Moore, *A Miracle and a Privilege* (Washington, D.C.: Joseph Henry Press, 1995), pp. 224–25. Also see "Into the Heart," part 2 of the Nova television series *Pioneers of Surgery.*

38. J. H. Gibbon, Jr., "The Army Doctor Comes Home and Looks at Civilian Practice," *Harper's* (February 1946): 175–80. The observation about socialized medicine was made by Ada Romaine-Davis in *John Gibbon and His Heart-Lung Machine,* p. 68.

39. *John Gibbon and His Heart-Lung Machine,* pp. 170–71.

40. Julius H. Comroe, *Exploring the Heart* (New York: W. W. Norton), 1983), p. 34.

41. Details of the machine's design are from Romaine-Davis. For anyone interested in a full account of the development of the heart-lung machine see her book *John Gibbon and His Heart-Lung Machine.*

42. "The Development of the Heart-Lung Apparatus," pp. 238–39.

43. John H. Gibbon, Jr., "Application of a Mechanical Heart and Lung Apparatus to Cardiac Surgery," *Minnesota Medicine* (March 1954): 176.

Although Gibbon is credited with having done "The first successful clinical operation performed with the aid of a completely mechanical pump oxygenator," Harris Schumacker writes in his book *The Evolution of Cardiac Surgery* that on August 7, 1951, in Turin, Italy, "Mario Dogliotti used the bubble oxygenator developed in his laboratories as a precautionary measure when resecting a large mediastinal tumor which was compressing the right side of the heart. The apparatus [which accomplished partial cardiopulmonary bypass] worked effectively during the period it was used, and the patient did well. No successful use of a heart-lung machine is known to have antedated Dogliotti's."

44. Stanton P. Nolan et al., "Reflections on the Evolution of Cardiopulmonary Bypass," *Annals of Thoracic Surgery* 64, no. 5 (1997): 1540–43.

45. John W. Kirklin, "The Middle 1950s and C. Walton Lillehei," *Journal of Thoracic and Cardiovascular Surgery* 98, no. 5, part 2, (1989): 823.

46. "The Development of the Heart-Lung Machine," p. 239.

47. Stephen L. Johnson, *The History of Cardiac Surgery, 1896–1955*, (Baltimore: Johns Hopkins University Press, 1978) pp. 151–2.

48. Lillehei recounts this story on Nova, *Pioneers of Surgery*, part 2, "Into the Heart," but does not name the source of the remark. Romaine-Davis identifies Haupt in *John Gibbon and His Heart-Lung Machine*, p. 143.

49. *The History of Cardiac Surgery, 1896–1955*, pp. 151–54.

50. Nova, *Pioneers of Surgery*, part 2, "Into the Heart."

51. Nova, *Pioneers of Surgery*, part 2, "Into the Heart." The one lawsuit involved a mother who suffered brief cardiac arrest and as a consequence some neurological deficit. Lillehei, who had malpractice insurance, advised her to sue, but instead of suing for several hundred thousand dollars, her lawyers raised the stakes to several million and the case went to court instead of being settled as planned. The woman lost and got nothing because the court ruled that she had been adequately warned of the risk.

52. Harry Minetree, *Cooley: The Career of a Great Heart Surgeon* (New York: Harper's Magazine Press, 1973), p. 132. Confirmed in a telephone interview with Cooley (February 4, 1998).

53. The coronary and bronchial blood that returned to the operating field could be aspirated away, but this damaged red cells.

Chapter 4: Groping in the Dark

1. Claude S. Beck, "My Life in Heart Surgery—1923–1969," *Geriatrics* 26 (February 1971):85–86.

2. Elliott C. Cutler and Claude S. Beck, "The Present Status of the Surgical

Procedures in Chronic Valvular Disease of the Heart—Final Report of All Surgical Cases," *Archives of Surgery* 403 (1929):413–16.

3. Beck, "My Life in Heart Surgery," p. 86.

4. Interview with Paul Corso Washington, D.C., December 16, 1996.

5. John W. Kirklin, "The Middle 1950s and C. Walton Lillehei," *Journal of Thoracic and Cardiovascular Surgery* 98 (1989):822–24. Four of the eight patients died.

6. Interview with Paul Taylor, Cleveland (May 29, 1996).

7. Interview with Tom Fogarty, Portola Valley, Calif. (November 12, 1996).

8. Beck, "My Life in Heart Surgery," pp. 88–92.

9. Jane Fitsch, "Cardiologists Say Portable Defibrillators Can Save Time and Lives," *New York Times* (April 16, 1997), p. A1.

10. Matthew L. Wald, "Airlines Prepare to Fight Heart Attacks Aloft," *New York Times* (June 7, 1998), p. TR3.

11. Jane E. Brody, "A $3,000 'Fire Extinguisher' to Put Out Heart Attacks" *New York Times* (April 13, 1999), p. D6.

12. Jay Katz, *Experimentation with Human Beings* (New York: Russell Sage Foundation, 1972), p. 727.

13. Beck, "My Life in Heart Surgery," p. 93.

14. J. Baldwin, J. Sanchez, and R. J. Bing, "Coronary Artery Surgery," in *Cardiology: The Evolution of the Science and the Art,* ed. R. J. Bing (Chur, Switz.: Harwood Academic Publishers, 1992), pp. 169–70.

15. Ibid.

16. Josephine Robertson, "Repairing the Human Pump," *Cleveland Plain Dealer* (February 26, 1956), Pictorial Magazine.

17. Ibid.

18. Rebecca M. Johnson and Steven D. Johnson, "Claude S. Beck (1894–1971)," manuscript in Case Western Reserve University archives, pp. 8–10.

19. Beck, "My Life in Heart Surgery," p. 94.

20. Interview with Laurence Groves, Cleveland (October 18, 1996).

21. J. R. Kitchell, R. P. Glover, and R. H. Kyle, "Bilateral Internal Mammary Artery Ligation for Angina Pectoris," *American Journal of Cardiology* 1 (1958): 46–50; D. E. Harken in L. B. Ellis, H. L Blumgart, D. E. Harken, H. S. Sise, and F. J. Stare, "Clinical Conference: Long-Term Management of Patients with Coronary Artery Disease," *Circulation* 17 (1958):945–52, and I. C. Brill, W. M. Rosenbaum, E. E. Rosenbaum, and J. R. Flannery, "Internal Mammary Ligation," *Northwest Medicine* 57 (1958):483–86.

22. Leonard A. Cobb et al., "An Evaluation of Internal-Mammary-Artery Ligation by a Double-Blind Technic," *New England Journal of Medicine* 260, no. 22 (1959): 1115–18.

23. J. D. Ratcliff, "New Surgery for Ailing Hearts," *Reader's Digest* 71 (1957): 70–73.

24. Cobb et al., p. 1118.

25. Personal communication with Jacob Eren, Altea, Spain (March 5, 1996).

26. Interview with Leonard A. R. Golding, Cleveland (May 29, 1996).

27. Beck, "My Life in Heart Surgery," p. 93.

28. Arthur Vineberg's reference is to M. J. Schlesinger and P. M. Zoll, "Inci-

dence and Localization of Coronary Artery Occlusion, *Archives of Pathology* 32 (1941): 170. He makes the reference in his own article "Experimental Background of Myocardial Revascularization by Internal Mammary Artery Implantation and Supplementary Technics, with its Clinical Application in 125 Patients: A Review and Critical Appraisal," *Annals of Surgery* 159, no. 2 (1964):185.

29. Ibid., p. 187.

30. Vineberg, *Annals of Surgery,* reporting on the work of James Walker of Boston and Charleston, West Virginia, who did forty-five Vineberg operations, and a physician named Bigelow (no first name given), who did eleven.

31. René G. Favaloro, *The Challenging Dream of Heart Surgery* (Cleveland: Cleveland Clinic Foundation, 1992), p. 24.

32. At the annual meeting of the American College of Cardiology in May 1959, and later that year at the American Heart Association meeting, F. Mason Sones reported on opacifying the coronary arteries by injecting dye into cavities near their openings. A four-paragraph abstract of this report titled "Cine-Coronary Arteriography" was published on pp. 773–74 of the abstracts of the 32nd Scientific Sessions of the American Heart Association. The first publication on injecting dye directly into the coronary arteries appeared in July 1962 in *Modern Concepts of Cardiovascular Disease* 31, no. 7:735–38. It was called "Cine Coronary Arteriography," without a hyphen, and the authors were F. Mason Sones, Jr., and Earl K. Shirey.

33. Golding, interview.

34. Ibid.

35. Reuters, Washington Post (April 23, 1997), p. A19.

36. Interview with Geraldine Sones, Solon, Ohio (October 18, 1996).

37. Ibid.

38. Interview with Elaine Clayton, Cleveland (October 17, 1996).

39. Willian L. Proudfit, "F. Mason Sones, Jr., M.D. (1918–1985):The Man and His Work," *Cleveland Clinic Quarterly* 53 (Summer 1986):121–22.

40. Sones interview.

41. Clayton interview.

42. Proudfit, "F. Mason Sones, Jr.," p. 122.

43. This quotation is as remembered by Roysten Lewis during an interview at his home in Shaker Heights, Ohio, on October 16, 1996. What Sones wanted Lewis to do was to give the patient enough digitalis to improve the muscular tone of the heart so it would pump more efficiently.

44. Ibid.

45. Ibid. The other two men Lewis said profoundly influenced his life were his father and William Proudfit, a former chief of cardiology at the Cleveland Clinic.

46. Ibid.

47. Ibid. I have not been able to find West By God, West Virginia, but it is the name—not easily forgotten—that Lewis remembers.

48. Favaloro, *The Challenging Dream of Heart Surgery,* p. 25.

49. Closed-chest cardiac massage and direct-current defibrillation were unknown at the time.

50. Lewis interview.

51. Interview with Earl K. Shirey, Cleveland (May 30, 1996).

52. Clayton interview.

53. Earl Shirey, interview of May 30, 1996, supplemented by a telephone interview on August 26, 1998.

54. Ibid. (May 30, 1996).

55. Lewis interview.

56. Ibid.

57. Sones interview.

58. Shirey interview.

59. Ibid.

60. Sones and Shirey, "Cine Coronary," pp. 735–38.

61. Interview with William Proudfit, Cleveland (May 29, 1996).

62. Clayton interview.

63. Favaloro, *The Challenging Dream of Heart Surgery*, p. 24.

64. Interview with David Sabiston, Durham, N.C. (January 29, 1997).

Chapter 5: Accidents and Innovations

1. René Favaloro, *The Challenging Dream of Heart Surgery* (Cleveland: Cleveland Clinic Foundation), 1992, p. 61.

2. Interview with Rosalind Talisman, Cleveland (May 29, 1996).

3. David C. Sabiston, Jr., "The Coronary Circulation," *Johns Hopkins Medical Journal* 134 (June 1974): 320–21.

4. Favaloro, *The Challenging Dream of Heart Surgery*, pp. 7–11. The biographical details of Favaloro's life come from this source unless otherwise noted.

5. Interview with Geraldine Sones, Solon, Ohio (October 18, 1996).

6. Talisman interview.

7. Dwight Harken advanced heart surgery in a number of ways, especially in the removal of projectiles from the heart. Harken also was among the first to operate on heart valves.

8. Interview with William Sheldon, former chief of cardiology at the Cleveland Clinic, Cleveland (May 30, 1996).

9. An internal mammary artery graft was first successfully used to supply blood to the heart muscle by Vasilii Kolessov in the Soviet Union in 1964 and reported in November 1966. George Green of New York University reported on similar work in 1968. This operation was more difficult than saphenous vein grafts, however, and it took a decade or more before it caught on generally, although surgeons at the Cleveland Clinic began doing it regularly in about 1970.

10. Favaloro, *The Challenging Dream of Heart Surgery*, p. 60.

11. These operations were done by David Sabiston at Johns Hopkins in 1962, a team led by Edward Garrett at Baylor in 1964, and Donald Kahn at the University of Michigan in 1966.

12. This operation was done in Leningrad (now St. Petersburg) by Vasilii Kolessov in 1964.

13. Favaloro, *The Challenging Dream of Heart Surgery*, p. 69.

14. Arthur M. Vineberg, *Myocardial Revascularization by Arterial/Ventricular Implants* (Boston: John Wright, 1982), p. 60.

15. Favaloro, *The Challenging Dream of Heart Surgery*, p. 70.

16. Interview with John Kirklin, Birmingham, Ala.: (May 15, 1996).

17. Interview with Paul Taylor, Cleveland (May 29, 1996).

18. One reason Garrett and his team did not repeat the operation might have been the fact that the patient suffered a postoperative heart attack, which they attributed to closing of the graft. But when the patient was studied by arteriography years later, at Favaloro's suggestion, the graft was found to be wide open.

19. René Favaloro "Coronary Artery Bypass Surgery Thirty Years Later: Some Social Implications," lecture at Leiden University, Netherlands (February 1997).

20. 1997 Heart and Stroke Statistical Update, American Heart Association, p. 28.

21. Henry A. Zimmerman, "The Dilemma of Surgery in the Treatment of Coronary Artery Disease," *American Heart Journal* 77, no. 5 (May 1969): 577.

22. Eugene Braunwald, "Direct Coronary Revascularization . . . A Plea Not to Let the Genie Escape from the Bottle," *Hospital Practice* (May 1971): 442–43.

23. M. L. Murphy et al., "Treatment of Chronic Stable Angina: A Preliminary Report of Survival Data of the Randomized Veterans Administration Cooperative Study," *New England Journal of Medicine* 297, no. 12 (1977): 621–27.

24. Eugene Braunwald, "Coronary-Artery Surgery at the Crossroads," *New England Journal of Medicine* 297, no. 12 (1977): 662.

25. The left main coronary artery is a stubby vessel rising out of the aorta and from which the left coronary arterial system branches. Survival rates are poor when this artery is significantly diseased.

26. See comment by Jay L. Ankeney in response to a paper presented by Raymond C. Read at the fifty-seventh annual meeting of the American Association for Thoracic Surgery, Toronto, April 18, 19, and 20, 1977. The paper, titled "Survival of Men Treated for Chronic Stable Angina Pectoris," was published in the *Journal of Thoracic and Cardiovascular Surgery* 75, no. 1 (1978): 1–16.

27. CASS Principal Investigators and Their Associates, "Coronary Artery Surgery Study (CASS): A Randomized Trial of coronary artery Bypass Surgery: Survival Data," *Circulation* 68 (1983): 939–50.

28. Gerald M. Lawrie and Michael E. DeBakey, "The Coronary Artery Surgery Study," *Journal of the American Medical Association* 252, no. 18 (1984): 2609–11.

Lawrie and Debakey cited a range of clinical indicators such as small number of diseased vessels, relatively good ejection fraction, little congestive heart failure, mild angina, and relative youthfulness (mean age of 51.2 years) to demonstrate the low-risk status of the CASS cohort.

29. CASS Principal Investigators and Their Associates, "Myocardial Infarction and Mortalty in the Coronary Artery Surgery Study (CASS)," *New England Journal of Medicine* 310, no. 12 (1984): 756.

30. The following studies support the hypothesis that patients with an ejection fraction greater than 34 percent but less than 50 percent have a better survival rate if they are treated surgically rather than medically: E. Passamani et al., "A Randomized Trial of Coronary Artery Bypass Surgery: Survival of Patients with a Low Ejection Fraction," *New England Journal of Medicine* 312, no. 26 (1985): 1665–71. E. A. Caracciolo, et al., "Comparison of Surgical and Medical Group Survival in Patients with Left Main Equivalent Coronary Artery Disease: Long-term CASS Experience," *Circulation* 91, no. 9 (1995): 2335–44. E. A. Caracciolo et al., "Comparison of Surgical and Medical Group Survival in Patients with Left Main Coronary

Artery Disease: Long-Term CASS Experience," *Circulation* 91, no. 9 (1995): 2325–34.

31. Lawrie and DeBakey, "The Coronary Artery Surgery Study," p. 2610.

32. European Coronary Surgery Study Group, "Long-Term Results of Prospective Randomized Study of Coronary Artery Bypass Surgery in Stable Angina Pectoris," *Lancet* 2: (1982) 1173–80.

At five years 92.4 percent of the patients in the surgery group were alive, compared to 83.1 percent in the drug-therapy group.

33. Edvardas Varnauskas and the European Coronary Surgery Study Group, "Twelve-Year Follow-up of Survival in the Randomized European Coronary Surgery Study," *New England Journal of Medicine* 319, no. 6, (1988): 332–37.

At twelve years, 70.6 percent of the patients in the surgery group were alive, compared to 66.7 percent in the drug-treated group.

34. Ibid., p. 332.

35. A meta-analysis of the three large surgery trials and four smaller trials reported the following: "A strategy of initial CABG [coronary artery bypass graft) surgery is associated with lower mortality than one of medical management [drug therapy] with delayed surgery if necessary, especially in high-risk and medium-risk patients with stable coronary heart disease. In low-risk patients, the limited data show a non-significant trend towards greater mortality with CABG." Salim Yusuf et al., "Effect of Coronary Artery Bypass Graft Surgery on Survival: Overview of Ten-Year Results from Randomised trials by the Coronary Artery Bypass Graft Surgery Trialists Collaboration," *Lancet* 344 (August 27, 1994): 563–70.

36. John Kirklin points out correctly that "the capability of using clinical experiences in a reasonably rigorous way to derive clinically important inferences" is so far extremely limited. (John W. Kirklin, "Technical and Scientific Advances in Cardiac Surgery Over the Past 25 Years," *Annals of Thoracic Surgery* 49 [1990]: 26–31.) Nonetheless, the amount of data collected from clinical experience between 1970 and 1990 overwhelmingly points toward significant survival benefits for surgically treated patients with serious coronary artery disease.

37. Robert M. Califf et al., "The Evolution of Medical and Surgical Therapy for Coronary Artery Disease: A 15-Year Perspective," *Journal of the American Medical Association* 261, no. 14 (1989): 2077–86. Also see Salim Yusuf et al., "Effect of Coronary Artery Bypass Graft Surgery on Survival," pp. 563–70.

The categories used to classify coronary artery disease are crude at best, not indicating, for example, the amount of myocardium that is jeopardized by a blockage. And John Kirklin, who generally supports Califf's view, points out that "a patient with a truly isolated 60 percent stenosis of the midportion of the anterior descending artery may have a very different natural history than one with a 90 percent stenosis of the proximal portion of this artery that also involves the origin of the second diagonal artery. Yet both patients would probably be characterized as having single-vessel disease." Kirklin et al., "Research Related to Surgical Treatment of Coronary Artery Disease," *Lancet* 60, no. 7 (1979): 1615.

38. Braunwald, "Coronary-Artery Surgery at the Crossroads," pp. 661–63.

39. See, among others, Sheldon et al., "Surgical Treatment of Coronary Artery Disease: Pure Graft Operations, with a Study of 741 Patients Followed 3–7 Yr.," *Progress in Cardiovascular Diseases* 18, no. 3 (1975): 237–53, and Loop et al.,

"Coronary Bypass Surgery Weighed in the Balance," *American Journal of Cardiology* 42 (July 1978): 154–56.

40. Califf et al., "Evolution of Medical and Surgical Therapy," p. 2082.

41. Maria G. M. Hunink et al., "The Recent Decline in Mortality from Coronary Heart Disease, 1980–1990," *Journal of the American Medical Association* 277, no. 7 (1997): 535.

42. With very few exceptions, the hundred or more cardiologists and cardiac surgeons interviewed for this book agreed that both bypass surgery and angioplasty were being done in cases where they shouldn't. Most would not quantify their judgment. Eugene Braunwald was fairly typical when he said in a December 9, 1997, interview in Boston: "I think there is overuse of both catheter-based and surgical revascularization. And I think some of it has a financial base, I am sorry to say. I wouldn't say it's blatant, but I think at the margins there is overuse. I think there are people who are being revascularized who don't need to be. I can't put a number on it." A 1997 study done by the RAND Corporation for the National Coalition on Health Care said that "In a study of patients who underwent coronary artery bypass graft surgery (CABG), 1.6 percent had surgery for inappropriate reasons." Projected nationally, this would represent more than fifty-five hundred patients who had bypass surgery without needing it.

43. Interview with Laurence K. Groves, Cleveland (October 18, 1996).

44. Interview with William Proudfit, Cleveland (May 29, 1996).

45. Braunwald, "Coronary-Artery Surgery at the Crossroads," p. 663.

Chapter 6: Surgeons

1. Interview with John W. Kirklin, Birmingham, (May 15, 1996).
2. Ibid.
3. Ibid.
4. Interview with Paul Taylor, Cleveland (May 29, 1996).
5. Kirklin interview.
6. Ibid.
7. Effler et al., *Journal of Thoracic and Cardiovascular Surgery* 62, no. 4 (1971): 506.
8. Taylor interview.
9. Interview with Laurence Groves, Cleveland (October 18, 1996).
10. Interview with Leonard A. R. Golding, Cleveland (May 29, 1996).
11. Interview with Stephen Oesterle, Palo Alto, Calif. (November 15, 1996).
12. Kirklin interview.
13. Ibid.
14. René G. Favaloro, "The Present Era of Myocardial revascularization—Some Historical Landmarks," *International Journal of Cardiology* 4 (1983): 334.

Chapter 7: Smart Operators

1. Interview with Wes Sterman, Redwood City, Calif. (November 15, 1996).
2. Ibid.
3. Robert G. Petersdorf, "Foreword," in *Biomedical Research: Collaboration and*

Conflict of Interest," ed. Roger J. Porter and Thomas E. Malone (Baltimore: Johns Hopkins University Press, 1992), p. viii.

4. Steven A. Rosenberg, "Secrecy in Medical Research," *New England Journal of Medicine* 334, no. 6 (1996): 392–94.

5. Ibid.

6. Beating-heart surgery, of course, also results in quick recovery, and is even cheaper because there is a $2,000 to $4,000 saving by avoiding use of a heart-lung machine. Beating-heart surgery is also faster than the arrested-heart operation, saving operating-room costs at about $60 a minute, and its kit, priced at about $2,000, is substantially cheaper than Heartport's, which sells for about $5,000.

7. Interview with Chuck Taylor, Cupertino, Calif. (March 28, 1997).

8. Ibid.

9. Cornelius Borst, et al., "Coronary Artery Bypass Grafting Without Cardiopulmonary Bypass and Without Interruption of Native Coronary Flow Using a Novel Anastomosis Site Restraining Device (Octopus)," *Journal of the American College of Cardiology* 27, no. 6 (1996): 1356–64.

10. Benetti reported 1 percent operative mortality and 4 percent morbidity on 700 cases done between May 1978 and March 1990. Benetti et al., "Direct Myocardial Revascularization Without Extracorporeal Circulation," *Chest* 100, no. 2 (1991): 312–16.

11. Buffolo reported on 1,274 cases of off-pump surgery from 1981 to 1994 with an in-hospital mortality of 2.5 percent. Enio Buffolo et al., "Coronary Artery Bypass Grafting Without Cardiopulmonary Bypass," *Annals of Thoracic Surgery* 61 (1996): 63–66.

12. Taylor interview.

13. Interview with Federico Benetti, Washington, D.C. (September 24, 1997).

14. Taylor interview.

15. David Cassak, "Be Still My Beating Heart: Can Heartport Deliver?" *In Vivo: The Business and Medicine Report* (February 1997): 37.

16. Bruce Lytle, "Minimally Invasive Cardiac Surgery," *Journal of Thoracic and Cardiovascular Surgery* 111, no. 3 (1996): 554–55.

17. Renée S. Hartz, "Minimally Invasive Heart Surgery," *Circulation* 94, no. 10 (1996): 2669–70.

18. The four potential causes of stroke are: cross clamping of the ascending aorta; puncture of the ascending aorta for arterial return of oxygenated blood from the heart-lung machine; puncture of the ascending aorta for cardioplegia delivery; and puncture of the left ventricle for draining blood from the heart.

19. Interview with Wes Sterman, Redwood City, Calif. (March 31, 1997).

20. Smith, Barney, "A Discussion of Small-Cap Cardiology" (November 21, 1996): 13.

21. Alex. Brown & Sons, Inc. Medical Device/Hospital Supply, "Minimally Invasive Cardiac Surgery" (February 20, 1997): 1.

22. Financial analysts would also take into account the fact that minimally invasive valve surgery can only be done using cardiopulmonary bypass, but that consideration is outside the scope of this book.

23. The Smith, Barney analysts were skeptical about minimally invasive surgery drawing many patients from the angioplasty cohort because "We don't believe that

the vast majority of interventional cardiologists will refer virgin cases of LAD and/or RCA disease to surgery without attempting PTCA/stenting first. . . . Referral patterns for PTCA and CABG are not currently objective, in that the interventional cardiologist is the physician diagnosing, referring and very often treating the disease. There is an obvious bias on the interventional cardiologists' part in that, if the case appears amenable to PTCA/stents, there will be a self-referral." P. 23.

24. Beating-heart bypass surgery goes back at least to 1964. The first report in English may have been V. L. Kolessov, "Mammary-Coronary Artery Anastomosis as a Method of Treatment for Angina Pectoris," *Journal of Thoracic and Cardiovascular Surgery* 54 (1967): 535–44.

25. Pfister, A. J., et al., "Coronary Artery Bypass Without Cardiopulmonary Bypass," *Annals of Thoracic Surgery* 54 (1992): 1085–91. The 3.1 percent mortality rate for 1995 is from the Summit National Database of the Society of Thoracic Surgeons.

26. In a comment on the Pfister paper, which was presented at the twenty-eighth annual meeting of the Society of Thoracic Surgeons in 1992, Dr. Steven R. Gundry of Loma Linda, Calif., said the following:

> Beginning in 1989 after the return of one of my colleagues from a fellowship in South America to learn these techniques, our group as a whole decided to attempt off-bypass revascularization in all patients undergoing coronary revascularization, and in fact in 1989 was able to accomplish this in 128 patients. We applied a mean number of three grafts per patient with a range of from one to five grafts. Anatomy was not considered a detriment to the performing of these arterial grafts, and in fact direct attacks on the circumflex and posterolateral systems was done using very novel techniques developed in South America.
>
> In perhaps our enthusiasm and excitement for this technique two of my colleagues reported our results last year, and indeed found very similar results to what Pfister and associates have found today, such as slightly less hospital stay, less blood loss, and a very good in-hospital mortality.
>
> Unfortunately, in the year after that experience, we have found in this patient cohort a number of quite early and late deaths, and an unfortunately large number of patients have returned to our institution with recent onset angina. Those patients who have had angiograms have had an inordinate number of graft stenoses at the sites of the stay sutures or loops placed around vessels to give a good operative field. Because of this finding we have totally abandoned this technique at Loma Linda University and I do not recommend it to our members.

27. Interview with Paul Corso, Washington, D.C. (December 16, 1996).
28. Ibid.
29. Ibid.
30. Interview with Rich Ferrari, Cupertino, Calif. (March 28, 1997).
31. Ruth SoRelle, "Minimally Invasive Heart Surgery," *Circulation* 96, no. 8 (1997): 2483–84.
32. Corso interview.

33. Seymour I. Schwartz, G. Tom Shires, and Frank Spencer, eds., *Principles of Surgery* (New York: McGraw-Hill, 1998).

34. In an interview in New York on April 28, 1997, Galloway said improvements in technology, such as biologically or heparin-coated surfaces in the plastic tubing that transports blood to and from the heart-lung machine, have made the use of cardiopulmonary bypass less traumatic.

35. Because the majority of bypass candidates are over sixty-five and covered by Medicare, they are free to choose a surgeon or a surgical procedure, unlike most of those under sixty-five, who are likely to have both choices limited by their HMO or other third-party payer.

36. Interview with Michael Mack, Washington, D.C. (September 24, 1997).

37. Although it is not certain what causes the cognitive loss associated with the use of the heart-lung machine, the prime suspect is microemboli that are dislodged from the aorta and migrate to the brain. The risk is higher with older patients because they are likely to have more atherosclerotic plaque, which is the source of the microemboli, in their aortas.

38. In mid-1997 John Stevens became Heartport's chief technical officer and ceased performing surgery, but by 1999 he was no longer a company officer and was performing surgery again.

39. See Thomas J. Moore, "Deadly Medicine" (New York: Simon & Schuster, 1995); also see Roger J. Porter, and Thomas E. Malone, eds., *Biomedical Research: Collaboration and Conflict of Interest* (Baltimore: Johns Hopkins University Press, 1992), 122.

40. See David Zinman, "Doctors as Stockholders," *Newsday* (September 29, 1987), Discovery Section, p. 1; René G. Favaloro, *The Challenging Dream of Heart Surgery* (Cleveland: The Cleveland Clinic Foundation, 1992), pp. 74–75, and Baruch A. Brody, *Ethical Issues in Drug Testing, Approval, and Pricing* (New York: Oxford University Press, 1995), p. 69.

41. Henry Thomas Stelfox, et al., "Conflict of Interest in the Debate Over Calcium-Channel Antagonists," *New England Journal of Medicine*, 338, no. 2 (1998) 101–06.

42. Telephone interview with Maurice Buchbinder (June 12, 1998).

43. Rex, Dalton, "2 at USCD Banned from Experiments on Patients," *San Diego Union-Tribune* (April 4, 1994), p. B-1.

44. William Boyd, *Brazzaville Beach* (London: Penguin Books, 1991), p. 266.

45. Brody, *Ethical Issues,* pp. 144–46. Brody offers the following examples of sensitive decisions that can influence the outcome of a clinical trial. The first group has to do with the design of clinical trials:

1. Which treatments will be tested in the proposed trial and which will not be tested?
2. Will there be a placebo control group as well, or will the treatments be tested against each other or against some active control group?
3. What will be taken as the favorable end points (the results that constitute the evidence of efficacy of the treatment) and what will be taken as the adverse end points (the results that constitute the evidence of dangerousness of the treatment)?
4. What will be the conditions for inclusion or exclusion of subjects from the trial?

5. What provisions will be made for informed consent, and what information will be provided as part of the informed consent process?

This second group deals with the conduct of trials:

6. Under what conditions will the trial be stopped or modified because there have been too many adverse end points in one or more arm of the trial or because the preliminary data have shown that one of the treatments is clearly the most favorable treatment?
7. Under what conditions will the trial be stopped or modified because of newly available results of other trials?
8. Which patients who meet the entry criteria will actually be enrolled and which will not?

46. Roger J. Porter, "Conflict of Interest in Research: Investigation Bias—The Instrument of Conflict," in *Biomedical Research: Collaboration and Conflict of Interest,* ed. Roger J. Porter and Thomas E. Malone (Baltimore: Johns Hopkins University Press, 1992), p. 155.

47. William C. Roberts, "Sensitive Areas Between Physicians and Pharmaceutical Companies," *American Journal of Cardiology* (June 1, 1989): 1421.

48. Bernadine Healy, et al., "Conflict-of-Interest Guidelines for Multicenter Clinical Trial of Treatment After Coronary-Artery Bypass-Graft Surgery," *New England Journal of Medicine* 320, no. 14 (1989): 949–51.

Chapter 8: A Momentous Decision

1. The patient's name and a few biographical and descriptive details have been changed to protect his privacy and the privacy of his family.

2. René G. Favaloro, citing the report in "Critical Analysis of Coronary Artery Bypass Surgery: A 30-Year Journey," *Journal of the American College of Cardiology* 31, no. 4, Supplement B (1998): 1B–63B.

3. This account was supplied by Hollander. Ramey did not return repeated telephone calls made to verify Hollander's version of his care and advice.

4. Thomas J. Ryan, "Revascularization: Reflections of a Clinician," *Journal of the American College of Cardiology* 31, no. 4, Supplement B (1998): 91B.

Chapter 9: Angioplasty: A Balloon on a Snake

1. This account of Charles Dotter's contribution to angioplasty is based largely on "Taking Catheters into Intervention," chapter 6 in *The Catheter Introducers* (Chicago: Mobium Press, 1993), by Leslie A. Geddes and LaNelle E. Geddes. Other sources include Richard L. Mueller and Timothy A. Sanborn, "The History of Interventional Cardiology: Cardiac Catheterization, Angioplasty, and Related Interventions," *American Heart Journal* 129, no. 1 (1995): 146–72, and Gary S. Roubin, "History of Cardiovascular Intervention," *Interventional Cardiovascular Medicine: Principles and Practices,* Gary. S. Roubin, ed. (New York: Churchill and Livingston, 1994), 1–15.

2. Roubin, "History of Cardiovascular Intervention."

3. Interview with Richard Myler, Carmel, Calif. (July 15, 1997).

4. Geddes and Geddes, *The Catheter Introducers,* p. 65.

5. Geddes and Geddes write that in 1951 Dotter began experimenting in dogs with a balloon-tipped catheter to measure right ventricular pressure. The procedure was not attempted in humans until 1970, when H. J. Swan and William Ganz developed a more easily guidable balloon-tipped catheter for the same purpose.

6. Gruentzig's early history as recounted in this paragraph and elsewhere in this chapter draws on several sources, but most importantly on interviews with Spencer B. King III and Richard K. Myler, and "Angioplasty from Bench to Bedside to Bench" by Spencer B. King III, which appeared in *Circulation* 93, no. 9 (1996): 1621–29. Other sources include Richard K. Myler and Simon H. Stertzer, "Coronary and Peripheral Angioplasty: Historic Perspective," *Textbook of Interventional Cardiology,* 2nd ed., ed. Eric J. Topol, (Philadelphia: W. B. Saunders, 1993), Roubin, and Mueller and Sanborn.

7. King, "Angioplasty," p. 1622, citing notes written by Gruentzig in 1985 for a book he was planning to write.

8. Ibid., p. 1623.

9. Interview with Richard Myler, San Mateo, Calif. (April 2, 1997).

10. Interview with John Abele, Natick, Mass., December 10, 1997.

11. Myler interview, San Mateo, April 2, 1967.

12. Ibid.

13. Roubin, "History of Cardiovascular Intervention," p. 6.

14. Spencer B. King III, "The Development of Interventional Cardiology," *Journal of the American College of Cardiology* 31, no. 4, Supplement B (1998): 64B–88B.

15. Roubin, "History of Cardiovascular Intervention," p. 9.

16. Andreas Gruentzig, "Transluminal Dilatation of Coronary-Artery Stenosis," *Lancet* (February 4, 1978): 263.

17. R. M. Wilson, *The Beloved Physician: Sir James Mackenzie* (New York: Macmillan, 1926), p. 177.

18. Salvatore Margiorre and Linda Z. Nieman, "Cardiac Ausculatory Skills of Internal Medicine and Family Practice. Trainees: A Comparison of Diagnostic Proficiency," *Journal of the American Medical Association* 278 no. 9 (1997), 717–22.

19. This account of what occurred in the catheterization laboratory at Peter Bent Brigham Hospital relies mainly on John Abele's recollection of what he was told later the same day by Gruentzig. The quotations are given as recollected by Richard Myler who also discussed the events in the lab with Gruentzig not long afterward. Simon Stertzer's account is taken from an interview in Palo Alto, Calif., on July 7, 1997. It was based on conversations with Gruentzig and others at Peter Bent Brigham Hospital and is essentially the same as Myler's, though less detailed. Grossman said in an interview on July 28, 1997, in San Francisco that he does not recall that the patient's artery closed, nor does he remember Gruentzig being especially upset by his trying to complete the case.

20. Interview with Spencer B. King III (May 15, 1996). My account of how Gruentzig came to join the medical faculty of Emory University is based largely on conversations with King and J. Willis Hurst, chief of medicine at Emory at the time. Others, including Richard Myler, contributed to the story.

21. Because their equipment was primitive and because there was a learning curve for the new procedure, Gruentzig was extremely cautious and often would

stop cases in midprocedure. These cases were carried on the books as unsuccessful, which in considerable part was responsible for the low success rate he reported.

22. Interview with J. Willis Hurst, Atlanta (May 16, 1996).

23. Interview with Simon Stertzer, Palo Alto, Calif. (July 11, 1997).

24. According to Willis Hurst, Gruentzig conducted four courses before leaving Zurich and ten while at Emory.

25. W. Bruce Fye, *American Cardiology: The History of a Specialty and Its College* (Baltimore: Johns Hopkins University Press, 1996), pp. 318–19.

26. Jack V. Tu et al., "Use of Cardiac Procedures and Outcomes in Elderly Patients with Myocardial Infarction in the United States and Canada," *New England Journal of Medicine* 336, no. 21 (1997): 1500–5.

27. Salim Yusuf, reporting to the forty-sixth annual scientific sessions of the American College of Cardiology and summarized by James J. Ferguson in *Circulation* 96, no. 2 (1997): 368–69.

28. King, "Angioplasty," p. 1626.

29. The following account is based on interviews with Stan Hinden in Washington, D.C. (May 6, 1997) and Sara and Stan Hinden in Rockville, Md. (May 22, 1997), and Stan Hinden's medical records provided by Emory University Hospital.

Chapter 10: The Interventionalist as Entrepreneur

1. Interview with Wil Sampson (April 1, 1997).

2. The quotation marks around John Simpson's words reflect his recollections of what he said at the time. They come from an interview conducted in Menlo Park, Calif., on December 1, 1997.

3. Interview with William Parmley, San Francisco (July 17, 1997).

4. Sampson interview.

5. Interview with Edward W. (Ned) Robert, Los Gatos, Calif. (November 25, 1997).

6. Interview with Ray Williams, Palo Alto, Calif. (April 1, 1997).

7. Sampson interview.

8. Ibid.

9. Spencer B. King III, "The Development of Interventional Cardiology," *Journal of the American College of Cardiology* 31, no. 4, Supplement B (1998): 64B–88B.

10. The Advisory Board Company of Washington, D.C., provided these figures based on reports from the National Center for Health Statistics and the American Heart Association.

Chapter 11: Trials and Errors

1. Interview with Spencer B. King III, Atlanta (May 15, 1996).

2. Peter Libby and Peter Ganz, "Restenosis Revisited—New Targets, New Therapies," *New England Journal of Medicine* 337, no. 6 (1997): 418–19.

3. Abigail Zuger, quoting Oxford University physician David L. Sackett in the *New York Times* (December 16, 1997), p. C1.

4. René G. Favaloro, "Critical Analysis of Coronary Artery Bypass Graft Surgery:

A 30-Year Journey," *Journal of the American College of Cardiology* 31, no. 4, Supplement B (1998): 1B–63B.

5. Nicolaus Reifart et al., "Randomized Comparison of Angioplasty of Complex Coronary Lesions at a Single Center: Excimer Laser, Rotational Atherectomy, and Balloon Angioplasty Comparison (ERBAC) Study," *Circulation* 96, no. 1 (1997): 91–98.

6. Eugene Braunwald, "Shattuck Lecture—Cardiovascular Medicine at the Turn of the Millennium: Triumphs, Concerns, and Opportunities," *New England Journal of Medicine* 337, no. 19 (1997): 1360–69. On p. 1365 Braunwald writes: ". . . the course of cardiovascular disease remains unchanged in the majority of patients who receive the optimal therapy in the most successful clinical trials."

7. John W. Kirklin, "The Future of Cardiac Surgery," *Heart Disease and Stroke* (July–August 1993): 361–64.

8. James Herrick, "An Intimate Account of My Early Experience with Coronary Thrombosis," *American Heart Journal* 27, no. 1 (1944): 1–18.

9. Committee for Evaluating Medical Technologies in Clinical Use, Institute of Medicine, *Assessing Medical Technologies* (Washington, D.C.: National Academy Press, 1985).

10. Spencer B. King III et al., "A Randomized Trial Comparing Coronary Angioplasty with Coronary Bypass Surgery," *New England Journal of Medicine* 331, no. 16 (1994): 1044–50.

11. Spencer B. King III, "Comparison of Angioplasty and Coronary Bypass Surgery: The Emory Angioplasty vs. Surgery Trial," in *The Practice of Interventional Cardiology*, 2nd ed., ed. John H. K. Vogel and Spencer B. King III (St. Louis: Mosby—Year Book, 1993), pp. 133–38.

12. Clinical exclusions for EAST were (1) revascularization not needed, (2) the presence of a noncardiac illness influencing survival, (3) heart attack within the past five days, (4) severe congestive heart failure, and (5) unavailability for follow-up. Angiographic criteria for exclusion were (1) a narrowing of the left main coronary artery of more than 30 percent, (2) total blockage of a major artery that supplies viable heart muscle and is judged to have occurred more than eight weeks before the evaluation, (3) total blockage of two or more major coronary arteries, (4) left ventricular ejection fraction of less than 25 percent, (5) coronary artery lesions longer than standard balloons (20mm), (6) coronary lesions complicated by blood clots, and (7) a need for other coronary surgery. These exclusions are listed in King, "Comparison of Angioplasty and Coronary Bypass Surgery" in Vogel and King.

13. William S. Weintraub et al., "A Comparison of the Costs of and Quality of Life After Coronary Angioplasty or Coronary Surgery for Multivessel Coronary Artery Disease," *Circulation* 92, no. 10 (1995): 2831–40.

14. King, "Randomized Trial," pp. 1044–50.

15. Ibid.

16. Ibid.

17. The BARI trial showed a statistically significant benefit for treating diabetic patients with bypass surgery rather than angioplasty, but EAST did not. Additional study is under way.

18. "Protocol for the Bypass Angioplasty Revascularization Investigation," *Circulation* 84, no. 6, Supplement 5 (1991): V-1.

19. The BARI investigators, "Comparison of Coronary Bypass Surgery with Angioplasty in Patients with Multivessel Disease," *New England Journal of Medicine* 335, no. 4 (1996): 217–25.

20. Stuart J. Pocock, et al., "Meta-analysis of Randomised Trials Comparing Coronary Angioplasty with Bypass Surgery," *Lancet* 346 (November 4, 1995): 1179–84.

21. Harvey D. White, "Angioplasty Versus Bypass Surgery," *Lancet* 346 (November 4, 1995): 1174–75.

22. Daniel B. Mark et al., "Continuing Evolution of Therapy for Coronary Artery Disease: Initial Results from the Era of Coronary Angioplasty," *Circulation* 89, no. 5 (1994): 2015–25.

23. Daniel B. Mark, "Coronary Artery Disease," an unpublished chapter originally intended for inclusion in the *Foundation for Accountability Guidebook for Performance Measurement*.

24. The Veterans Administration Cooperative Trial of Angioplasty Compared with Medicine (ACME) was reported by Alfred F. Parisi et al., "A Comparison of Angioplasty with Medical Therapy in Single-Vessel Coronary Artery Disease," *New England Journal of Medicine* 326, no. 1 (1992): 10–16.

25. Spencer B. King III, "The Development of Interventional Cardiology," *Journal of the American College of Cardiology* 31, no. 4, Supplement B (1998): 73–74B.

26. Edwin L. Alderman and Javier Botas, "Selection of Revascularization for Patients with Stable Angina Pectoris," *Coronary Artery Disease* 4, no. 12 (1993): 1061–67.

27. Ibid.

Chapter 12: Interventional Cardiology Expands

1. Eric J. Topol, "Coronary-Artery Stents—Gauging, Gorging and Gouging," *New England Journal of Medicine* 339, no. 23 (1998): 1702–4.

2. Interview with Julio Palmaz, Washington, D.C. (September 26, 1997). My account of Palmaz's work is based principally on this interview.

3. The word "stent" apparently derives from the name of a nineteenth-century London dentist named Charles Stent, who developed a splint to stabilize skin grafts that has similarities to coronary stents. Ulrich Sigwart, "Introduction," *Endoluminal Stenting*, ed. Ulrich Sigwart (London: W. B. Saunders, 1996), p. 2.

4. Palmaz interview.

5. Ibid.

6. Ulrich Sigwart, "Introduction," *Endoluminal Stenting*, p. 2.

7. In 1991 Serruys et al. reported in the *New England Journal of Medicine* 324, no. 1 (1991): 13–17 that the device Sigwart used was associated with a high rate of blood clots.

8. The Belgium-Netherland Stent (Benestent) investigators reported their results in the *New England Journal of Medicine* 331, no. 8, (1994): 489–95. The Stent Restenosis Study (STRESS) was reported in same issue, pp. 496–501.

9. In 1992 the Gianturco-Roubin stent was approved for emergency use if an artery closed abruptly during angioplasty.

10. Spencer B. King III, "The Development of Interventional Cardiology,"

Journal of the American College of Cardiology 31, no. 4, Supplement B (1998): 77B.

11. Topol, "Coronary-Artery Stents," p. 1703.

12. Ron Winslow, "Missing a Beat: How a Breakthrough Quickly Broke Down for Johnson & Johnson," *Wall Street Journal* (September 18, 1998), p. 1.

13. Interview with Valentin Fuster, New York (October 1, 1997).

14. The quoted material appeared in Gina Kolata, "When Marketing and Medicine Meet," *New York Times* (February 10, 1998) p. 14. During a telephone conversation on April 7, 1998, Nissen confirmed that the quotation was accurate and used in proper context. He added that treatment choices for hundreds of thousands of patients are affected adversely when industry has too much influence on what physicians learn about new therapies.

15. Stephen S. Hall, "Success Is Like a Drug," *New York Times Magazine* (November 23, 1997), p. 66.

16. Interview with Stephen Oesterle, Palo Alto, Calif. (November 15, 1996). Oesterle was chief of interventional cardiology at Stanford when this interview was conducted.

17. David Gunnell, Ian Harvey, and Lee Smith, "The Invasive Management of Angina: Issues for Consumers and Commissioners," *Journal of Epidemiology and Community Health* 49 (1995): 335–43, and Jack V. Tu et al., "Use of Cardiac Procedures and Outcomes in Elderly Patients with Myocardial Infarction in the United State and Canada," *New England Journal of Medicine* 336, no. 21 (1997): 1500–1505.

18. Baruch A. Brody, *Ethical Issues in Drug Testing, Approval and Pricing* (New York: Oxford University Press, 1995), p. 150.

19. Fuster interview.

20. King, "The Development of Interventional Cardiology," p. 80B.

21. Valentin Fuster and Ira S. Nash, "The Generalist/Cardiovascular Specialist: A Proposal for a New Training Track," *Annals of Internal Medicine* 127, no. 8 (part 1) (1997): 630–34.

22. See George A. Beller and Robert A. Vogel, "Are We Training Too Many Cardiologists?" *Circulation* 96, no. 2 (1997): 372–78.

Chapter 13: How Healing Can Harm

1. Lewis Thomas, *Late Night Thoughts on Listening to Mahler's Ninth Symphony* (New York: Viking Press, 1984), p. 67.

2. Valentin Fuster, Lewis Connor Memorial Lecture delivered at the American Heart Association's sixty-sixth scientific sessions, November 8, 1993, in Atlanta, and published as "Mechanisms Leading to Myocardial Infarction : Insights from Studies of Vascular Biology," *Circulation* 90, no. 4 (1994): 2126–46. Fuster speaks here only of thrombolytic drugs, but the alternative use of emergency angioplasty is unlikely to have a large impact on the number of survivors. René Favaloro, writing in the March 15, 1998 Supplement B to the *Journal of the American College of Cardiology,* says, "the absolute reduction in mortality with our current thrombolytic therapy ranges between 2 percent and 4 percent."

3. Spencer B. King III, "The Development of Interventional Cardiology," *Journal of the American College of Cardiology* 31, no. 4, Supplement B (1998): 74B.

4. Figure supplied by the American Hospital Association, Washington, D.C.

5. Marcus DeWood et al., "Prevalence of Total Coronary Occlusion During the Early Hours of Transmural Myocardial Infarction," *New England Journal of Medicine* 303, no. 16 (1980): 897–902.

6. A detailed account of the development of thrombolytic therapy can be found in Baruch A. Brody, *Ethical Issues in Drug Testing, Approval and Pricing: The Clot-Dissolving Drugs* (New York: Oxford University Press, 1995), pp. 5–98. The brief narrative on thrombolytics in this chapter is based largely on Brody's excellent account.

7. The cardiologist Thomas N. James writes that "both thrombolysis and angioplasty are increasingly performed 'electively' in clinical circumstances in which an acute progression of events is not happening, and in many of these cases, choosing nature's balancing course can be an attractive alternative decision." "Complex Causes of Fatal Myocardial Infarction," *Circulation* 96, no. 5 (1997): 1696–1700.

8. David C. Sane and William C. Little, "Is Time Running Out on Streptokinase?" *Journal of the American College of Cardiology* 31, no. 4 (1998): 780–82.

9. Interview with Valentin Fuster, New York (January 29, 1998).

10. See Rudolph Virchow, *Phlogose und thrombose in gefassystem gesammelte abhandlungen zur wissenschaftlichen medizin* (Frankfurt-am-Main, Ger.: Meindinger Sohn, 1856), p. 458, and C. von Rokitansky, *A Manual of Pathological Anatomy*, vol. 4, trans. G. E. Day, (London: Sydenham Society, 1852), p. 261. Virchow hypothesized that fat was deposited in the arterial wall, and von Rokitansky hypothesized fibrin deposits and secondary deposits of fats.

Russell Ross, "The Pathogenesis of Atherosclerosis—an Update," *New England Journal of Medicine* 314, no. 8 (1986): 488–500.

11. Ronald S. Freudenberger and Valentin Fuster, "Fifty Years of Experience with Antithrombotic Therapy in Cardiac Disease: A 1996 Approach Based on Pathogenesis and Risk," *Mount Sinai Journal of Medicine* 63, nos. 5, 6 (1996): 344.

12. King, "The Development of Interventional Cardiology," p. 79B.

13. Interview with Valentin Fuster, New York (October 1, 1997).

14. Arteries may dilate to compensate for a narrowing caused by plaque formation, leaving a channel that on angiography looks round, smooth, and completely normal.

15. Interview with Paul Yock, April 1, 1997.

16. This definition is taken from a paper by Zahi A. Fayad et al., "Noninvasive In Vivo High Resolution Magnetic Resonance Imaging of Atherosclerotic Lesions in Genetically Engineered Mice," *Circulation* 98 (1998): 1541–47.

17. Shankar Vallabhajosula and Valentin Fuster, "Atherosclerosis: Imaging Techniques and the Evolving Role of Nuclear Medicine," *Journal of Nuclear Medicine* 38, no. 11 (1997), 1788–96.

18. Mark Brezinski et al., "Optical Coherence Tomography for Optical Biopsy: Properties and Demonstration of Vascular Pathology," *Circulation* 93, no. 6 (1996): p. 1211.

19. Ibid.

20. André J. Duerinckx, "MR Angiography of the Coronary Arteries," *Topics in Magnetic Resonance Imaging* 7, no. 4 (1995): 267–85.

21. A. P. Burke, et al., "Coronary Risk Factors and Plague Morphology in Men with Coronary Disease Who Died Suddenly," *New England Journal of Medicine* 336, no. 18 (1997) 1276–82.

22. Interview with Valentin Fuster, New York (January 29, 1998).

23. Matthias Maass et al., "Endovascular Presence of Viable Chlamydia Pneumoniae Is a Common Phenomenon in Coronary Artery Disease," *Journal of the American College of Cardiology* 31, no. 4 (1998) 827–32. Viable virus was detected in 16 percent of the plaques and chlamydial DNA in 30 percent.

24. K. L. Gould, "Reversal of Coronary Atherosclerosis: Clinical Promise as a Basis for Noninvasive Management of Coronary Artery Disease," *Circulation* 90, no. 3 (1994): 1558–71.

Chapter 14: What Shall We Make of All This?

1. Edmund D. Pellegrino, "The Goals and Ends of Medicine: How Are They to Be Defined?" unpublished paper delivered at the Kennedy Institute of Ethics, Georgetown University, Washington, D.C. (April 28, 1998).

2. Roy Porter, The Greatest Benefit to Mankind: A Medical History of Humanity (New York: W. W. Norton, 1998), p. 718.

3. Sherwin B. Nuland, "Medicine Isn't Just for the Sick Anymore," *New York Times* (May 10, 1998), sec. 4, p. 1.

4. Mark A. Schuster, Elizabeth A. McGlynn, and Robert H. Brook, *Why the Quality of U.S. Health Care Must Be Improved.* (Santa Monica, Calif.: RAND Corporation, 1997), pp. 13–14.

5. Nuland, "Medicine Isn't Just for the Sick Anymore," p. 1.

6. Jon Jeter, "With House Calls and Humanity, Doctor Wins Iowa Town's Heart," *Washington Post* (June 30, 1998), p. A1.

7. Donald C. Swain, "The Rise of a Research Empire: NIH, 1930 to 1950," *Science* 138, no. 3546 (1962): 1233–37.

8. Harold Varmus, "Shattuck Lecture—Biomedical Research Enters the Steady State," *New England Journal of Medicine* 333, no. 12 (1995): 811–16.

9. William F. May, "Money and the Medical Profession," *Kennedy Institute of Ethics Journal* 7, no. 1 (1997): 2.

10. Schuster, McGlynn, and Brook, *Why the Quality of U.S. Health Care Must Be Improved*, p. 45.

11. Gina Kolata, "Broader Benefit Found in Drug for Cholesterol," *New York Times* (May 27, 1998), p. A1.

12. The RAND report *Why the Quality of U.S. Health Care Must Be Improved* concludes, "A large part of our quality problem is the amount of inappropriate care that is provided in this country. If such useless and potentially harmful care were eliminated, there would be a large savings in human and financial costs."

13. Eric Topol, "Coronary-Artery Stents—Gauging, Gorging and Gouging," *New England Journal of Medicine* 339, no. 23 (1998): 1703.

14. Stephen G. Ellis, "Analysis and Comparison of Operator-Specific Outcomes in Interventional Cardiology. From a Multicenter Database of 4,860 Quality Controlled Procedures," *Circulation*, 93, no. 3 (1996) 431–39.

15. Edmund L. Erde, "Conflicts of Interest in Medicine: Philosophical and Ethical Morphology," in *Conflicts of Interest in Clinical Practice and Research,* ed. Roy G. Spece, Jr., David S. Shimm, and Allen E. Buchanan (New York: Oxford University Press, 1996), p. 21.

16. Jay Katz, "Informed Consent to Medical Entrepreneurialism," in *Conflicts of Interest in Clinical Practice and Research,* p. 294.

17. The Orphan Drug Act defines a rare disease as one that affects fewer than two hundred thousand people.

18. Stephen A. Sherwin, M.D., chief excutive of Cell Genesys of Foster City, Calif., in a telephone interview (August 8, 1998).

19. The most recent statistics on NIH funding for rare-disease research were released in February 1989 by the National Commission on Orphan Diseases, Office of the Undersecretary for Health, Department of Health and Human Services, Washington, D.C. According to the Commission report (GPO: 241–256/00401) 18.7 percent of the NIH research budget goes for rare diseases (pp. 41–44), but 57.6 percent of this is for various forms of cancer, each of which affects fewer than two hundred thousand persons annually (p. 44). This translates to about 8.5 percent of the budget. Stephen A. Groft, who heads the NIH's rare-disease office, says he believes this percentage changed little if at all between 1988 and 1998.

20. Telephone interview with Belinda Seto, senior adviser to the director for extramural research, National Institutes of Health (June 8, 1998).

21. National Heart, Lung, and Blood Institute, National Institute of Health, *NHLBI Cardiovascular Clinical Trials, 1985 to Present—by Start Date* (September 27, 1996).

22. David S. Shimm, Roy G. Spece, Jr., and Michelle Burpeau DiGregorio, "Conflicts of Interests in Relationships Between Physicians and the Pharmaceutical Industry," in *Conflicts of Interest in Clinical Practice and Research,* p. 323.

23. Robert Pear, "Study Finds Risks to Patients in Drug Trials," *New York Times* (May 10, 1998), p. A9.

24. Telephone interview with Gary Ellis (June 10, 1998).

25. Milt Freudenheim, "Insurers Tighten Rules and Reduce Fees for Doctors," *New York Times* (June 28, 1998), p. A1.

26. Edmund D. Pellegrino argues that "The physician is . . . bound by a covenant of trust which must not be compromised by other roles, e.g., as gatekeeper, entrepreneur, guardian of social resources, or economic pressures to undertreat." This quotation is from Pellegrino's unpublished paper "The Goals and Ends of Medicine: How Are They to Be Defined?"

Appendix A: Designing and Mounting Clinical Trials

1. National Heart, Lung, and Blood Institute, National Institutes of Health, *Fact Book Fiscal Year 1995,* p. 85.

2. Kenneth F. Schulz, "Subverting Randomization in Controlled Trials," *Journal of the American Medical Association* 274, no. 18 (1995): 1456–58.

3. Ibid.

4. "Protocol for the Bypass Angioplasty Revascularization Investigation," *Circulation* 86, no. 6, Supplement (1991): V-1, V-2. Patients eligible for the trial had multivessel disease and angina or compromised blood flow to the heart muscle.

5. If a clinical trial is being mounted by a drug company, as is often the case, funding will be provided by the company.

Index